Classical Anesthesia Files

Classical Anesthesia Files

DAVID M. LITTLE, JR., M.D.

Editor, Classical File
Survey of Anesthesiology
1957–1981

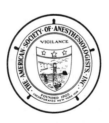

WOOD LIBRARY-MUSEUM OF ANESTHESIOLOGY
SPONSORED BY
THE AMERICAN SOCIETY OF ANESTHESIOLOGISTS
515 BUSSE HIGHWAY, PARK RIDGE, ILLINOIS 60068

Copyright © 1985
Wood Library-Museum of Anesthesiology
Sponsored by
The American Society of Anesthesiologists
515 Busse Highway
Park Ridge, Illinois 60068

Made in the United States of America

Library of Congress Cataloging-in-Publication Data

Main entry under title:

Classical anesthesia files.

 Consists of abridged articles previously published 1955–1980 in the classical file
pages of Survey of anesthesiology.
 1. Anesthesia—History—Addresses, essays, lectures. I. Little, David M, (David
Mason), 1920–1981. II. Survey of anesthesiology. [DNLM: 1. Anesthesia—history.
WO 211.1 C614]
RD79.C53 1985   617'.96   85-12088
ISBN 0-9614932-0-8

Composed and printed at the
Waverly Press, Inc.

Preface

In years past the Board of Trustees of the Wood Library-Museum of the American Society of Anesthesiologists have made available to persons interested in the origin and evolution of anesthesiology selected publications and reprints relating to its history. These Trustees believe that the legacy to historians left by Dr. David M. Little, Jr., in his bimonthly contributions to the Classical File of *Survey of Anesthesiology* over a period of 25 years, should be collected in a single volume for preservation, and for availability and education of the present and future generations. Dr. Little culled medical literature from the 18th century through the 1960's for seminal papers which led to landmark changes in the evolution of anesthesiology. Identifying these important contributions was only the beginning. What evoked genuine awe of Dr. Little's achievements was his originality of concept, breadth of treatment, and depth of knowledge apparent in each of his introductory comments preceding each reprint of an historical contribution. His clear flowing style of a storyteller transformed his pleasure in writing to pleasure in reading. The Subcommittee which assembled this volume has left Dr. Little's brilliant introductions untouched. Although most of the historical papers have been abridged to conserve pages, the reader has not been deprived of their source.

The medical profession is indebted to the Wood Library-Museum, the Williams and Wilkins Company, publishers, and to the Waverly Press for their forbearance and cooperation in assembling this volume. Nobody who delves into it will be disappointed. From Dr. Little's descriptions of the American Revolution to his "Fable of Anesthesia for Our Times", he regales our heritage with fervor and pride.

SUBCOMMITTEE

BETTY J. BAMFORTH, M.D.
S. G. HERSHEY, M.D.
K. GARTH HUSTON, M.D.

ARTHUR S. KEATS, M.D.
C. R. STEPHEN, M.D.
CHARLES C. TANDY, M.D.

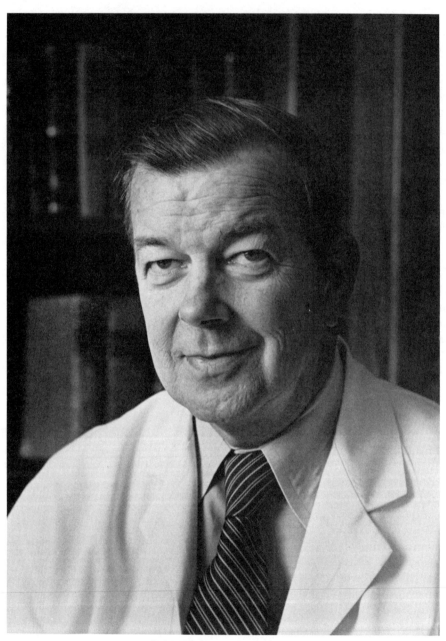

DAVID M. LITTLE, JR.
1920–1981

David M. Little, Jr.

D M L, a New Englander first and always, but blessed with just enough extroversion and unfailing humor to confound any stereotype, was born in Boston in 1920. After attending Middlesex School and Princeton University, he graduated from Harvard Medical School in 1944. During his internship at Hartford Hospital and military service in the U.S. Navy, he developed a primary interest in obstetrics which he pursued at the Boston Lying-In Hospital. However, his enthusiasm in this area soon waned, and later in 1947 he began and completed a residency in Anesthesiology under Dr. Ralph Tovell at Hartford Hospital. A period of private practice in Stamford, Connecticut followed, but, with his scholarly background, it was inevitable that he test his academic talents. So he traveled to nearby Yale University School of Medicine where he was an Assistant Clinical Professor of Anesthesiology for four years. By 1955 he knew where he wanted to be and what he wanted to achieve. He returned to Hartford Hospital as a Senior Staff Anesthesiologist and remained there until his untimely death on November 17, 1981.

To picture in words a man of diverse talents is difficult: throughout his too-short span of time D M L was a teacher, a scholar, an educator, an explorer, a friend to many, and always a family man.

Dave was a sensitive and demanding teacher, as those who moved through the residency program at Hartford Hospital know full well. He loved nothing better than to have a student or resident with him "at the head of the table", indoctrinating, questioning and teaching the art and science of anesthesia.

Yet he never abandoned scholarly pursuits. He read widely, and particularly explored the realm of the development of Anesthesiology, which he unfolded, six times a year, in the Classical File pages of "Survey of Anesthesiology". Through his fascinating and erudite introductions, as seen in the following pages, he earned the distinction of bringing the past into the orientation of the present. And it was not all pedantic: his personal puckish humor allowed him to forge a legacy which will not be forgotten.

In the decade following the Second World War, D M L sensed in his breadth of vision that the national organizations of Anesthesiology needed support. He believed that he could aid in the education and upgrading, not only of his fellow anesthesiologists, but of the specialty of Anesthesiology in the eyes of other medical disciplines and the public. So he became involved and soon emerged in a leadership role. At various times in his career he was President of the American Society of Anesthesiologists, Secretary and President of the American Board of Anesthesiology, President of the Academy of Anesthesiology, and President of the New England Society of Anesthesiologists. In 1979, with the unanimous approval of his peers, he was presented with the American Society of Anesthesiologists' Distinguished Service Award.

Throughout his brilliant and varied career, D M L never wavered from his loving and caring role as a husband and father. Those of us who were privileged to visit his home, and there were many, were always royally entertained by his wife, "Skippy", and their fine children. (However, before going "home", one usually was detoured to make a pilgrimage to the lifelike sculpture of Horace Wells in the downtown Hartford park!)

The only thing that was little about Dave was his name.

C. R. Stephen, M.D., C.M., F.F.A.R.C.S.

Twenty-five Year Cumulative Index. 1957–1981

VOLUME 1 (1957)

February

BIGELOW, H. J.
"Insensibility during Surgical Operations Produced by Inhalation"
Boston Medical and Surgical Journal, *35:* 309, 1846.

April

GRIFFITH, H. R., AND JOHNSON, G.E.
"The Use of Curare in General Anesthesia"
Anesthesiology, *3:* 418, 1942

June

SISE, L. F.
"Pontocain-Glucose Solution for Spinal Anesthesia"
Surgical Clinics of North America, *15:* 1501, 1935.

August

BANNISTER, F. B., AND MACBETH, R. G.
"Direct Laryngoscopy and Endotracheal Intubation"
Lancet, *2:* 660, 1944.

October

HAGGARD, H. W.
"The Absorption, Distribution, and Elimination of Ethyl Ether"
Journal of Biological Chemistry, *59:* 737, 1924.

December

HAGGARD, H. W.
"The Absorption, Distribution, and Elimination of Ethyl Ether"
Journal of Biological Chemistry, *59:* 737, 1924.

VOLUME 2 (1958)

February

WELLS, H.
"A History of the Discovery of the Application of Nitrous Oxide Gas, Ether, and Other Vapors, to Surgical Operations"
J. Gaylord Wells, corner of Main and Asylum Streets, Hartford, Connecticut, 1847.

April

LUNDY, J. S.
"Intravenous Anesthesia: Preliminary Report of the Use of Two New Thiobarbiturates"
Proceedings of the Staff Meeting of the Mayo Clinic, *10:* 536, 1935.

June

COMROE, J. H., JR., AND BOTELHO, S.
"The Unreliability Of Cyanosis in the Recognition of Arterial Anoxemia"
American Journal of Medical Sciences, *214:* 1, 1947.

August

EDWARDS, W. B., AND HINGSON, R. A.
"Continuous Caudal Anesthesia in Obstetrics"
American Journal of Surgery, *57:* 459, 1942.

October

COURVILLE, C. B.
"Asphyxia as a Consequence of Nitrous Oxide Anesthesia"
Medicine, *15:* 129, 1936.

December

COURVILLE, C. B.
"Asphyxia As a Consequence of Nitrous Oxide Anesthesia"
Medicine, *15:* 129, 1936.

VOLUME 3 (1959)

February

Annotation
"Fatal Application of Chloroform"
Lancet, *1:* 161, 1848.

April

STILES, J. A., NEFF, W. B., ROVENSTINE, E. A., AND WATERS, R. M.
"Cyclopropane as an Anesthetic Agent: A Preliminary Clinical Report"
Current Researches in Anesthesia and Analgesia, *13:* 56, 1934.

June

HALL, R. J.
"Hydrochlorate Of Cocaine" (Letters To The Editor)
New York Medical Journal, *40:* 643, 1884.

August

COURTIN, R. F., BICKFORD, R. G., AND FAULCONER, A., JR.
"The Classification and Significance of Electroencephalographic Patterns Produced by Nitrous Oxide-Ether Anesthesia during Surgical Operations"
Proceedings of the Staff Meetings of the Mayo Clinic, *25:* 197, 1950.

1775

Published February, 1976

The year 1775 was one full of momentous events for America since they led directly to the American Revolution. But they did not occur suddenly and independently: they were the results of other events which had gone before.

Every schoolchild knows the story of these other events. The British Parliament passed a series of laws which laid direct taxes on the colonists, stationed troops among them, regulated their trade, and closed their frontiers to settlement. The colonies resisted, the British passed even sterner measures, and fighting finally broke out at Lexington and Concord to start the war.

All true.

But the laws which the Parliament had passed and which had caused the colonies to revolt also applied to other British colonies which did *not* resist, so the simple explanation is not sufficient for the serious historian.

No, there were deeper causes. It is necessary to go back to the beginning.

In the course of the 150 years since the first settlements, the British colonies along the Atlantic seaboard had developed from a starving band of pilgrims to a prosperous body of farmers, merchants, planters, and laborers. The rice and tobacco civilizations of the South were thriving enterprises. New England shipmasters docked at every wharf in the Western Hemisphere. Colonists in New York and Pennsylvania had grown rich supplying flour for bread to the British Empire. Land-hungry farmers, planters, and land-speculators looked longingly toward the West, and were impatient that further expansion was blocked by the French and Indians in those territories. The French and Indian War was thus almost inevitable; and when it was over, the French empire in America had been destroyed.

This event also destroyed the strongest tie which remained between Britain and the colonies, for the colonies and the mother country had grown further apart than either had realized in the 150 years since the landing at Plymouth Rock. In fact, although the colonists still felt "loyal" to England, their only important need of the British was for protection: the British Navy protected American trade on the high seas, and British troops helped to guard the colonists' homes from attack by the French and Indians.

Furthermore, there were aspects of life in the colonies which were quite frankly inimical to strong ties with England. Strong political assemblies had developed in nearly every colony, which had won more and more control over their own internal affairs to the point that many colonies were, for practical purposes, almost self-governing. The British Parliament tried by taxation and in other ways to regulate the trade of the colonies and thereby maintain control of what went on, but the colonists paid little attention to trade laws: many kinds of customs duties were freely avoided; and, in fact, often the British themselves made no serious attempt to collect them.

Another strain on the loyalty to the crown were the perquisites of royalty. The best offices in the colonies were always given to friends of the King, for only in a few of the colonies could the people themselves elect their governors and counselors, and this was a continuing source of irritation and complaint. In addition, the Anglican Church, which was the state church of England, had become firmly established in the South and exerted the state's influence there; and those in the other colonies—with their own church allegiances—feared its incursion into their way of life and religion.

Finally, there were areas of the colonies where there were no ties to be strained because there were no ties to England at all. Thousands of immigrants, attracted by the opportunities of the New World and

1

driven by unhappy conditions at home, poured into the colonies from Germany and Ireland. They had no attachment whatsoever to Great Britain, and they built up a sturdy, independent life in newly developed areas behind the seaboard settlements.

It is against all of this background of increasing independence of the colonies from their ties to England that the schoolboy version of the causes of the Revolution can be accepted. For, indeed, at the end of the French and Indian War, the British found themselves in great debt from the war, and with vast new captured territories to protect. When George Grenville became the British Prime Minister in 1763, he reasoned that the best way to handle the many colonial problems that peace had brought was to effect a moratorium on settlement in the new territories until a sound plan for governing them and protecting them could be evolved; and he also thought that, since the colonies would get the most benefit from both, it was only fair that they should pay part of the cost. His plan made no great change in the *legal* relationship between Great Britain and the colonies, but it made a very great change in their *real* relationship: *i.e.*, he proposed not only to levy taxes but to collect them. In short, the colonists, who had become almost self-governing, suddenly found that the British proposed to rule them in fact as well as in law, and this aroused immense resentment—particularly since the first thing hit was the colonial pocketbook.

The immediate causes of the war began with Grenville's legislative program. The first of these was the Proclamation of 1763, which closed the territory west of the Allegheny mountains to settlement, to the great chagrin of both settlers and land promoters. This pronouncement was followed almost immediately by the *Revenue Act of 1764*, which was an interesting law in that it, in fact, lowered the tax on molasses from sixpence to threepence a gallon. However, the law also provided that the tax should actually be collected, instead of ignored as in the past; and since it additionally placed duties on a number of other commodities, it roused the wrath of New England trad-

ers, who argued that it would ruin both the shipping and fishing interests, and raise the price of goods in America so much that the colonists could not buy them. The next offensive law was the *Quartering Act*, which not only provided for stationing troops in America, but at the expense of the colonists. This law caused little joy in either New York or Boston, where it was proposed to station the troops. The fourth law was the infamous *Stamp Act* which was passed in the spring of 1765. It was the most devastating in that, while the first 3 had aroused the ire of individual groups of colonists, the Stamp Act affected all of the colonies simultaneously. It required that every newspaper, every pamphlet, every deed or other legal paper, every license, even every college diploma, must carry a stamp costing from a halfpenny to ten pounds. Stamp taxes had long been in effect in England, and it was not anticipated that any particular opposition should be expected from the colonies. Indeed, Benjamin Franklin, who represented the interests of the colonies in London, did not even bother to protest about it. But the opposition to the Stamp Act in America was both immediate and violent. The colonists' cry became, "Taxation without representation is tyranny," and they burnt the stamps publicly. Parliament responded by repealing the Act in March of 1766—although declaring that it had the right to bind the colonies "in all cases whatsoever"—and the news was greeted with celebrations all over the colonies.

But England still had to find the money for the defense of its American colonies, and within a year a new revenue act had been passed. Charles Townshend, the Chancellor of the Exchequer, persuaded Parliament to pass 3 bills which came to be known, not unreasonably, as the *Townshend Acts*.

The first of these placed import duties on tea, glass, paper, and painter's colors which were brought into the colonies, and the proceeds were to be used to pay the salaries of local officials and for the cost of maintaining troops in America; the second law created a new board of customs commissioners to enforce the revenue act; and the third one abolished the legislature in New York for its failure to obey the Quartering Act!

The colonial resentment of these laws was swift and vicious. Richard Henry Lee of Virginia said of the act suspending the legislature of New York that it "hangs like a flaming sword over our heads and requires by all means to be removed." Samuel Adams and James Otis, the foremost leaders of the opposition in New England, wrote a circular letter which was adopted by the Massachusetts assembly, and which urged all the other assemblies to resist the acts. A boycott of British goods was a common form of resistance, and sometimes entire colonies adopted the boycott formally through their legislature.

Given these conditions, a fight between the colonists and the redcoats could hardly have been avoided; and on the night of March 5, 1770, it occurred in the form of the "Boston Massacre" on King's Street (now Washington Street, most appropriately) in Boston. Some mischievous boys threw snowballs at a British sentry; an uproar followed; a mob formed and threatened the British soldiers with clubs and stones; and when the troops had finished firing at the crowd, 5 of the latter were dead or dying and 6 others were wounded.

The opposition, the violence, and the threat to British trade were enough to cause the repeal of the notorious Townshend Acts, but the duty on tea was maintained because "there must always be one tax to keep up the right" (to tax). It led to one of the more romantic events precipitating the Revolution, the Boston Tea Party on December 16, 1773, in which a band of citizens disguised as Indians and armed with tomahawks, threw the contents of 342 chests of tea from British ships into Boston Harbor.

Thus the stage was set for the fighting to start in earnest by 1775, a year of supreme importance in American history.

For the anesthesiologist, the year 1775 has another significance, for that was the year during which Joseph Priestly published the results of his experiments leading to the discovery of oxygen. Section III,

entitled "Of Dephlogisticated Air, and of the Constitution of the Atmosphere," from his "Experiments and Observations on Different Kinds of Air," is republished below.

EXPERIMENTS AND OBSERVATIONS ON DIFFERENT KINDS OF AIR
VOLUME II

SECTION III
OF DEPHLOGISTICATED AIR, AND THE CONSTITUTION OF THE ATMOSPHERE

JOSEPH PRIESTLEY, L.L.D., F.R.S.

London, 1775

The contents of this section will furnish a very striking illustration of the truth of a remark, which I have more than once made in my philosophical writings, and which can hardly be too often repeated, as it tends greatly to encourage philosophical investigations; viz. that more is owing to what we call *chance*, that is, philosophically speaking, to the observation of *events arising* from *unknown causes*, than to any proper *design*, or preconceived *theory* in this business. This does not appear in the works of those who write *synthetically* upon these subjects; but would, I doubt not, appear very strikingly in those who are the most celebrated for their philosophical acumen, did they write *analytically* and ingenuously.

* * * *

On the 8th of this month I procured a mouse, and put it into a glass vessel, containing two ounce-measures of the air from mercurius calcinatus. Had it been common air, a full-grown mouse, as this was, would have lived in it about a quarter of an hour. In this air, however, my mouse lived a full half-hour; and though it was taken out seemingly dead, it appeared to have been only exceedingly chilled; for, upon being held to the fire, it presently revived, and appeared not to have received any harm from the experiment.

Published April, 1976

There are, for some, no more thrilling words in American literature than those by Henry Wadsworth Longfellow in his poem entitled, "Paul Revere's Ride":

> "Listen, my children and you shall hear
> Of the midnight ride of Paul Revere,
> On the eighteenth of April in Seventy-five;
> Hardly a man is now alive
> Who remembers that famous day and year.
> He said to his friend, 'If the British march
> By land or sea from the town tonight,
> Hang a lantern aloft in the belfry arch
> Of the North Church tower as a signal light—
> One, if by land, and two, if by sea;
> And I on the opposite shore will be,
> Ready to ride and spread the alarm
> Through every Middlesex village and farm,
> For the country folk to be up and to arm,'
> Then he said, 'Good-night!' and with muffled oar
> Silenty rowed to the Charlestown shore."

The poet's license is abundant. Paul Revere's own account of his ride, contained in a letter he wrote to Dr. Jeremy Belknap in 1798, is somewhat less romantic, since in point of fact Revere was captured by the British and never did reach Concord.

"I set off on a very good horse; it was then about eleven o'clock and very pleasant. After I had passed Charlestown Neck . . . I saw two men on horseback under a tree. When I got near them, I discovered they were British officers. One tried to get ahead of me, and the other to take me. I turned my horse very quick and galloped towards Charlestown Neck, and then pushed for the Medford Road. The one who chased me, endeavoring to cut me off, got into a clay pond near where Mr. Russell's Tavern is now built. I got clear of him, and went through Medford, over the bridge and up to Menotomy. In Medford, I awakened the captain of the minute men; and after that, I alarmed almost every house, till I got to Lexington. I found Messrs. Hancock and Adams at the Rev. Mr. Clark's; I told them my errand and enquired for Mr. Daws; they said he had not been there; I related the story of the two officers, and supposed that he must have been stopped, as he ought to have been there before me.

"After I had been there about half an hour, Mr. Daws came; we refreshed ourselves, and set off for Concord. We were overtaken by a young Dr. Prescott, whom we found to be a high Son of Liberty . . .

"We had got nearly half way. Mr. Daws and the doctor stopped to alarm the people of a house. I was about one hundred rods ahead when I saw two men in nearly the same situation as those officers were near Charlestown. I called for the doctor and Mr. Daws to come up. In an instant I was surrounded by four. They had placed themselves in a straight road that inclined each way; they had taken down a pair of bars on the north side of the road, and two of them were under a tree in the pasture. The doctor being foremost, he came up and we tried to get past them; but they being armed with pistols and swords, they forced us into the pasture. The doctor jumped his horse over a low stone wall and got to Concord.

"I observed a wood at a small distance and made for that. When I got there, out started six officers on horseback and ordered me to dismount. One of them, who appeared to have the command, examined me, where I came from and what my name was. I told him. He asked me if I was an express. I answered in the affirmative. He demanded what time I left Boston. I told him, and added that their troops had catched aground in passing the river, and that there would be five hundred Americans there in a short time, for I had alarmed the country all the way up. He immediately rode towards those who stopped us, when all five of them came down upon a full gallop. One of them, whom I afterwards found to be a Major Mitchel, of the 5th Regiment, clapped his pistol to my head, called me by name and told me he was going to ask me some questions, and if I did not give him true answers, he would blow my brains out. He then asked me similar questions to those above. He then ordered me to mount my horse, after searching me for arms. He then ordered them to advance and to lead me in front. When we got to the road, they turned down towards Lexington. When we had got about one mile, the major rode up to the officer that was leading me, and told him to give me to the sergeant. As soon as he took me, the major ordered him, if I attempted to run, or anybody insulted them, to blow my brains out.

"We rode till we got near Lexington meeting-house, when the militia fired a volley of guns, which appeared to alarm them very much. The major inquired of me how far it was to Cambridge, and if there were any other road. After some consultation, the major rode up to the sergeant and asked if his horse was tired. He answered him he was—he was a sergeant of grenadiers and had a small horse. 'Then,' said he, 'take that man's horse.' I dismounted, and the sergeant mounted my horse, when they all rode towards Lexington meeting-house.

"I went across the burying-ground and some pastures and came to the Rev. Mr. Clark's house, where I found Messrs. Hancock and Adams. I told them of my treatment, and they concluded to go from that house towards Woburn. I went with them and a Mr. Lowell, who was a clerk to Mr. Hancock.

"When we got to the house where they intended to stop, Mr. Lowell and myself returned to Mr. Clark's to find what was going on. When we got there, an elderly man came in; he said he had just come from the tavern, that a man had come from Boston who said there were no British troops coming. Mr. Lowell and myself went towards the tavern, when we met a man on a full gallop, who told us the troops were coming up the rocks. We afterwards met another, who said they were close by. Mr. Lowell asked me to go to the tavern with him, to get a trunk of papers belonging to Mr. Hancock. We went up chamber, and while we were getting the trunk, we saw the British very near, upon a full march. We hurried towards Mr. Clark's house. In our way we passed through the militia. There were about fifty. When we had got about one hundred yards from the meeting-house, the British troops appeared on both sides of the meeting-house. In their front was an officer on horseback. They made a short halt; when I saw, and heard, a gun fired, which appeared to be a pistol. Then I could distinguish two guns, and then a continual roar of musketry; when we made off with the trunk."

Across the ocean in England in that same year of 1775, when the colonists were engaged in their struggle for independence, Joseph Priestley published his epic work leading to the discovery of oxygen. Section III of Volume II of his *Experiments and Observations on Different Kinds of Air* was republished in February, 1976, in "Classical File"; Section IV is republished below.

SECTION IV
A MORE PARTICULAR ACCOUNT OF SOME PROCESSES FOR THE PRODUCTION OF DEPHLOGISTICATED AIR

Joseph Priestly, L.L.D., F.R.S.

London, 1775

* * * *

I took half an ounce of *lead-ore*, and having saturated it with spirit of nitre, I dried it as before, put it into a gun-barrel, filled up to the mouth with pounded flint, and placed vessels filled with water to receive the air. The consequence was, that as soon as this mixture began to be warm, air was generated very fast, insomuch that, being rather alarmed, I stood on one side; when presently there was a violent and loud explosion, by which all the contents of the gun-barrel were driven out with great force, dashing to pieces the vessels that were placed to receive the air, and dispersing the fragments all over the room; so that all the air which I had collected, and which was about a pint, was lost.

It is sufficiently evident from these experiments, that dephlogisticated air is produced from all kinds of earth mixed with spirit of nitre, only that a greater quantity of air is produced from some than from others; the advantage in this respect being on the side of the metallic and calcareous earths.

*   *   *   *

Published June, 1976

Thomas Fleming, an eminent and highly literate historian, has recently written of the mythology which has developed over the years on the subject of the American Revolution:

"1. Lexington-Concord was a vicious, unjustified assault on a peaceful, unprepared people, proving that the British intended to enslave and humiliate all Americans.

"2. Both battles—(*i.e.*, Lexington-Concord and Bunker Hill)—were victories of amateurs over professionals, of courageous farmers over cowardly regulars, of spirited patriots over robot mercenaries.

"3. Patriotism, enthusiasm for the cause, was the key to Revolutionary Victory, assuring the Americans of overwhelming military superiority."

Fleming continues about these myths: "George Washington and the men around him eventually freed themselves of these illusions. Many other Americans of the Revolutionary era remained trapped in them to the end of their lives. More than a few contemporary Americans are still troubled by them. They think wistfully of the Revolution as a golden age of effulgent patriotism in comparison with our own era of dull, mediocre brass. The cure for this malaise is a strong dose of historical realism."

Perhaps the biggest myth of all was about the Battle of Bunker Hill, which took place just 201 years ago this month.

In the first place, it was the Battle of Breed's Hill, not the Battle of Bunker Hill. General Artemus Ward, the senior General of the Massachusetts Army, had ordered that Bunker Hill, the higher of the twin hills where Messrs. Breed and Bunker grazed their cattle, be fortified. Through either misunderstanding or stupidity, the detail dispatched from Cambridge spent the entire night of June 16, 1775, fortifying Breed's Hill, the lower of the peaks. It was a military mistake, since Breed's was closer to the water, closer to the guns of the Royal Navy and the batteries in Boston itself, and also to beaches where British troops could land. Nevertheless, the militia dug all night, and when dawn came the British in Boston were at first incredulous, and then awestruck, that the Charlestown peninsula, which had been a green, unpeopled knob the night before, now swarmed with men and showed fresh-turned brown earth in the form of fortifications thrown up in a surprisingly short time.

In the second place, it was a military disaster for the colonials the next day—June 17th—when the battle was actually fought, because they lost the battle despite what the history books say. But the history books are not entirely wrong, because the farmers actually did achieve a moral victory of sorts. These were, after all, green and untested troops—if indeed they could even be called troops. Across the harbor on the Boston waterfront there was a pageant of sight and sound as redcoated regulars and the blue-and-red-clad men of the Royal Regiment of Artillery swarmed into barges and longboats to the sound of pounding drums and the shrilling of fifes in the warm air of the brilliant June morning. As the first wave of red and white moved up Breed's Hill, they were greeted by a strange and disturbing quiet. Not a shot was fired from the hilltop redoubt until the British troops, with bayonets flashing in the bright sunlight, were within 15 paces of the lines. This was the true miracle of June 17th: instead of a ragged scattered volley and a panicked and frantic retreat, there was a spontaneous trigger-discipline until every shot counted; and *then* a ripping volley that decimated the invaders and sent them pounding back to the beaches and waiting longboats. A second assault later in the day proved an equal slaughter for the British forces (their casualty lists that day included 1,054 dead and wounded of the 2,300 troops involved). In the smoky dusk, the British launched an incredible third assault. This time, there was no ripping volley to tear them asunder, and waves of light infantry, Grenadiers, and line companies, with bayonets ready and eager for the seemingly inevitable massacre, stormed the hilltop redoubt, which by now was virtually abandoned by the ammunition-less colonials. This was the second miracle of June 17th, as miraculous as the fire control of the first two assaults—the orderly retreat of spent, untrained colonial militia to the safety of the mainland.

In the third place, then, was the myth of the spontaneous qualities of leadership of the colonial commanders. Not only had they sent their men to fortify the wrong hill; they had done so with no provision for their relief; with no supplies of food and water; and, worst of all, with no reserves of ammunition. One cannot win wars without munitions; and by the time of the third British assault on Breed's Hill on June 17th, the colonials had exhausted their powder supplies. There was absolutely no alternative to retreat. "Don't fire until you see the whites of their eyes" has come down through the ages as an order given before the first British assault on Breed's. This is unquestionably part of the myth, because those Yankee farmers knew how many rounds they had in their cartridge pouches when they started the day—not many— and they knew that supply was all that they were going to have.

Amos Farnsworth, a Massachusetts militiaman, has left an account of the Battle of Bunker Hill:

"*Friday June 16.* Nothing done in the forenoon; in the afternoon we had orders to be redy to march. At six agreable to orders our regiment preadid and about sun-set we was drawn up and herd prayers; and about dusk marched for Bunkers Hill under command of our own Col. Prescott. Just before we turned out of the rode to go up Bunkers-Hill, Charlestown, we was halted; and about sixty men was taken out of our battalion to go into Charlestown, I being one of them. Capt. Nutten heded us down to the town house; we sot our centres by the waterside; the most of us got into the town house house but had orders not to shut our eyes. Our men marched to Bunker-Hill and begun thair intrenchment and careed it on with the utmost viger all night. Early in the morning I joined them.

"*Saturday June 17.* The enemy appeared to be much alarmed on Saturday morning when thay discovered our operations and immediately began a heavy cannonading from a batery on Corps-Hill, Boston, and from the ships in the harbour. We with little loss continued to carry on our works till 1 o'clock when we discovered a large body of the enemy crossing Charles-River from Boston. Thay landed on a point of land about a mile eastward of our intrenchment and immediately disposed thair army for an attack, previous to which thay set fire to the town of Charlestown. It is supposed that the enemy intended to attack us under the cover of the smoke from the burning houses, the wind favouring them in such a design; while on the other side their army was extending northward towards Mistick-River with an apparent design of surrounding our men in the works, and of cutting of(f) any assistance intended for our relief. Thay ware however in some measure counteracted in this design, and drew their army into closer oreder.

"As the enemy approached, our men was not only exposed to the attack of a very numerous musketry, but to the heavy fire of the battery on Corps-Hill, 4 or 5 men of war, several armed boats or floating batteries in Mistick-River, and a number of field pieces. Notwithstanding we within the intrenchment, and at a breast work without, sustained the enemy's attacks with great bravery and resolution, kiled and wounded great numbers, and repulsed them several times, and after bearing, for about 2 hours, as sever and heavy a fire as perhaps was ever known, and many having fired away all their ammunition, and having no reinforsement, althoe thare was a great boddy of men nie by, ware overpowered by numbers and obliged to leave the intrenchment, retreating about sunset to a small distance over Charlestown Neck.

"N.B. I did not leave the intrenchment untill the enemy got in. I then retreated ten or fifteen rods; then I received a wound in my rite arm, the bawl gowing through a little below my elbow breaking the little shel bone. Another bawl struck my back, taking a piece of skin about as big as a penny. But I got to Cambridge that night. The town of Charlestown supposed to contain about 300 dwelling-houses, a great number of which ware large and elegant, besides 150 to 200 other buildings, are almost laid in ashes by the barbarity and wanton cruelty of that infernal villian Thomas Gage.

"Oh, the goodness of God in preserving my life althoe thay fell on my right and and on my left! O, may this act of deliverance of thine, O God, lead me never to distrust the(e); but may I ever trust the(e) and put confodence in no arm of flesh! I was in great pane the first night with my wound."

The year 1775 saw not only the Battles of Concord and Lexington, and of Bunker (Breed's) Hill, but also the publication of Joseph Priestley's epic work leading to the discovery of oxygen, *Experiments and Observations on Different Kinds of Air*. Section III of Volume II was published in February issue of *Survey of Anesthesiology* this year, and Section IV in the April issue. Section V is republished below.

SECTION V
MISCELLANEOUS OBSERVATIONS
ON
THE PROPERTIES OF
DEPHLOGISTICATED AIR

JOSEPH PRIESTLY, L.L.D., F.R.S.

London, 1775

It is pleasing, however, to observe how readily and perfectly dephlogisticated air mixes with phlogisticated air, or air injured by respiration, putrefaction, etc. each tempering the other; so that the purity of the mixture may be accurately known from the quantity and quality of the two kinds of air before mixture. Thus, if one measure of perfectly noxious air be put to one measure of air that is exactly twice as good as common air, the mixture will be precisely of the standard of common air.

*   *   *   *

It may hence be inferred, that a quantity of very pure air would agreeably qualify the noxious air of a room in which much company should be confined, and which should be so situated, that it could not be conveniently ventilated; so that from being offensive and unwholesome, it would almost instantly become sweet and wholesome. This air might be brought into the room in casks; or a laboratory might be constructed for generating the air, and throwing it into the room as fast as it should be produced.

*   *   *   *

The dipping of a lighted candle into a jar filled with dephlogisticated air is alone a very beautiful experiment. The strength and vivacity of the flame is striking, and the heat produced by the flame, in these circumstances is also remarkably great. But this experiment is more pleasing, when the air is only a little more than twice as good as common air; for when it is highly dephlogisticated, the candle burns with a crackling noise, as if it was full of some combustible matter.

*   *   *   *

My reader will not wonder, that, after having ascertained the superior goodness of dephlogisticated air by mice living in it, and the other tests above mentioned, I should have the curiosity to taste it myself. I have gratified that curiosity, by breathing it — — —. The feeling of it to my lungs was not sensibly different from that of common air; but I fancied that my breast felt peculiarly light and easy for some time afterwards. Who can tell but that, in time, this pure air may become a fashionable article in luxury. Hitherto only two mice and myself have had the privilege of breathing it.

1777

Published August, 1976

Every area of human endeavor has its status symbols—it has its Tiffany's, or its Chippendale, or its Beethoven, or its Stanley Cup Winners—and the American Revolution was no different: it had its prestige battles.

These were, of course, the Battle of Lexington and Concord, and the Battle of Bunker Hill. They are the sentimental favorites, treasured in folklore and mythology.

But neither was, in fact, important to the final outcome of the war. Consider, if you will, the fact that the Colonials lost both of these encounters. History books to the contrary, the rebels really did not do too well at either "the rude bridge which arched the flood" (*i.e.*, Lexington-Concord) or at Breed's Hill (*i.e.*, Bunker Hill). They *did* prove their adaptability, their obstinacy, their self-discipline, and their fortitude; but they did not win either of these contests.

People think of the American Revolution as a collection of episodes which include the likes of the Boston Tea Party, Paul Revere's Ride, The Battle of Lexington and Concord, the Battle of Bunker Hill, Valley Forge, and then July Fourth, the Declaration of Independence, the Constitution, and, wow, The United States of America.

It wasn't like that at all.

It was a long, dirty, painful war, lasting a dreary 7 years.

And the turning point, the landmark battle, was one that nobody ever speaks about very much: The Battle of Saratoga.

The Battle of Saratoga was the really crucial, really decisive, battle of the American Revolution. Crucial because it was the first major American victory—and they needed one, badly—and decisive because it brought France into the war on the side of the colonies, and this kept the sea lanes open.

The Battle of Saratoga was of massive design, the brain-child of flamboyant Major General John Burgoyne. Except that it did not work out the way that he had planned it.

It was an extravagant campaign to seal off New England from the rest of the colonies, which would result in "the tons of supplies and thousands of men that flowed out of those . . . states (to) dry to a trickle, and the spine of the revolution would be snapped." It was an ambitious plan, bold in concept, and requiring perfect execution and timing by 3 separate forces: those of General Burgoyne in Canada, those of Lieutenant Colonel Barry St. Leger on Lake Ontario, and those of Sir William Howe in New York City.

General Burgoyne was to go from Quebec down Lake Champlain, capturing Fort Ticonderoga (which was weakly held by 2000 American troops, known to be definitely substandard in morale, health and equipment) on the way, and then cross the narrow land bridge that separated the lake from the upper Hudson River to push gloriously on to Albany. At Albany, Burgoyne would be joined by St. Leger's mixed body of British, Hessians, Tories, and Indians, who would have stormed down the Mohawk River valley from St. Leger's base at Oswego on Lake Ontario. And then, this united force of Burgoyne's and St. Leger's troops would act as the anvil for a smashing sledgehammer blow that Sir William Howe's army was to launch up the Hudson River from New York City. When these forces combined at Albany, the British would have complete control of the great waterway that ran from New York Harbor to the St. Lawrence River, and New England would no longer be a factor in the war.

But some funny things happened on the way to Albany.

The first was that St. Leger panicked when scouts reported that Major General Benedict Arnold was marching up the Mohawk River valley with 3500 Continentals. St. Leger broke camp and started a hasty retreat west for his Oswego base.

The second was that Sir William Howe, rather than coming north up the Hudson River valley, decided to head for Pennsylvania to engage George Washington's forces and smash the Valley Forge army. Howe wrote Burgoyne a nice note, saying, almost as an afterthought, "My intention is for Pennsylvania, where I expect to meet Washington, but if he goes northward . . . and you can keep him at bay, be assured I shall soon be after him to relieve you. After your arrival at Albany, the movements of the enemy will guide yours. Success be ever with you." This was enough to rock any general back on his heels. Not only was Howe not coming north unless Washington moved there, but Burgoyne was supposed to bear the brunt of the American blow until Howe, never noted for speed, came to help out.

The third was that "Gentleman Johnny" Burgoyne was having a pretty poor time himself.

Saratoga was never part of the game plan. It just happened. As a matter of fact, the Battle of Saratoga was really a long series of encounters that went all of the way from Quebec City to Saratoga itself, and included the capture of Fort Ticonderoga; the 26 day march through the 20 miles of steamy, mosquito infested "Drown'd Lands" south of Fort Ticonderoga, across which the British had to build 40 wilderness bridges to transport their massive artillery; the Battle of Bennington (as the twin engagements attempting to take the vast masses of Rebel stores and horses at Bennington came to be known); and the 2 battles of Freeman's Farm.

The latter were the true Battle of Saratoga. Freeman had a farm and clearing whose open acres seemed like a gift from heaven to Burgoyne, a place where his troops could operate in the open in true European fashion, without ambushes and rifle fire from deep forests and impenetrable woods. But that was an illusion. Because Freeman's Farm was surrounded by woods;

and out of them, on 2 occasions—September 19th and October 7th—the victories that were the Battle of Saratoga were fired. Burgoyne could not break out of the fields and clearings of Freeman's Farm; and as he began to withdraw his tattered forces toward entrenchment at Saratoga, his forces were now outnumbered by the Rebels in a ratio of 3:1. The final result was the surrender of the 5000 crack British and German troops under Burgoyne's command.

This was the military significance of the Battle of Saratoga, the total surrender of a major British force. But the true significance of Saratoga was the impetus given to the momentous decision of Louis XVI officially to recognize the new republic and to sign a treaty pledging full military support to the United States.

That same year of 1777 found another Frenchman involved in *two* other revolutions, one the French Revolution (which eventually caused him to be guillotined because he was a tax-collecting official of the government), and the other the scientific revolution that was to become the discipline of chemistry. He was Antoine-Laurent Lavoisier, born in Paris on August 26, 1743. He had an embracing education, which included the Law, Astronomy, Botany, Chemistry, and Geology. In 1772 he began to study combustion; and after Joseph Priestley discovered "dephlogisticated air," Lavoisier (who called it "oxygen") demonstrated that it is the element that is absorbed by metals when they form "calces" (oxides). He reported his work in a presentation before the Paris Academy of Sciences on September 5, 1777, under the title of "General Considerations on the Nature of Acids," which is reprinted below.

GENERAL CONSIDERATIONS OF THE NATURE OF ACIDS

Antoine-Laurent Lavoisier

Comptes Rendus,
Paris Academy of Sciences, 1777

I have in earlier memoirs demonstrated to you as far as it is possible to demonstrate in physics and chemistry that the purest air, that to which M. Priestley has given the name of "dephlogisticated air", enters as a constituent part into the composition of several acids, notably of phosphoric vitriolic and nitric acids.

*   *   *   *

In consequence of these facts, —I shall henceforth call dephlogisticated air or air most suitable for respiration, when it is in a state of combination of fixity, by the name of "the acidifying principle", or, if one prefers the same meaning in a word from the Greek, "the principle Oxygine".

*   *   *   *

Published October, 1976

In July of 1775, a remarkable document was sent to King George III of England from his American Colonies.

It began:

"To the King's most excellent Majesty

"Most gracious sovereign

"We your majesty's faithful subjects of the colonies of New Hampshire, Massachusetts Bay, Rhode-island and Providence plantations, Connecticut, New York, New Jersey, Pennsylvania, the counties of New Castle, Kent & Sussex on Delaware, Maryland, Virginia, North Carolina and South Carolina in behalf of ourselves and the inhabitants of these colonies, who have deputed us to represent them in general Congress, entreat your Majesty's gracious attention to this our humble petition . . . ."

This was the introductory paragraph to the famous Olive Branch Petition, a fluent and obsequious document which was written at the behest of those many who, while not Tories, were genuinely distressed by the thought of a split from the Mother country. It was signed after the Battles of Concord and Lexington, and Bunker hill, and the historic document was the colonists' final effort to settle their differences with England amicably.

And it was signed by all of the members of the Second Continental Congress in a show of unanimity, although the "Independence men" realized that in signing it they were wagering that Britain would refuse to accept it and that this would swing the conciliatory minority over to the movement for separation from the Mother country.

It was a worthwhile gamble on the part of the "Independence men," because even though the loquacious and placative petition was hand-carried to England by William Penn's grandson Richard, the King refused either to see him or to accept the document. This was therefore the first step on the road to the Declaration of Independence.

It was not an easy road.

The Tories were not a factor in the equation at all, since they were utterly loyal to the King and had no part in any discussions concerning separation. It was within the rebel movement itself that the division was felt. The Conservatives maintained that the colonies could not possibly survive if separated from England; it would be "like a child being thrust violently out of his father's house." The "Independence men," on the other hand, followed their leader, John Adams, completely when he said, over and over, "Nothing can save us but discipline in the army, governments in every Colony and a confederation of the whole . . . . A Union and a confederation of Thirteen States, independent of Parliament, of Minister, and of King."

But it was an Englishman who turned the philosophical battle in the direction of independence.

Thomas Paine's little 47 page tract, "Common Sense," was the spark which ignited the Revolution toward independence. It was addressed "To The Inhabitants of America," and spoke out "On the following interesting Subject":

"I. Of the Origins and Design of Government in General, with Concise Remarks on the English Constitution.

"II. Of Monarchy and Hereditary Succession.

"III. Thoughts on the Present State of American Affairs.

"IV. On the Present Ability of America, with some Miscellaneous Reflections"

Paine was a torrid and volatile writer, and some of his thoughts made even the most radical colonists wince; but some of his phrases also echoed in the minds of the time with a vibrant beat: "T'is not the affair of a city, a county, a province, a kingdom, but of a continent . . . Now is the seed-time of continental union, faith and honor . . . Time hath found us. Time hath found us! O! Ye that love mankind, stand forth . . . Ye that dare oppose not only tyrany but the tyrant, stand forth! O! receive the fugitive, and prepare . . . an asylum for mankind."

The last page of Paine's little pamphlet carried the following sentence in stark, black letters: "THE FREE AND INDE-PENDENT STATES OF AMERICA."

The debate between Conservative and Independent roiled and riled, but the tide toward Independence was at flood; and in the early summer of 1776, as couriers from the grass-roots Provincial Congresses rode mud-splattered into Philadelphia with resolutions for the consideration of the Continental Congress, it became increasingly evident that the *people* wanted independence. And perhaps it was the latter which ultimately produced The Democracy: the *people* wanted Independence, and the Continental Congress listened to them.

The Congress appointed a Committee to collate in coherent, proper legal terms the separate resolutions of the 13 colonies. And a top-drawer committee it was, too: Benjamin Franklin of Pennsylvania, John Adams of Massachusetts, Roger Sherman of Connecticut, Robert Livingston of New York, and Thomas Jefferson of Virginia. They all labored, they all consulted among themselves and with the other delegates to the Congress, but it was the young Virginian, Thomas Jefferson—who, according to John Adams, wrote "ten times better than any other man present"—to whom the brunt of the burden of penning the Declaration of Independence fell.

It began by saying:

"When in the course of human events it becomes necessary for one people to dissolve the political bonds which have connected them to another, and to assume among the powers of the earth the separate and equal station to which the laws of nature and nature's god entitles them, a decent respect to the opinions of mankind requires that they should declare the causes which impells them to the separation.

"We hold these truths to be self-evident: that all men are created equal; that they are endowed by their creator with certain inalienable rights; that among these are life, liberty, and the pursuit of happiness."

And it ended by saying:

"And for the support of this declaration, with a firm reliance on the protection of Divine Providence, we mutually pledge to each other our lives, our fortunes, and our sacred honor."

Jefferson labored for 18 days during the warm Philadelphian June at his task, and when he had finished, he had created a masterpiece of simple beauty which warmed the hearts of men from New Hampshire to Georgia. Naturally, the Continental Congress took its turn at changing some sentences and paragraphs, cutting others, and even adding a few. But when the debates were concluded and the final vote was taken on July 4, 1776, John Adams could write to his beloved Abigail:

"Yesterday, the greatest question was decided, which ever was debated in America, and a greater, perhaps, never was nor will be decided among men. A resolution was passed without one dissenting colony, 'That these United Colonies are, and of right ought to be free and independent States, and as such they have, and of right ought to have, full power to make war, conclude peace, establish commerce, and do all other acts and things which other States may rightfully do.' You will see in a few days a Declaration setting forth the causes which have impelled us to this mighty revolution, and the reasons which will justify it in the sight of God and man. A plan of confederation will be taken up in a few days."

While these momentous events were unfolding on this side of the Atlantic Ocean, equally important events—although of an entirely different nature and embracing an entirely different area of human activity—were occurring on the other side of the Atlantic. These were, of course, the studies of the great French scientist, Antoine-Laurent Lavoisier, on oxygen, oxygenation, and respiration which laid the cornerstones for our knowledge of all three subjects.

The last issue of *Survey* reprinted a first section of Lavoisier's work under the title of "General Considerations on the Nature of Acids," which he had reported in a presentation before the Paris Academy of Sciences on September 5, 1777. A second section, entitled "Experiences sur la respiration des animaux, et sur les changements qui arrivent à l'air en passant par leur poumon", was published in *Histoire de l'Academie Royale des Sciences* for the year 1777 and is republished in translation below.

OXYGENATION, HEMOBLOGIN AND CARBON DIOXIDE

Antoine-Laurent Lavoisier

Histoire de l'Academic Royale des Sciences, Paris, France, 1777

Here, then, is the most complete kind of proof that can be calculated by Chemistry: the decomposition of air and its recomposition. Evidently it comes about, then, 1) that five-sixths of the air that we breathe is, as I have already stated in a previous Report, in a mephitic state, which is to say, incapable of supporting the respiration of animals, or the ignition or combustion of matter; 2) that the remainder, meaning only a fifth of the volume of atmospheric air, is respirable; 3) that in the process of calcination of mercury this metallic substance absorbs the healthful fraction of air, leaving behind the mephitic one; and 4) that bringing together these two fractions of air thus separated — the respirable fraction and the mephitic fraction — results in a reconstitution of air so that it becomes similar to the air of the atmosphere.

*　　*　　*　　*

Does it not follow from all these facts that eminently respirable air has the property of combining with blood; and that it is this combination which is responsible for the red coloring of the blood? In addition, whichever one of the two opinions one chooses to embrace — whether the portion of respirable air combines with the blood or whether it is changed into aeriform chalky acid (carbon dioxide) in its passage through the lung — I am inevitably led to believe that both phenomena occur during the act of respiration.

*　　*　　*　　*

Published December, 1976

In the end, it was the French Navy which won the American Revolutionary War for the colonists.

This is an unpatriotic, unsentimental, unromantic, and heretical statement. It ignores the sacrifices, the bravery, the suffering, the raw courage, and the almost superhuman tenacity against overwhelming odds of 6 years of dirty, painful struggle. It completely overlooks the carnage on Lexington Green, the bloody assaults on Breed's Hill, the guileful capture of Fort Ticonderoga, the shivering winter of starvation at Valley Forge, the smarting defeat at Brooklyn Heights and the American disaster on Long Island (which almost was the war, right there), the inspired crossing of the Delaware for the victories at Trenton and Princeton, the twin defeats at Brandywine and Germantown which allowed the British to occupy Philadelphia, the sweet triumph of the "Green Mountain Boys" at Bennington, the crucial surrender of Gentleman Johnny Burgoyne at Saratoga, the disastrous confusion at Monmouth, the furious charges on King's Mountain, the important triumph at Guilford Court House, and literally hundreds of other skirmishes, fights and battles.

The ultimate encounter of the American Revolution, however, was the Siege of Yorktown; and the victory at Yorktown was entirely dependent upon the French Fleet.

The story of Yorktown properly begins with the signing of the Treaty of Alliance between France and the Colonies at Paris in February, 1778, because this document immediately changed both the nature and the complexion of the war. Britain was now fighting a World War with France, and the

Thirteen States were merely one theater of action; and for the next two and a half years, the fight between England and her enemies (Spain had joined the French-American Alliance in 1779, and Holland came in later) was for control of the seas and was waged in European waters and in the West Indies, where the Caribbean Islands represented the richest trading area in the world.

On the continent of North America, the British shifted their attention to the southern colonies. There have been many good reasons put forward for this. One was that General Washington's main forces were tied up on the Hudson watching the army of Sir Henry Clinton in Manhattan, and the military strength of the Colonies in the southern states was far less than that which the British command could mount there. A second was the fact that the Southern Colonies, and particularly Virginia, were vital cogs in the maintenance of the economic machinery of the Thirteen States. A third was the real possibility of knocking the 4 southernmost states out of the war entirely, leaving the other 9 states to "go it alone." And a fourth was undoubtedly the need which the British felt to have their main forces closer to the important actions in the West Indies.

Savannah was taken by the British in December of 1778; Augusta soon fell and in May of 1780, General Benjamin Lincoln was forced to surrender his 5,000 Continental troops in the besieged city of Charlestown, South Carolina. In the meantime, strong amphibious forces were sent from New York by Sir Henry Clinton to devastate the Tidewater area of Virginia, which they did with great success. Encouraged by these and other forays, Clinton turned his attention south in earnest—and the stage was being set for the Siege of Yorktown.

Clinton sent the despised American traitor, Benedict Arnold (who was now a full-fledged *British* Brigadier General) and 1,200 men down to Virginia (Clinton had control of the sea along the American coast, and could move troops at will) to establish a raiding base along the James River in January of 1781. At first they had things all their own way, since Virginia could offer as little resistance as it had been able to mount against the earlier raiding forces of Matthew and Collier. But now General Washington, who was immobilized in his winter quarters at Tappan on Hudson by the aforementioned necessity of keeping a close eye on Clinton in New York, saw a chance to kill two birds with one stone by trapping the British forces against the James River and at the same time capturing the traitor, Arnold, "an event particularly agreeable to this country." In February of 1781, therefore, he ordered the young French Marquis de Lafayette south to Virginia with a picked force of 1,200 New England and New Jersey troops, to be backed up by 1,200 French troops under convoy by Admiral Destouches and the French fleet from Newport, Rhode Island.

Bad weather at sea and the British Fleet foiled the master plan, however, and Lafayette was alone in Virginia with 1,200 troops against a British array of forces along the James which had swollen to 7,200 men. All that Lafayette could do was parry and spar. He wrote to Washington, "Were I to do battle, I should be cut to pieces, the militia dispersed and the arms lost . . . I am therefore determined to skirmish, but not to engage too far."

It was on August 14, 1781, that the turning point came, and the end of the war was fore-ordained—almost. On that day a courier arrived at Washington's headquarters with the news that the French Admiral Francois Joseph Paul de Grasse "had cleared the French West Indies with 28 ships of the line and a cloud of transports which carried the Agenais, Gatinais and Touraine regiments under General the Comte de St. Simon."

This news sent the sodium pumps in George Washington's internuncial neurones working overtime. Lord Charles Cornwallis, who had become the overall British commander in Virginia, could be pinned against the sea *if* de Grasse's fleet could reach the waters of Chesapeake Bay and control them against the British Navy, thus preventing Cornwallis' escape by sea; *if* Washington himself, with his French compatriot Comte de Rochambeau (with 5,000 crack French troops), could force-march to Virginia in time; *if* General Clinton could be persuaded to stay and defend Manhattan (he was: Washington ostentatiously built a complex system of baking ovens on the north Jersey shore which could obviously bake enough bread for a massive and prolonged assault on Manhattan); and *if* the money could be found to support the march south, since Washington was almost entirely without funds (it was: Rochambeau generously contributed half of his own remaining war chest); and (the final if) *if* Cornwallis could be prevented from crossing the York River in small boats (assuming de Grasse had taken care of the British fleet) from Yorktown to Gloucester Point, which would have provided the British with a land-escape route.

All of the "if's" were affirmative, but the crucial one was de Grasse's control of the sea lanes. The laconic de Grasse reported to General Washington before dawn on September 15 (1781) that he was now back in Chesapeake waters; that he had met the British Admirals, Hood and Graves; that they had broken off the engagement and scudded north; and that the convoy of West Indies regiments was headed for James River anchorages.

Historians have noted, "That one sea action, so tersely reported and so little noted save in detailed histories, unseen save by the relatively few participants, was actually the one decisive engagement of the war. It is ironic that not a single American soldier had taken part in the sudden climax of six years of bitter fighting. Yet there the record stands. The French had seized that one all-important factor that America had lacked from the start, control of the seas, and had been able to hold it just long enough."

The rest was all downhill for the Americans. The Gloucester Point escape route was slammed shut for good by a combination of the siege lines on Yorktown, the Duc De Lauzan's flashy lancers and hussars, and the Marquis de Choisy's overall leadership. There was fighting left to do—and bloody fighting, at that (bayonet fighting almost always produces gore)—but the siege was essentially over. It was mostly a matter of the pomp and panoply of the Surrender at Yorktown, the last really meaningful event of the American Revolution, described in the following account by James Thacher, a Massachusetts surgeon in the Continental Army:

"(October) 19th.—This is to us a most glorious day, but to the English, one of bitter chagrin and disappointment. Preparations are now making to receive as captives that vindictive, haughty commander and that victorious army, who, by their robberies and murders, have so long been a scourge to our brethren of the Southern states. Being on horseback, I anticipate a full share of satisfaction in viewing the various movements in the interesting scene.

"The stipulated terms of capitulation are similar to those granted to General Lincoln at Charleston the last year. The captive troops are to march out with shouldered arms, colors cased and drums beating a British or German march, and to ground their arms at a place assigned for the purpose. The officers are allowed their side-arms and private property, and the generals and such officers as desire it are to go on parole to England or New York. The marines and seamen of the king's ships are prisoners of war to the navy of France; and the land forces to the United States. All military and artillery stores to be delivered up unimpaired. The royal prisoners to be sent to the interior of Virginia, Maryland and Pennsylvania in regiments, to have rations allowed them equal to the American soldiers and to have their officers near them. Lord Cornwallis to man and despatch the *Bonetta* sloop-of-war with despatches to Sir Henry Clinton at New York without being searched, the vessel to be returned and the hands accounted for.

"At about twelve o'clock, the combined army was arranged and drawn up in two lines extending more than a mile in length. The Americans were drawn up in a line on the right side of the road, and the French occupied the left. At the head of the former, the great American commander, mounted on his noble courser, took his station, attended by his aides. At the head of the latter was posted the excellent Count Rochambeau and his suite. The French troops, in complete uniform, displayed a martial and noble appearance; their bands of music, of which the timbrel formed a part, is a delightful novelty and produced while marching to the ground a most enchanting effect. The Americans, though not all in uniform, nor their dress so neat, yet exhibited an erect, soldierly air, and every countenance beamed with satisfaction and joy. The concourse of spectators from the country was prodigious, in point of numbers was probably equal to the military, but universal silence and order prevailed.

"It was about two o'clock when the captive army advanced through the line formed for their reception. Every eye was prepared to gaze on Lord Cornwallis, the object of peculiar interest and solicitude; but he disappointed our anxious expectations; pretending indisposition, he made General O'Hara his substitute as the leader of the army. This officer was followed by the conquered troops in a slow and solemn step, with shouldered arms, colors cased and drums beating a British march. Having arrived at the head of the line, General O'Hara, elegantly mounted, advanced to his excellency the commander-in-chief, taking off his hat, and apologized for the nonappearance of Earl Cornwallis. With his usual dignity and politeness, his excellency pointed to Major-General Lincoln for directions, by whom the British army was conducted into a spacious field, where it was intended they should ground their arms.

"The royal troops, while marching through the line formed by the allied army, exhibited a decent and neat appearance, as respects arms and clothing for their commander had opened his store and directed every soldier to be furnished with a new suit complete, prior to the capitulation. But in their line of march we remarked a disorderly and unsoldierly conduct, their step was irregular, and their ranks frequently broken.

"But it was in the field, when they came to the last act of the drama, that the spirit and pride of the British soldier was put in the severest test: here their mortification could not be concealed. Some of the platoon officers appeared to be exceedingly chagrined when giving the word 'ground,' and I am a witness that they performed this

duty in a very unofficer-like manner; and that many of the soldiers manifested a *sudden temper*, throwing their arms on the pile with violence, as if determined to render them useless. This irregularity, however, was checked by the authority of General Lincoln. After having grounded their arms and divested themselves of their accoutrements, the captive troops were conducted back to Yorktown and guarded by our troops till they could be removed to the place of their destination.

"The British troops that were stationed at Gloucester surrendered at the same time and in the same manner to the command of the Duke de Luzerne (Lauzun).

"This must be a very interesting and gratifying transaction to General Lincoln, who, having himself been obliged to surrender an army to a haughty foe for the last year, has now assigned him the pleasing duty of giving laws to a conquered foe in return, and of reflecting that the terms which were imposed on him are adopted as a basis of the surrender in the present instance."

When, at precisely 2 P.M. on October 18, 1781, the British bands struck up the "British march" to which Thacher refers (it was a popular air of the day, wildly and appropriately titled, "The World Turned Upside Down"), the sullen redcoats quit their defenses and marched between the lines of American and French troops to stack their arms, it was all over at Yorktown. That evening an American officer "noticed that the allied officers and soldiers could scarcely talk for laughing, and they could scarcely walk for jumping and dancing and singing as they went about."

But was it all over elsewhere? George Washington, for one, was not at all sure that Yorktown was the end. He wrote, "My only apprehension is lest the late important success, instead of exciting our exertions . . . should produce such a relaxation in the prosecution of the war, as will prolong the calamities of it."

It was indeed over elsewhere.

There were occasional encounters and ragged volleys, but the war was essentially over with the surrender at Yorktown. The British had no stomach for a continuation of the conflict. Theirs was a war-weary nation; and when the staggering news of Cornwall's disaster arrived in London, the people called for peace. Commons declared that it "would consider as enemies of his majesty and the Country all those who should advise . . . or attempt the further prosecution of offensive war on the Continent of North America." Sir Guy Carleton replaced Clinton as the Commanding General in America, and promptly proceeded to evacuate the cities of Savannah and Charleston "in consequence of an unsuccessful war."

Peace negotiators were appointed by both sides (*i.e.*, the British and the allies), and these commissioners labored through the summer and fall of 1782 in Paris. The American Commissioners came to agreement with the British in November of that year; and when England finally came to terms with France and Spain, the formal agreement was signed on September 3, 1783. Thus, more than 8 years after Paul Revere's Ride, after more than 6 years of bitter fighting, and after more than 2 years of prolonged negotiations, America had won her freedom.

More than a century earlier, one of the bulwarks of the conduct of today's anesthetic management came into being when Richard Lower, of Oxford, laid the basis for the transfusion of blood in his communication, "The Method observed in Transfusing the Blood out of one Animal into another", a summary of which was contained in the Philosophical Transactions of the Royal Society, Monday, December 17, 1666 (*Philosophical Transactions, 1:* 353–358, 1666) and is reprinted below.

THE METHOD OBSERVED IN TRANSFUSING THE BLOOD OUT OF ONE ANIMAL INTO ANOTHER

R. LOWER

Philosophical Transactions, 1: 353–358, 1666

This method was promised in the last of these Papers. It was first practised by Doctor *Lower* in Oxford, and by him communicated to the Honourable *Robert Boyle*, who imparted it to the *Royal Society*.

(There follows a detailed description of transfusing blood from the carotid artery of one dog into the jugular vein of another dog, using quills to connect the two vessels).

*   *   *   *

1800

Published February, 1968

It is usual for those writing about the history of anesthesia to point to the Old Testament as the first written reference to surgical anesthesia, and to quote the twenty-first verse of the second chapter of Genesis: "And the Lord God caused a deep sleep to fall on Adam, and he slept: and he took one of his ribs and closed up the flesh instead thereof." Following this, mentions are generally made of Aesculapius in 1200 B.C., who used a potion called *nepenthe* to produce insensibility in his surgical patients; of Helen of Troy, whose tears contained the drug, *helenium*, which, taken in wine, would "assuage suffering, dispel anger, and produce forgetfulness of all sorrow"; of Pien Ch'iao, the Chinese physician who performed major operations on patients drugged with wine to which hemp had been added; of Dioscorides, the Greek army surgeon in the service of Nero, who employed henbane "prepared for lotions to take away pain, and for sharp and hot rhume, and for ear pains and griefs about the matrix"; of Pliny the Elder, who recognized the narcotic properties of mandragora wine; and of Hua T'o the famous Chinese surgeon, who administered wine containing a soporific effervescent powder to patients before major operations to produce complete insensibility. But the first true seeds of modern anesthesia as it is known and practiced today sprouted in the brilliant and inquiring mind of Sir Humphry Davy.

Davy was born at Penzance in Cornwall on December 17, 1778, the first of five children born to his parents, Robert and Grace Millett Davy. He was a bright, imaginative boy with a photographic memory, but he spent his early years at an undistinguished—if not, indeed, a thoroughly poor—school, the Penzance Grammar School. As a result, when his father died in 1794 and Davy's formal schooling was brought to an end by financial necessity, he was forced to begin the task of self-education. This he did during his apprenticeship to John Bingham Borlase, "an apothecary and surgeon"; for although Davy was determined to become medically qualified at Edinburgh, he was indentured to the Penzance surgeon on February 10, 1795, at the age of 16.

His first major area of studious effort was poetry, and his verses were surprisingly good, being acclaimed by both Southey and Coleridge. Indeed, the former published some of them in the "Annual Anthology" in both 1799 and 1800; and the latter is said to have remarked that if Davy had not been the premier chemist he would have been the premier poet of his age.

Then, in the winter of 1797–1798, Davey began the study of chemistry. He had the most primitive of apparatus and access to only two textbooks, Nicholson's *Dictionary of Chemistry* and Lavoisier's *Elements*; yet within 20 months he had conducted the experiments on the nature of light and heat which led him to his extraordinary theory of light. In the spring of 1798 he became interested in nitrous oxide and embarked on the studies which were to take him to Bristol, then to London, and, finally, to the Chair of the Royal Society and to a Baronetcy.

Bristol was the site of the Pneumatic Medical Institution run by Dr. Thomas Beddoes, although the practice of pneumatic medicine had passed its peak before the Pneumatic Institution had opened its doors. Beddoes had heard of Davy, through a mutual friend, as "a very ingenious young chemist," and he negotiated to have Davy released from his indentures to Borlase to become an assistant at the Pneumatic Institution. Davy arrived there in October 1798; and since there were no patients as yet, he plunged to work in the well-equipped laboratory, experimenting with nitrous oxide and perfecting its manufacture, testing the application of this and other gases in disease, trying their effects on animals and fish, breathing them himself and inducing his friends to breathe them, and recording the sensations that he felt and the sensations that his friends described to him. At the end of almost two years, the results of his work were published in the 600-page treatise, *Researches, Chemical and Philosophical; Chiefly Concerning Nitrous Oxide or Dephlogisticated Nitrous Air and Its Respiration*. It was not his most important work—that was to follow later—but it was of outstanding significance in relation to anesthesia, as will be seen.

Davy's work, both that on nitrous oxide and that on light and heat, had brought him to the attention of the scientific world, and in 1801 he was called to the Royal Institution of Great Britain as assistant lecturer in chemistry. His style of lecturing was brilliant, designed to make science of interest to the many; and since the object of the Royal Institution was "the promotion of science, art and manufactures," this pleased the Managers of the Institution and led to Davy's election to Professor of Chemistry in 1802. The following year, when he was not yet twenty-six, he was honored again by election as a Fellow of the Royal Society. From that time onward, he added some important new achievement or discovery almost every year until his position as the foremost chemist of the day was beyond doubt. Among his most important contributions were the development of the chemical action of the voltaic battery, the discoveries of sodium and potassium, the identification of chlorine, and the invention of the miner's lamp. His meteoric career was recognized when the honor of a knighthood was conferred on Davy by the Prince Regent on April 8, 1812, at the age of 34.

Three days later, Davy married. Lady Davy was a wealthy widow and a brilliant woman; but it was not a happy marriage, and Davy's researches suffered from the domestic discomfort. It is true that the invention of the safety lamp occurred in the period after his marriage, but Davy's character was changing for the worse and Science was becoming far less of a driving force in his life. Travel and sport, made possible by his new wealth, claimed an ever-increasing proportion of his time, although honors still continued to come to him. In 1817, the coal owners and miners of the north of England presented him with a service of plate, valued at some 1500 pounds, as a token of gratitude for his great gift of the safety lamp to their industry. The following year, in recognition for this same great benefit to humanity, he was created a baronet—which, as Cartwright has pointed out, was a somewhat empty honor to a childless man. In 1820, he was elected the President of the Royal Society by a huge majority, and then was reelected to the Chair in 1826. But Davy's health was failing and his career was at an end. He delivered his last discourse to the Royal Society after his reelection to the Chair in 1826 with great effort, and he was so unwell afterwards that he was unable to attend the annual dinner. Two weeks later he suffered a stroke which left him with a partial right hemiplegia. He recovered sufficiently to go abroad for most of the last year and a half of his life, but he suffered a second stoke and died in Geneva on May 29, 1829. In accordance with the terms of his will (dated, incidentally, one day before his death), he was buried there on June 1: "I wish to be buried where I die *natura curat suas reliquias.*"

Many of Davy's chemical discoveries have affected anesthesia, if only indirectly; but the studies on nitrous oxide have a direct pertinence, and in *Researches, Chemical and Philosophical; Chiefly Concerning Nitrous Oxide or Dephlogisticated Nitrous Air and Its Respiration* (London, J. Johnson, 1800, pp. 451–465 and 548–559), he clearly reports the analgesic properties of the gas in the first of the excerpts reprinted below and equally clearly suggests its use for the prevention of the pain of surgical operations in the second of the excerpts reprinted below.

RESEARCH IV. RELATING TO THE EFFECTS PRODUCED BY THE RESPIRATION OF NITROUS OXIDE. DIVISION 1. HISTORY OF THE DISCOVERY— EFFECTS PRODUCED BY THE RESPIRATION OF DIFFERENT GASES. DIVISION III. OBSERVATIONS ON THE EFFECTS OF NITROUS OXIDE BY DR. BEDDOES— CONCLUSION.

HUMPHREY DAVY

Superintendant of the Medical Pneumatic Institution
London, England
in

RESEARCHES, CHEMICAL AND PHILOSOPHICAL: CHIEFLY CONCERNING NITROUS OXIDE
OR
DEPHLOGISTICATED NITROUS AIR
AND ITS RESPIRATION.

HUMPHREY DAVY

(London, J. Johnson, pp. 451–465 & 548–559, 1800)

A narrative first person account of Davy's first experiments in breathing nitrous oxide and its subjective effects, as well as his thoughts on its potential usefulness.

1824

Published February, 1966

In 1960, Dr. W. Stanley Sykes published the first of two volumes entitled *Essays On The First Hundred Years of Anaesthesia* (E. & S. Livingston Ltd., Edinburgh). It was a unique book: scholarly, witty, original, thoughtful, and a delight to read. There had not been before—and has not been since—anything quite like it written on the subject of the history of anesthesia. Sykes was dedicated to his subject, unsparing in his research, and fluent and facile with his pen. In 1961, the second volume appeared; and at the time of Sykes' premature death, he had sufficient essays on hand for five more volumes. The literature on anesthesia is a great deal poorer for the fact that these planned volumes never reached printer's ink. (Volume three is now available, *Ed.*)

One of the most fascinating of the eight essays comprising the first volume (which boasts perhaps the only illustrated preface to a book) is concerned with the men and the momentous events which they effected during the period from 1799 to 1847, and which culminated in the introduction of clinical anesthesia. Sykes has listed the seven pioneers of anesthesia in chronological order (Davy, Hickman, Long, Wells, Morton, Jackson, and Simpson); and then arranged them in what he considers to be their order of merit for the credit of the discovery of anesthesia (Hickman, Wells, Morton, Davy, Long, Simpson, and "a long way last," Jackson). His arguments are cogent and perceptive.

Charles Thomas Jackson is dismissed easily by Sykes: "He did not have the idea of anaesthesia in the first place. All he did was try to cash in upon it when it proved successful. He did no work upon it himself, and there is little evidence that he ever used ether at all, although he wrote a book about it. He did not even take the trouble to see an anaesthetic given until five weeks after Ether Day. It is almost incredible that a man who claimed, or was about to claim, an important part in such an obviously revolutionary idea, should take so little interest in its development. It tends to prove that his part in the whole affair was very small indeed, and that it only assumed importance in his eyes when it showed signs of being successful, and possibly lucrative."

Sykes did not give very high marks to Sir James Young Simpson, either, although he recognized that Simpson had at least worked, and in an enlightened manner, for the cause of anesthesia: "There was no originality about him—not as regards anaesthesia, anyway. He had nothing to do with its introduction, which was entirely due to others. His mind was receptive enough, though, and he welcomed the new idea at once. He began to use ether in his obstetric practice as soon as the news reached him, and liked it. But he did not consider it was perfect, and his enquiring mind soon began to look around for something better. He deserves every credit for this. Moreover he tested drugs on himself, helped by his assistants Keith and Matthew Duncan. So he was not deficient in courage. The amount of this work, however, was not large . . . No, Simpson's outstanding service to anaesthesia was not his use of chloroform, that beautiful, easy and treacherous drug, but his energy as a propagandist. Pamphlet after pamphlet poured from his vituperative pen in defence of chloroform."

Of Crawford W. Long, Sykes says, "[a] pioneer who could easily have held a much higher place. He had only himself to blame . . . Long's place in the ranking order is low simply because of this extraordinary reticence . . . surely very little vision was required to realise what a tremendous discovery he had made . . . He was beyond doubt the first successful practical anaesthetist the world had ever seen, antedating Wells by two years and Morton by four, but, if it had not been for the efforts of these two men, anaesthesia would have died, as it was born, with Crawford W. Long."

Sir Humphrey Davy was a chemist, and he inhaled nitrous oxide on many an occasion, as well as trying it on animals, birds, insects and fish (he was one of the few investigational scientists of the pioneers). He noted well its analgesic properties, and made his now famous suggestion that it could be used for surgical operations. But, as Sykes points out, "Having made the suggestion he dropped the matter and took no further steps to follow it up . . . what is surprising is that his suggestion was ignored by the very people whom it should have interested most; that surgeons could have continued, for nearly fifty years longer, to operate upon screaming, struggling patients in full consciousness. Surely a lasting testimonial to their thickheadedness. If he had only taken a little more trouble, not to experiment with it in surgery himself, but to see that somebody else did so, then the whole credit of anaesthesia would have belonged to him. He would have gone straight to the top of the list without question. But he did not do it, and his idea remained stillborn, which explains his lowly place in the merit order."

William T. G. Morton has to be credited as the first to publicly demonstrate the clinical efficacy of anesthesia during surgical operation. He took the idea of anesthesia itself from Wells, with whom he had been in partnership in the practice of dentistry; and his choice of ether was due to luck, having been suggested either by Jackson or his own knowledge of student "ether frolics." But in any event, Morton learned from Wells' genius and Wells' impatient failure; he then persisted through experiments upon animals, himself, some private dental patients, and some private surgical patients of Dr. Henry J. Bigelow; and he came to the Massachusetts General Hospital on October 16, 1846 with a sufficiently powerful drug, enough experience, and enough confidence to carry the thing out. As Sykes says, "To Morton belongs the undoubted credit of introducing successful anaesthesia with sufficient publicity to ensure that it immediately achieved worldwide acceptance . . . (but he) does not take a high place for originality."

Horace Wells, the Hartford dentist, Sykes ranks next to the top, because, "he gets almost full marks for the originality of his idea, but not quite, say seven out of ten . . . he did not think of anaesthesia at all until he had seen Colton's public exhibition of the effect of inhaling nitrous oxide . . . but, given this stimulus and the sight of a man partly under the influence of gas failing to notice an injury, he saw the possibilities of it at once, as no one else had done. So much so that he arranged for a personal trial of it for the very next day . . . after his personal experience of anaesthesia and a very small practice in administering it to patients—about fifteen cases—he went off at halfcock and gave his disastrous public demonstration at the Massachusetts General Hospital in January, 1845 . . . his luck was bad, in that he used a weak and technically difficult anaesthetic, and used it prematurely . . . but nothing can rob Wells of the honour of being the first person to use anaesthesia effectively, who at the same time tried to introduce his discovery to the world. The fact that he failed hardly matters."

But it was to Henry Hill Hickman that Sykes awarded the highest merit for the development of anesthesia. Some Americans, noting that the British eventually claim almost all innovations and advances in anesthesia for their own shores, might argue the point in favor of Wells, or Morton, or Long (it is doubtful that *anyone* would argue for Jackson) depending upon individual geographical sympathies and sentiment; but alas, we have no Sykes. Sykes' case for Hickman was simply that, "he above all others had the idea of anaesthesia most deeply and spontaneously engrained in him, and hence he had the most originality of mind . . . he alone conceived the idea without external stimulus of any kind."

Henry Hill Hickman was born in the hamlet of Lady Halton, in the parish of Bromfield, Shropshire, on January 27th, 1800. He was the third child of the four born to Sarah and John Hickman, and the only one to survive infancy. He was baptized in the Parish Church of Bromfield three days later, and then was lost to history's view until he was admitted as a medical student in Edinburgh. He qualified as M.R.C.S. from Edinburgh before he was twenty-one years of age, and that same year he married Eliza Hannah Gardner of Leigh Court near Worcester and returned to his native county of Shropshire. There he and his bride settled down to the life of a country practitioner, and the card that hung outside of his surgery proclaimed, "At home, every Tuesday, from 10 o'clock until 4, for the purpose of giving advice, gratis, to the poor and labouring classes." He remained in practice at Ludlow, which was only two miles from his birthplace, for about two years. It was in this country town that the main part of Hickman's experimental work was done during March and April of the year 1823; he moved to the village of Shifnal some time between January and August 1824. In that same year, he published his pamphlet entitled, "A Letter on Suspended Animation, Containing Experiments Showing That It May Be Safely Employed During Operations On Animals, With The View of Ascertaining Its Probable Utility in Surgical Operations On The Human Subject, Addressed To T. A. Knight, Esq., of Downton Castle, Herefordshire, One Of The Presidents Of The Royal Society," which is reprinted below.

Hickman waited three years for encouragement or practical help from his colleagues, and then took off for France to try again, for at that time it was Paris, rather than London or Edinburgh, which was the center of medical and scientific thought. Once there, he addressed himself to King Charles X, in a letter that is also republished below.

Both Hickman's famous pamphlet and his letter to Charles X are contained in the souvenir volume of the Henry Hill Hickman Centenary Exhibition at the Wellcome Historical Medical Museum in 1930, and are reprinted here with the kind permission of the Wellcome Foundation and the Wellcome Historical Medical Museum.

A LETTER ON SUSPENDED ANIMATION, CONTAINING EXPERIMENTS SHOWING THAT IT MAY BE SAFELY EMPLOYED DURING OPERATIONS ON ANIMALS, WITH THE VIEW OF ASCERTAINING ITS PROBABLE UTILITY IN SURGICAL OPERATIONS ON THE HUMAN SUBJECT,

ADDRESSED TO T. A. KNIGHT, ESQ., OF DOWNTON CASTLE, HEREFORDSHIRE, ONE OF THE PRESIDENTS OF THE ROYAL SOCIETY

* * * *

A LETTER, ETC.

Sir,

The facility of suspending animation by carbonic acid gas, and other means, without permanent injury to the subject, having been long known, it appears to me rather singular that no experiments have hitherto been made with the object of ascertaining whether operations could be successfully performed upon animals whilst in a torpid state; and whether wounds inflicted upon them in such a state would be found to heal with greater or less facility than similar wounds inflicted on the same animals whilst in posssession of all their powers of feeling and suffering. Several circumstances led me to suspect that wounds made on animals whilst in a torpid state, would be found, in many cases, to heal most readily; and the results of some experiments which I have made lead me to think that these conjectures are well founded, and to hope that you will think the results sufficiently interesting to induce you to do me the honour to lay them before the Royal Society. The experiments were necessarily made upon living animals, but they were confined to animals previously condemned to death; and as their lives were preserved, and their suffering very slight, (certainly not so great as they would have sustained if their lives had been taken away by any of the ordinary methods of killing such animals) I venture to hope that they, in the aggregate, rather received benefit than injury. Subjects of different species were employed, chiefly puppies of a few weeks or months old, and the experiments were often repeated, but as the results were all uniform, and as my chief object is to attract the attention of other medical men to the subject, I wish to do little more than state the general results.

Experiment 1st. Dogs of about a month old were placed under a glass cover, surrounded by water, so as to prevent the ingress of atmospheric air, where their respiration in a short time ceased, and a part of one ear of each was then taken off; there was no hemorrhage, and the wounds were healed at the end of the third day, without any inflammation having taken place, or the Animals having apparently suffered any pain or inconvenience from the operation.

Experiment 2nd. After the same animals had fully recovered their powers of feeling, a similar part of the other ear was taken off; a good deal of blood now flowed from the wounds, and some degree of inflammation followed, and the wounds did not heal till the fifth day.

Experiment 3rd. An experiment was made similar to No. 1, in every respect, except that the suspension of animation was much more suddenly brought on by the agency of sulphuric acid and carbonate of Lime. The results in this case were not so satisfactory; some blood escaped from the wounds, and a slight degree of inflammation followed and the wounds did not heal so rapidly as the first experiment.

Experiment 4th. Mice, having been confined in a glass tube of a foot long, were rendered insensible by carbonic acid gas slowly introduced in small quantities, and one foot from each was taken off; no hemorrhage took place upon the return of sensation, and the wounds appeared quite healed on the third day, without the animals having apparently suffered pain, when they were given their liberty.

Experiment 5th. An adult dog was rendered insensible by means similar to the preceding, and the muscles and blood vessels of one of its legs were divided. There was no hemorrhage from the smaller vessels; a ligature which secured the main artery came away on the fourth day, and the animal recovered without having at any period shown any material symptom of uneasiness. In this experiment animation was suspended during seventeen minutes, allowing respiration occasionally to intervene by means of inflating instruments.

Experiment 6th. A dog was rendered insensible by the means employed in experiment first, and an incision was made through the muscles of the loin, through which a ligature was passed, and made tight; no appearance whatever of suffering occurred upon the return of animation, nor till the following day, when inflammation came on with subsequent suppuration. The ligature came away on the seventh day, and on the twelfth the wound was healed.

As the recital of such experiments as those preceding must be as little agreeable to you, as the repetition of them has been to myself, I shall not give a detail of any others, but shall only state the opinions which the aggregate results have led me to entertain. I feel perfectly satisfied that any surgical operation might be performed with quite as much safety upon a subject in an insensible state as in a sensible state, and that a patient might be kept with perfect safety long enough in an insensible state, for the performance of the most tedious operation.

*   *   *   *

I remain, Sir,
Your obedient Servant,
H. H. HICKMAN.

Shiffnal, Aug. 14th, 1824.

1831–1832

Published December, 1970

The history of the development of intravenous therapy—the modality which is so completely essential to the modern day practice of anesthesiology—is a fascinating one.

The story undoubtedly begins in Oxford, England, in 1659, but there are those who would start the tale several hundred miles away and almost two centuries earlier—on the banks of the Riber Tiber in

1492. It seems that the Pope, Pope Innocent VIII, had suffered a cerebrovascular accident the previous year, and for some time had fallen into a kind of somnolency, which was occasionally so profound that the whole court believed him to be dead. All means to awaken his exhausted vitality had been resorted to in vain, when a Flemish doctor proposed to do so by transfusion of blood from a younger person, an experiment which had hitherto only been made on animals. Accordingly, the blood of the decrepit old Pontiff was passed into the veins of a youth, whose blood was then transferred back into the veins of the old man. The experiment was tried three times, and at the cost of the lives of three boys, probably due to air embolism. The good Pope continued his downhill course and died anyway.

The tale is almost certainly apocryphal, since it is difficult to conceive how blood transfusion, as the procedure is understood today, could have been practiced at a time when the circulation of the blood was not recognized—and, of course, it was not recognized until William Harvey published his landmark book, *De Motu Cordis*, in 1628. In any event, so the tale continues, the three boys and the Pope having died, the Flemish physician quickly disappeared!

The far more certain fact is that the major foundation for intravenous therapy was laid, as noted above, in 1659 by Sir Christopher Wren, undoubtedly England's most famous architect. He was the man who was responsible for the reconstruction of St. Paul's Cathedral following The Great Fire of London in 1666, and, in addition, he designed a further 52 churches and many other buildings in London, including the additions to both Kensington and Hampton Court Palaces. Sir Christopher was a man of many parts, however, and far more than just an architect. He held the degrees of Bacheolor of Arts, Master of Arts, Doctor of Civil Law, and Doctor of Law; and he was at one time a Professor of Astronomy at Oxford. He invented a corn planter; he prepared microscopically enlarged drawings of insects for Charles II; he evolved a scheme for the graphic construction of solar and lunar eclipses; he solved a problem in geometry which had

been posed by no less a mathematician than Pascal; he wrote extracts on the cycloid; he worked on the graphic determination of a comet's path; and he even proposed ways by which to predict the weather.

Like many a genius, Sir Christopher Wren was not a modest man, and in 1665 he wrote in *The Philosophical Transactions of the Royal Society of London* as follows:

"Whereas there have lately appeared in publick some *Books*, printed beyond the Seas, treating of the Way of *Injecting liquors into Veines*; in which Books the *Original* of that *Invention* seems to be adscribed to others, besides him, to whom it really belongs . . . . 'Tis notorious, that at least six years since (a good while before it was heard off, that any one did pretend to so much as thought of it) the Learned and Ingenious Dr. *Christopher Wren* did propose in the *University of Oxford* (where he is now the Worthy Salivian Professor of *Astronomy*, and where very many curious persons are ready to attest this relation) to that Noble Benefactor to Experimental Philosophy, Mr. *Robert Boyle*, Dr. *Wilkins*, and other deserving Persons, That he thought, he could easily contrive a Way to conveigh any liquid thing immediately into the Mass of Blood; *videl*: By making Ligatures on the Veines, and then opening them on the side of the Ligature towards the Heart, and by putting into them slender . . . . Quills, fastened to bladders (in the manner of Clysterpipes) containing the matter to be injected . . . ."

Thus was the hypodermic needle, the basis for all intravenous therapy, invented.

The second great milestone in the history of intravenous therapy occurred on the moors of Scotland during the epidemic of asiatic cholera in the summer of 1831, when Thomas Latta, of Leith, first used the intravenous route to replace lost water and salts in order to save life. An editorial in the June 2nd, 1832, issue of *The Lancet* commented—and with remarkable clarity, when one remembers that the year was 1832—upon the effects of dehydration on all the body tissues:

"Now when we contemplate the phenomenon of cholera, when we see the plump vigorous limbes of youth and adolescence wither in a few hours to the shrunken dimensions of emaciated old age, it is impossible not to conclude that not only has the blood lost much of its water as chemistry has so satisfactorily ascertained, but that all the living solids of the form, the muscles, the nerves, its vascular tunics, and the membranes have been robbed of the bulk of fluid essential to the due discharge of their functions—to the preservation of their vital condition. The quantity of water to be replaced is therefore immense and bears no relation to the presumed quantity of blood which the human body naturally contains."

This comment pertained to the letter from Dr. Latta, "Relative to the Treatment of Cholera by the Copious Injection of Aqueous and Saline Fluids into the Veins," which was published in the same issue (*Lancet, 2:* 274–277, 1831–1832) and is reprinted below.

RELATIVE TO THE TREATMENT OF CHOLERA BY THE COPIOUS INJECTION OF AQUEOUS AND SALINE FLUIDS INTO THE VEINS

LATTA, T.

Lancet, 2:274–277, 1831–1832.

A narrative account of Dr. Latta's treatment of an unstated number of terminal cholera patients with dehydration and circulatory collapse by injection of six pints of water containing sodium chloride and bicarbonate at 112°F at no more than three ounces per minute. During the course of the injections, patients roused and had complete relief of symptoms – until the diarrhea resumed.

1847

Published February, 1957

In the beginning there was ether. Many men and many events contributed to the eventual dawning of anesthesia, but Morton's classical public demonstration of its efficacy on October 16th, 1846, remains the significant landmark. The chronicles of the incident were not long in appearing. The Wednesday, November 18th, 1846, issue of the *Boston Medical and Surgical Journal* contained, in addition to a dissertation on "The Fevers Of The Champlain Valley," an account of "Insensibility During Surgical Operations Produced By Inhalation" by Henry Jacob Bigelow, M.D., a surgeon of the Massachusetts General Hospital. Ten days later, a copy of the *Boston Daily Advertiser*, containing an extract of Bigelow's paper was sent by his father, Jacob Bigelow, Professor of Materia Medica at the Harvard Medical School, to an old friend in London, Dr. Francis Boott. Dr. Bigelow's letter was three weeks in transit,

but it took Boott only moments to appreciate the implications of the contained news. He wrote immediately to the *Lancet*, enclosing both the elder Bigelow's letter and the extract of the son's paper; he wrote also to Robert Liston, Professor of Clinical Surgery in the University of London (who promptly and successfully employed the inhalation of ether during two of his operations); and he arranged the performance of an operation under ether anesthesia in the study of his own home (for the extraction of a molar tooth from one Miss Lonsdale, by Mr. Robinson, "without the least sense of pain, or the movement of muscle").

The issue of the *Lancet* that was published on January 2nd, 1847 contained, under the title of "Surgical Operations Performed During Insensibility, Produced By The Inhalation of Sulphuric Ether," a remarkable documentation of the discovery of anesthesia. It included an extract of

Henry Jacob Bigelow's original paper from the *Boston Medical and Surgical Journal* on the first use of ether anesthesia; Boott's own description of the first anesthetic administration of ether in England; Liston's prompt appraisal of the success of anesthesia in alleviating pain during operation; and a letter from James A. Dorr, Morton's newly-appointed British agent, which was prophetic of the tragic patent fight which was to bring ruin to the lives of so many of the principals involved in one of man's greatest triumphs—the triumph over pain.

SURGICAL OPERATIONS PERFORMED DURING INSENSIBILITY PRODUCED BY THE INHALATION OF SULPHURIC ETHER.

Lancet, 1: 5–8 (Jan. 2) 1847

(Communicated by Francis Boott, M.D.)

To the Editor of The Lancet.

Sir, –I beg to call your attention to the report of an anodyne process, by means of which surgical operations have been performed without pain. I think it would be interesting to the profession if published in The Lancet, I also send a letter from Dr. Bigelow, bearing date more than three weeks after the report drawn up by his son. I wish to add, that Dr. Bigelow is one of the first physicians of Boston, a professor of the Medical School of Harvard College, and a man of great accomplishment. – Yours sincerely, Gower Street, Bedford Square, Dec 1846   F. Boott

Extract from a private letter from Dr. Bigelow to Dr. Francis Boott.

Boston, Nov. 28, 1846.

"My Dear Boott, –I send you an account of a new anodyne process lately introduced here, which promises to be one of the important discoveries of the present age. It has rendered many patients insensible to pain during surgical operations, and other causes of suffering. Limbs and breasts have been amputated, arteries tied, tumours extirpated, and many hundreds of teeth extracted, without any consciousness of the least pain on the part of the patient.

"The inventor is Dr. Morton, a dentist of this city, and the process consists of the inhalation of the vapour of ether to the point of intoxication. I send you the Boston Daily Advertiser, which contains an article written by my son Henry, and which is extracted from a medical journal, relating to the discovery.

"Let me give you an example. I took my daughter Mary, last week, to Dr. Morton's rooms, to have a tooth extracted. She inhaled the ether about one minute, and fell asleep instantly in the chair. A molar tooth was then extracted, without the slightest movement of a muscle or fibre. In another minute she awoke, smiled, said the tooth was not out, had felt no pain, nor had the slightest knowledge of the extraction. It was an entire illusion.

"The newspaper will give you the details up to its date, since which other operations have been performed with uniform success.

"Dr. F. Boott."

The extract of Henry Jacob Bigelow's original paper from the *Boston Medical and Surgical Journal* then followed.

Published February, 1970

Estimation of the depth of anesthesia has been a problem ever since that landmark day in 1844 when Horace Wells demonstrated the efficacy of nitrous oxide to produce unconsciousness and analgesia for operation. In fact, it was Wells' inaccurate assessment of the depth of anesthesia, in front of John Collins Warren's surgical class at the Harvard Medical School the following February, which cost him the credit for the discovery of anesthesia. And, despite two undoubted scientific additions to the art, it is not very much easier today to decide how deeply the patient is anesthetized than it was a century and a quarter ago.

The first of these scientific additions was the measurement of the actual level of the anesthetic drug in the arterial blood. Howard W. Haggard, in a brilliantly conceived and meticulously executed series of studies, set the stage for such measurements. He injected a 5 per cent solution of ether in saline into the carotid artery of a dog at a rate which was adjusted so that about 0.5 gm. of ether per minute was delivered uninterruptedly into the blood stream to the head. This infusion produced all of the signs and indications of general anesthesia. Blood levels of the anesthetic, immediately upon completion of the infusion, showed that the venous return from the head contained 0.9 gm. of ether per liter, whereas arterial blood drawn from the femoral artery at the same time contained only 0.03 gm. of ether per liter. This experiment convinced Haggard that the concentration reached in the central nervous system was the determining factor in the anesthetic action of ether. It was only one step further to show that the ether content of the arterial blood was the critical factor in determining the concentration of ether in the central nervous system, and this Haggard did by drawing samples simultaneously from the femoral artery, the internal jugular vein, and the right heart.

The measurement of the actual level of the anesthetic drug in arterial blood correlates well with the clinical symptoms and signs of the syndrome of general anesthesia, and it is unquestionably the most accurate gauge of the different depths of general anesthesia. It has never progressed from the confining bounds of a research tool to widespread usage as a routine clinical estimate, however, for, although arterial puncture is far more commonplace than it was just a few years ago and although gas chromatography is many-fold faster than the former chemical analyses of blood levels of anesthetics, the techniques remain formidable in terms of the day-to-day administration of clinical anesthesia at the operating room level.

The second scientific addition to the art of the estimation of the depth of anesthesia has been the electroencephalogram. Caton had demonstrated the occurrence of electric potentials in the brains of rabbits and monkeys as early as 1875, but it was not until 1929 that Hans Berger, the "father of electroencephalography," showed that these electrical potentials could be recorded by external electrodes placed upon the surface of the head, and it became possible to study the effects of anesthetic drugs by electroencephalography in the human subject. Several groups of research workers—including Berger himself, who studied the effects of chloroform anesthesia—investigated the effects of anesthetics upon cortical action potentials, but it was Gibbs and his associates who systematically studied some 20 drugs known to effect the central nervous system and described the effects of sedatives and anesthetics on the electroencephalogram: "Sedatives cause changes similar to those observed in normal sleep. In place of the fast and rather steady activity characteristic of the waking state, there are slow, large voltage fluctuations with occasional bursts of fast activity and also short periods in which there are almost no fluctuations. If sedation is so heavy that the patient cannot be aroused, the bursts of fast activity disappear, and the slow components become slower, of larger voltage and almost continuous. Ether produces, first, a decreased voltage of the lower frequencies in the normal record and an increased voltage of the higher frequencies and, later, large voltage, slow waves with a 10 a second rhythm superimposed."

Gibbs and his colleagues also were the first to suggest that electroencephalography might be useful as an estimation of the depth of anesthesia during surgery: "A practical application of these observations might be the use of the electroencephalogram as a measure of the depth of anesthesia during surgical operations. The anesthetist and surgeon could have before them on tape or screen a continuous record of the electrical activity of both heart and brain." This prediction remained just that, a prediction, until the 1950's when Bickford, Courtin, Faulconer and their colleagues at the Mayo Clinic undertook detailed studies and classifications of the electroencephalographic changes produced by ether, thiopental and cyclopropane under actual surgical conditions. Furthermore, in the case of both ether and cyclopropane, the various electroencephalographic patterns were correlated with blood levels. They were always at pains to point out, however, that they were not measuring "depth of anesthesia," but only "estimating the degree of cortical electric alteration associated with the action of anesthetic drugs."

The work of the Mayo Clinic group precipitated a great deal of clinical interest in electroencephalography as a guide to the depth of anesthesia for a period of several years, but although the method is still pursued avidly by certain anesthesiologists, widespread clinical use has dropped off quite precipitously during the past decade. Faulconer and Bickford themselves, writing in 1960, have stated their position on the value of electroencephalography during anesthesia:

"It is our opinion that electroencephalography may make an important contribution to anesthesiology when it is applied for the following special purposes and others like them:

"1. The maintenance of a steady state in laboratory investigations in which variations in depth of anesthesia are undesirable.

"2. The early detection of inadequate cerebral perfusion during whole body perfusion with extracorporeal circulation.

"3. The teaching of anesthesiology and the clinical evaluation of new anesthetic agents.

"4. The assessment of damage and recovery after severe anoxic accidents during anesthesia or cardiac arrest.

"5. The detection of critical changes in amplitude of cortical potentials during hypothermia.

"6. The maintenance of a steady state of anesthesia in the operating room when all other signs of anesthesia are unavailable."

Today, most practicing clinical anesthesiologists still rely on time honored signs to estimate the depth of anesthesia. These include the type, rate and depth of respiration; pupillary size and eyeball activity; corneal, conjunctival, pharyngeal, laryngeal, carinal, cutaneous, peritoneal, and various types of autonomic reflexes; pulse rate; blood pressure; and muscle tone. By the use of these signs as guides, it has been possible to develop various classifications of the depth of general anesthesia. Indeed, the first of these, developed on the basis of subjective criteria, was published just 3½ months following Morton's classical public demonstration of ether anesthesia at the Massachusetts General Hospital on October 16, 1846. It was contained in a letter to the editor, written by Dr. Francis Plomley on the subject of "Operations Upon The Eye," and published on pages 134 and 135 in the January 30, 1847, issue of *The Lancet.*

OPERATIONS UPON THE EYE

PLOMLEY, F.

Lancet 1:134, January 30, 1847

Dr. Plomley describes three successful ether anesthetics for operations about the head. He then assures the readers that ether works well on dogs and describes his own experiences with ether inhalation. Based on his own inhalations he describes an early pleasurable "half intoxication" stage, followed by one of extreme pleasure with consciousness but with indifference to pain. "The third stage, the only one, I think, for performing operations is one of profound intoxication and insensibility."

Published February, 1971

The phenomenon of the doctor turned popular author is really a fairly common one, and a number of examples of popular books written by physicians come to mind readily. Each reader's list of such books will differ, of course, but in this day of women's liberation probably the most recent on many such lists would be Dr. David Reuben's "Everything You Always Wanted to Know about Sex (But Were Afraid to Ask)." Another recent entry would be Dr. Michael Crichton's "The Andromeda Strain," a remarkable achievement for a man who was a full time medical student while he wrote it. That Crichton could then follow with another title on the best seller list, "Five Patients," within a couple of years and while still a house officer produces awe that is beyond description.

My own list necessarily has to include a book written a generation ago by a medical school classmate, Dr. David Bradley, and titled, "No Place To Hide," which was the log of a doctor assigned to duty with Operation Crossroads, the atom bomb tests at Kwajalein Harbor in the Bikinis. My list would also have to include two of the most famous of the many books popularizing science and medicine, Paul DeKruif's, "Microbe Hunters," and Hans Zinsser's, "Rats, Lice, and History." My favorite, however, is "Safe Deliverance," written by Dr. Frederick C. Irving, Professor of Obstetrics at Harvard, while he was a medical student.

"Safe Deliverance" was the fourth volume to receive a $2500 Life-in-America award from Houghton Miflin Company, and was both a history of the Boston Lying-In Hospital and the story of Fritz Irving, who was a living legend in his time. It contains a chapter titled, "The Gentleman in the Beaver Hat," which is devoted to the subject of anesthesia and is worth quoting at some length:

"Possibly Dr. Channing's love of fast driving was an escape from the strain of being a New Englander. He was born in Providence, his maternal grandfather having been one of the signers from Rhode Island of the Declaration of Independence, and all his life was spent between the shores of Narrangansett and Massachusetts Bays. He entered Harvard College in 1804; but in April 1807, with a group of other students he was expelled because he took part in an incipient riot over the quality of the food. On this occasion the University authorities reported that the conduct of the students was 'disorderly, indecent, an insult to the authority of the college, and a violation of the Laws made for the preservation of order and decorum, which ought not to be passed over in silence.' Later, however, when he became eminent, the College forgave him and awarded his A.B. as of 1808. He studied under Rush, Wistar, and Physick at the University of Pennsylvania Medical School, from which he received his M.D. in 1809; and he was given the same degree *ad eundem* by Harvard in 1812. For a while he was a pupil of James Jackson in Boston.

"As was the rule in those days for young physicians of means who hoped to rise in their profession, Channing went to Europe to complete his education. After some time, largely devoted to obstetrics, spent in the hospitals of London and Edinburgh, he returned in 1812 and entered practice in Boston, where at that time midwifery was at a particularly low ebb. There were no hospital clinics where the young physician could see and study obstetrical cases—or for that matter any cases of a medical or surgical nature. Practical experience, for those who had not been abroad, was derived solely through the apprentice system whereby the youthful doctor, acting as an assistant in private practice to an older practitioner, learned what he could of the art and science of medicine from his preceptor. The knowledge and special training acquired by Channing in Europe soon brought him recognition as the ablest obstetrician in the city. In 1815 he was appointed lecturer in obstetrics in Harvard Medical School, and in 1818 he became its first professor of midwifery and medical jurisprudence, a position that he held for 36 years.

"One cannot but speculate upon the curious association of apparently unrelated subjects indicated by Dr. Channing's title. Medical jurisprudence, or legal medicine, has had to do with that wide common ground where law and medicine meet. It concerns not only injuries to the person, deaths from violence, insanity, and malingering, but in addition it embraces subjects involving the sex relations, such as pregnancy, illegitimacy, rape, and criminal abortion—matters which alone in this entire field can have any possible bearing on obstetrics. It is likely that the faculty, having decided that someone should teach medical jurisprudence to the students, selected Dr. Channing, a comparatively young man and the first incumbent of a newly created chair, as the person who might offer the least-spirited resistance to such an assignment. If one may judge from a student's notebook of that day, medical jurisprudence was always with him distinctly a side issue.

"His outstanding public appearance as a medicolegal expert was in 1833 at the trial of Ephraim K. Avery, a revivalist minister, for the murder of Sarah Maria Cornell, a mill worker who was found hanging on a haystack on a farm in Tiverton, Rhode Island. Dr. Channing appeared for the defense; and he was instrumental in securing an acquittal by testifying that the fetus found in Sarah Maria's uterus was of such an advanced gestational development that Avery, who had known the girl only a short time, could not have been its father. Most people, however, did not agree with Dr. Channing. The newspapers were filled with accounts of the trial, broadsides were written about it, and poems were devoted to the piteous plight of the poor working girl and the brutality of the fiendish revivalist.

"To his teaching Dr. Channing brought the enthusiastic interest of an unusually bright and intelligent mind. In those days, now happily past, medical students were not all intellectual paragons; some were indolent and indifferent. The professor was a stimulating lecturer; at times he was clear and concise, on other occasions somewhat discursive, but he never failed to hold the attention of his listeners. One of his pupils describes him in 1832:

> He came fresh from his morning's drive, bright, cheery, and in the best of spirits. The first impression was a favorable one. He was a fluent, at times an eloquent speaker. He graphically described the bones of the female pelvis and clothed them with flesh and blood; he was full of anecdote; his manner was pleasant and interesting. The lecture reminded one of a fresh easterly breeze on a dry, hot summer day. The hour passed rapidly away; he briskly put on his coat and disappeared as suddenly as he came, leaving us almost spellbound.

"One summer morning Dr. Channing was in the midst of a lecture when an organ-grinder took his station beneath an open window. Presently the strains of a popular air began to mingle with the professor's description of puerperal convulsions. For a while the battle was evenly contested, the honors going first to the organ-grinder and then to Dr. Channing, who, completely drowned out at last, sat down and said, 'Gentlemen, Apollo was the god of music as well as physic.'

"The catalogue of the Medical School for 1830 states that the department of midwifery was provided with 'models from Florence to illustrate the practice and teach the anatomy of this branch of the profession. Besides these it is well supplied with plates and preparations to aid its study.' On occasions Dr. Channing produced the models from Florence, dusted them off, and invited members of his classes to diagnose the presentation and position of the artificial fetus in the imitation uterus. For the most part, however, instruction was entirely didactic; and although a few students acquired some practical experience under the preceptorial wings of practitioners, most of them not only graduated in medicine but even attended their first confinement without ever having seen a baby born.

"Dr. Channing was not only the attending physician but also the moving spirit in the establishment of the Boston Lying-In Hospital. The members of the Massachusetts Charitable Fire Society and the first trustees were his familiar friends. Among them was George Hayward, who with Bigelow, Gorham, John C. Warren, and Ware formed a medical club of which Channing was a member.

"Dr. Channing made two outstanding contributions to medicine. In his article entitled 'Notes on Anhaemia, principally in its connection with the Puerperal State', published in the October, 1842, issue of the *New England Quarterly Journal of Medicine*, he described for the first time the pernicious-like type of anemia which on rare occasions complicates pregnancy; and he reported ten such patients, all of whom succumbed. Modern treatment, which includes the use of liver, iron, and blood transfusion, has so improved the outlook that today few women die of the disease. Moreover, once the baby is born the anemia disappears and the patient again becomes normal. In Channing's day transfusion had never been successfully performed; for not only was there no method to prevent the blood from clotting during its transfer to the patient, but before 1910 nothing was known about blood grouping, which enables blood from a donor to be given to a recipient without causing its red cells to adhere and lose their hemoglobin, thus causing death or serious injury to the person whom it was designed to benefit. Channing's prophetic instinct was shown in this article when he said: 'The question of transfusion has often occurred to me. But of what possible benefit would be such a supply of blood? In a disease so fatal some risk might be incurred. But is transfusion an operation which our present knowledge of it would authorize? If safe in itself, however, might not time be gained by the operation of such functional changes to occur as would supply healthy blood?'

"Channing's most important contribution to medicine, however, was the use of anesthesia in childbirth, for he was the earliest prominent American advocate of the employment of ether to assuage the pains of labor and to produce unconsciousness during normal or operative deliveries. His name stands in history beside that of James Young Simpson of Edinburgh, who about six months before had applied this great discovery, used first in surgery, to the same purpose."

In fact, the first obstetric operation under anesthesia in America was performed by Dr. Channing on May 5, 1847, less than 7 months after Morton's classic public demonstration of ether anesthesia at the Massachusetts General Hospital on October 16, 1846; and in the following year, 1848, Channing published his book, *A Treatise on Etherization in Childbirth*, reporting the results in 581 cases gathered from his own experiences and from those of his friends.

Channing was to obstetric anesthesia in this country what Simpson had been to obstetric anesthesia abroad.

But despite the prominent part played by Channing, the credit for the introduction of obstetric anesthesia in America must go to a dentist, Nathan Colley Keep, who was the first dean of Harvard's School of Dentistry where he had been one of Morton's teachers and, before that, had very probably been the man to whom Horace Wells had been apprenticed for the study of dentistry. Keep's letter, addressed to the editor of the Boston Medical and Surgical Journal on April 10, 1847, was the first American report of obstetric anesthesia (*Boston Med. & Surg. J. 36:* 226 (April 14) 1847). It was also, more importantly, the initial description of an attempt to provide a technique of anesthesia particularly adapted to obstetrics, synchronizing the intermittent administration of the anesthetic with the regularly recurring contractions; and for this reason it is reprinted below.

LETTER TO THE EDITOR

KEEP, N.C.

Boston Med. & Surg. J. 36:226, 1847

A brief letter describing ether administration to one patient in labor and concluding with "Number of inhalations, five. No unpleasant symptoms occurred, and the result was highly satisfactory."

Published December 1980

The bottom line in the accounting to sum up the worth of any anesthetic agent or technique is necessarily the mortality associated with its use; and the subtotal, of course, is necessarily the morbidity.

The latter is difficult to quantitate. Certain complications such as nausea and vomiting, postspinal headache, nerve injuries, muscle pains, phlebitis, sore throat, aspiration of gastric contents, embolism, and so forth and so on, have been the subjects of an inordinate number of retrospective— and even some fairly imaginative prospec-

tive—investigations, but we really know surprisingly little about postoperative problems resulting from anesthesia.

On the other hand, we know quite a good deal, indeed, about mortalities following anesthesia and surgery from innumerable reviews on a subject which is one of intense interest, not only to anesthesiologists, but to surgeons, the medical profession in general, public health officials, even the general public, and, perhaps particularly, to the ubiquitous lawyers.

The incomparable John Snow, in his classic, *On the Inhalation of the Vapour of Ether*, which was published in 1847, reported the first such series of mortalities, having encountered 6 deaths in 78 administrations of ether. Of these he wrote, "It is very evident, that in none of the six cases that end fatally, out of the foregoing two lists, can the event have been caused, or in any degree promoted by the inhalation of ether, since there are very sufficient and well-recognized causes to account for the result."

Eleven years later, in the posthumous publication, *On Chloroform and Other Anaesthetics*, Snow recorded 50 deaths associated with the administration of chloroform. This time there was no question whatsoever that the anesthesia had been involved, and the usual mechanism of death was cardiac syncope. Many of these cases were reported by word of mouth or in the literature, and were therefore not always as well documented as Snow's own personal cases of ether administration had been. Nevertheless, it was an important study—and the first study—of deaths associated with anesthesia.

During the past quarter of a century, several important investigations into the incidence of anesthetic deaths and the factors involved have been undertaken.

A major review titled, "Study of Deaths Associated with Anesthesia and Surgery," was published in the *Annals of Surgery* for July, 1954, and was a survey of the deaths associated with anesthesia and surgery as they occurred in 10 University Medical Centers in the United States between January 1, 1948, and December 21, 1952. It contained data on 599,548 anesthesias administered at the University Hospitals involved in the study. The study was concerned with the role that anesthesia might have played in the total surgical care of the patients involved and in particular with the extent to which anesthesia contributed to mortality in the surgical patient. The death rate, when anesthesia was considered to have been the primary cause, was 1 : 2,680; and the death rate when anesthsia was *either* the primary cause or was an important contributory factor in death was 1 : 1,560.

These were the most authoritative figures up to that time because of the large size of the sample.

Another major study was carried out by the Committee studying deaths associated with anesthesia which had been appointed by the Council of the Association of Anaesthetists of Great Britain and Ireland. The Committee scrutinized voluntary and anonymous reports of deaths submitted to it on special forms provided by the Association; and by April, 1955, at the end of 5½ years, it had been notified of 1000 deaths. Out of this number, 598 were concluded to rank as anesthetic deaths. It was quite impossible, of course, with this anecdotal methodology, to learn anything about death rates, but a tremendous number of important points concerning mechanisms of anesthetic death were highlighted. Fatal regurgitation and vomiting, for instance, occurred in 110 of the 598 deaths; and of the 29 deaths from obstetric anesthesia, 15, or 52 per cent, were due to regurgitation or vomiting. These are sobering statistics. In the series, 107 cases died from circulatory failure immediately following iv. barbiturate injection, and on 72 occasions death took place at the onset of induction. Postoperative respiratory obstruction due to pharyngeal relaxation was the cause of death in 23 instances, and probably the cause in 11 more. Of considerable interest were 5 cases of death attributed to the anesthetic apparatus, since this was the first time in a large series that any mention at all was made of any death where faulty equipment was considered a major factor. It must be borne in mind, of course, that this study came at a time when anesthetic equipment was beginning to become a great deal more sophisticated and complex than in an earlier day.

All of the reviews of deaths associated with anesthesia point to the indisputable fact that human error is *the* cause of most anesthesia-related mortality, but that what Gordon Wyant has so elegantly phrased as the "mechanical misadventures of anesthesia" account for a solid 8 per cent of these deaths. Furthermore, the piece of equipment most commonly involved has been a simple piece of equipment indeed—an endotracheal tube. Indeed, it is the simple things which are not in functioning order—or, perhaps more importantly, have not been checked beforehand to ascertain that they are in functioning order—which cause many of the mishaps encountered in anesthetic practice. Mechanical mishaps and machine failure have been a part of the anesthetic scene since the introduction of ether in 1846, when it was related that the second attempt to induce anesthesia in London that year failed because of a faulty expiratory valve; Morton himself, within 8 months of his classic demonstration of the efficacy of ether anesthesia at the Massachusetts General Hospital on October 16, 1846, gave up the use of formal apparatus entirely. He related this in a letter to the *Lancet* on June 30, 1847, in a communication which is cited simply as, "Letter from Dr. Morton" (*Lancet, ii:* 80, 1847) and which is republished below.

LETTER FROM DR. W. T. G. MORTON OF BOSTON, U. S.

Lancet, 2: 80, 1847

"As in everything else new, I had to find my way along slowly and cautiously, after discovering the new properties of ether, and was for some time greatly embarrassed in procuring a suitable apparatus. My first attempts were made with a sponge; next, I used a simple conical glass tube, with a sponge in the large end; and after that, other instruments, none of which however, affording but partial success."

Later in the letter, Dr. Morton expresses his dissatisfaction with any type of apparatus and describes his return to the sponge. "I have found the result more sure and satisfactory, and the difficulty of inhalation very much reduced, or entirely removed. – – – The beauty and importance of this means is its perfect simplicity."

Published February, 1958

Announcement of the introduction of clinical anesthesia electrified the medical world of 1846. In retrospect, the astonishment seems somewhat unjustified; for, as has been true of so many great discoveries and events, the time was ripe and the way had been paved. The thought did not occur as a single flash of inspired genius in the mind of one man, but lay dormant in many minds conditioned by the march of the civilization of the day and a variety of human activities prior to that time. Joseph Priestley prepared and described nitrous oxide gas in 1777, and diethyl ether had been described by Valerius Cordus, an assistant of Paracelsus, as early as 1540. The inhalations of both substances were employed, during the early forties of the nineteenth century, at strange parties called "frolics" to produce an exhilaration, bordering on semi-inebriation, by medical students both in the United States and abroad. It is therefore perhaps more indicative of the inevitable progression of civilization than of coincidence that Crawford Long's use of ether in surgery in 1841, and Horace

Wells' use of nitrous oxide in dentistry in 1844, both followed upon the observations of the numbing effects of the inhalation of these agents at such "frolics". Long received no encouragement from either the local population or the medical profession in his area, and he failed to even publish his work until after the classic public demonstration of ether anesthesia by Morton in 1846. Wells, on the other hand, employed nitrous oxide anesthesia more than a dozen times with great success in his own practice, and decided to give a clinical demonstration of the method before Dr. Warren's medical class at the Massachusetts General Hospital. The event turned out to be a total fiasco, for Wells failed to secure adequate anesthesia, and he was hissed out of the room as a fraud with shouts of mingled scorn and derision.

It is one of the fallacies of human nature to understand only that which it is convenient to understand, and none of the principals involved in the introduction of anesthesia comprehended that its discovery was inevitable. Following Morton's public demonstration of ether anesthesia in 1846, they all struggled long and bitterly for the honors (and the patents!). Crawford Long's original administrations were belatedly brought to public attention, and in 1847 Horace Wells' "A History of the Discovery of the Application of Nitrous Oxide Gas, Ether, and Other Vapors, to Surgical Operations" was published by J. Gaylord Wells, corner of Main and Asylum Streets in Hartford. Wells' pamphlet is of tremendous interest as the presentation of the man's case in relation to the celebrated controversy. It is of further great interest in that it describes Wells' appreciation of the fact that general anesthetic agents produce an excitement stage before inducing depression, although he wrongly attributed the depression to stimulation, rather than attributing the stimulation to early depression.

A HISTORY OF THE DISCOVERY OF THE APPLICATION OF NITROUS

OXIDE GAS, ETHER, AND OTHER VAPORS, TO SURGICAL OPERATIONS

HORACE WELLS

Published in Hartford by J. Gaylord Wells, Corner Main and Asylum Streets, 1847

"I propose, in the briefest manner possible, to give, in the following pages, a true and faithful history of the discovery which is at present causing an unparalleled excitement throughout the whole medical world. I refer to the administering of exhilarating gas, or vapor, to prevent pain in surgical operations. It is very unfortunate that there should be more than one claimant for the honor of the discovery; but so it is: and the only alternative now is, for the man who considers himself entitled to this honor to present his proofs, that a discriminating and impartial public may "give credit to whom credit is due".

There follows a lengthy discussion of why Wells believed he should be treated as the discoverer of anesthesia.

Published February, 1961

James Simpson was born in 1811 at the little town of Bathgate, in Linlithgowshire County, Scotland, the seventh son and eighth child of the village baker. He died 59 years later in Edinburgh (of the doctor's disease, coronary occlusion), after having served as one of the University of Edinburgh's foremost professors, after having been knighted by the Queen of England, and after having become one of Scotland's most celebrated sons. In very large measure, these honors and fame were due to chloroform.

Simpson was a bright and able schoolboy, and the family determined to combine their resources to send him on to a higher education. Consequently, he enrolled in the arts classes at the University of Endinburgh at the age of 14 (!), graduated as a doctor of medicine at 21, and promptly accepted an assistantship at his alma mater.

Obstetrics was regarded as an almost vulgar profession in those days, and was hugely derided by other practitioners and, particularly, surgeons—who conveniently forgot that they themselves had not so long before been recognizable by a barber's pole. Nonetheless, when James Hamilton, Professor of Midwifery at the University of Endinburgh, died, Simpson set his cap for the vacant chair. Today, a professor is usually *chosen* for the job; but in that age, the man *sought* the job, and Simpson made application for the Professorship. In that age, also, the town council had as much—if not, indeed, more—say in the filling of the Professorship than did the faculty. The professors all opposed Simpson, and perhaps for that reason the councilors supported him. The contest for the vacant chair resembled nothing as much as it did a modern political campaign, with a small fortune being expended on printing, postage, posters and leaflets. Vituperation was rife, and a common charge against Simpson was the fact that he was only 28 years of age. The many who thought him too young referred to him as Young Simpson, and there is the (perhaps apocryphal) tale that Simpson obtained immediate revenge by promptly adding a middle name and signing himself James *Young* Simpson. In any event, the town council prevailed over the faculty, and on February 4, 1840, Simpson was able to write to his mother-in-law: "I was elected Professor today by a majority of one. Hurrah!!!"

Simpson was worshipped by women and his practice flourished—so, too, did his active medical mind. When news of Morton's triumph with ether reached the British Isles, he hailed the American discovery as "a glorious thought" and on January 17, 1847, became the first to employ ether in obstetric practice. His avowed purpose was to banish pain from the lying-in chambers of the world, and he was not discouraged from his task even by "the murdered spirit of Lady Eufame Macalyene, who in this very city of Edinburgh had been burnt at the stake by the ecclesiastics for attempting to assuage the pangs of labor by artificial means". He was discouraged, however, by the slow, uncertain and irritating qualities of ether, and he began a comprehensive search for a more energetic anesthetic drug. His method of search was a simple one, known to generations of anesthetists: self-experimentation. He and his two assistants, George Keith and Matthews Duncan, met in Simpson's dining room each evening after their day's work to inhale the vapor of iodoform, benzene, chloride of hydrocarbon (ethylene dichloride, or Dutch Liquid), and various oils and gases, to test for themselves the anesthetic properties of these substances; each morning, James Miller, the Professor of Surgery and Simpson's next door neighbour, would look in at breakfast time, "just to inquire if everyone was still alive."

It was a fellow Scotsman, David Waldie, like Simpson born in the Royal Burgh of Linlithgow, and at the time chemist at the Apothecaries Hall in Liverpool, who suggested that the experimenters try "perchloride of formyle," or chloroform. Indeed, Waldie even offered to prepare some of the liquid and send it to Simpson for trial, but the sending of the sample was delayed, and on November 4, 1847, the impatient Simpson determined on a trial of a sample prepared in the Department of Chemistry at the University of Edinburgh. Miller, Simpson's surgical colleague who lived next door, has described the scene: "They inhaled the vapour and their conversation became very bright. But suddenly there was a talk of sounds being heard like those of a cotton mill, louder and louder; a moment more, then all was quiet, and then—a crash. On awakening, Dr. Simpson's first preception was mental, 'this is far stronger and better than ether' . . . he saw Dr. Duncan snoring loudly; and then his eyes overtook Dr. Keith's feet and legs making valorous efforts to overturn the supper table . . . Later on, Simpson having regained his seat, Duncan having finished his unrefreshing slumber, and Keith having come to an arrangement with the table and its contents, the session was resumed . . . each expressed himself delighted with this new agent and its inhalation was repeated many times—one of the ladies gallantly taking her place and turn at the table—until the supply of chloroform was fairly exhausted."

For many of the particulars in the above story of the discovery of the anesthetic properties of chloroform, *Survey of Anesthesiology* and its readers are indebted to Dr. W. H. F. Boyd, of Edinburgh; the story of the first surgical uses of chloroform as an anesthetic is best told by Simpson himself, and was published in *Lancet* (Simpson, J. Y.: *Lancet 2*: 549–550, November 20, 1947), under the title, "On a new anaesthetic agent, more efficient than sulfuric ether."

ON A NEW ANAESTHETIC AGENT, MORE EFFICIENT THAN SULFURIC ETHER

J. Y. SIMPSON, M.D.

Professor of Midwifery in the University of Edinburgh, Physician-Accoucheur to Her Majesty in Scotland, etc.

Lancet, 2: 549–550, 1847

* * * *

"This new anaesthetic agent is chloroform, chloroformyle, or perchloride of formyle. Its composition is expressed by the chemical formula C_2HCl_3.

*   *   *   *

"As an inhaled anaesthetic agent, it possesses, I believe, all the advantages of sulphuric ether, without its principal disadvantages.

"1. A greatly less quantity of chloroform than of ether is requisite to produce the anaesthetic effect.

*   *   *   *

"2. Its action is much more rapid and complete, and generally more persistent.

*   *   *   *

"3. Most of those who know, from previous experience, the sensations produced by ether inhalation, and who have subsequently breathed the chloroform, have strongly declared the inhalation and influence of chloroform to be far more agreeable and pleasant than those of ether.

*   *   *   *

"4. I believe that, considering the small quantity requisite, as compared with ether, the use of chloroform will be less expensive than that of ether.

"5. Its perfume is not unpleasant, but the reverse, and the odour of it does not remain, for any length of time, attached to the clothes of the attendant, or exhaling, in a disagreeable form, from the lungs of the patient, as so generally happens with sulphuric ether.

*   *   *   *

"6. Being required in much less quantity, it is much more portable and transmissible than sulphuric ether.

*   *   *   *

"7. No special kind of inhaler or instrument is necessary for its exhibition.

*   *   *   *

"I have had an opportunity of using chloroform with perfect success in several surgical operations, (removal of tumours, of necrosed bone, partial amputation of the great toe,) and in tooth-drawing, opening abscesses, for annulling the pain of dysmennorrhoea and of neuralgia, in two or three cases where I was using deep and otherwise very painful galvano-puncture for the treatment of ovarian dropsy, and in removing a very large fibrous tumour from the posterior wall of the uterus by enucleation, &c.

"I have employed it also in obstetric practice, with entire success."

1848

Published February, 1959

There is, today, a salutary trend toward a dispassionate evaluation of the factors involved in deaths during anesthesia. Committees to study anesthesia morbidity and mortality have been set up in many areas; and in a number of such studies the anesthesiologist has been joined by his surgical colleagues—as well as pathologists, obstetricians, pediatricians, internists, and, of course, the ubiquitous statisticians—in the quest for answers. It has become apparent that a great many deaths that occur during anesthesia are in no way related to anesthesia *per se,* and it has become equally apparent that a great many deaths that occur in the postoperative period can trace their origins, directly or indirectly, to the anesthesia *per se*. These realizations have led to significant progress in terms of better preoperative preparation, correctly timed premedication, cautious anesthetic induction, cognizance of the effects of the duration and the depth of anesthesia, adequate replacement therapy, and meticulous, detailed postoperative care. In short, the concept of the "surgical team" is ceasing to be merely a textbook aphorism, and is becoming, at last, a reality.

It was not ever thus. For many years the prevalent attitude was that all deaths that occurred during operations were anesthesia deaths and could be attributed to the anesthetist. When old Blood and Guts plunged knife into belly with a roar and came out with a severed cystic artery, who was to demur that this was scarcely an anesthetic death? And if, perchance, some enterprising intern, showing more zeal than common sense, then went off on his own and obtained permission for an autopsy, the ultimate rejoinder to the pathologist's findings at the surgical death review would surely be, "well, what do you expect of a man—trying to operate on a moving target like that?" This attitude (that all operating room deaths were due to anesthesia) led in time to the ludicrous practice, when catastrophe threatened, of hastily moving the dying (or dead) patient to the corridor, where death (or the pronouncement of death) ensued.

There was a still earlier time, soon after the introduction of clinical anesthesia, when anesthesia was the domain of the surgeon: and death during anesthesia was regarded as a complication that could be laid at the door of no man, but, rather, was caused by the anesthetic agent itself. The first recorded death during anesthesia occurred on the 28th day of January, 1848, and was reported on page 161 of the first volume of *Lancet* for that year under the title, "Fatal Application of Chloroform."

FATAL APPLICATION OF CHLOROFORM

Lancet, 1: 161, 1848

"An inquest was held on Tuesday last, at Winlaton, about five miles from Newcastle-upon-Tyne, on view of the body of HANNAH GREENER, a girl of 15 years of age, who died on the Friday, under the influence of chloroform. The case excited great interest.

"JOHN RAYNE said, the deceased suffered a great deal in her feet, and about four months ago she became an inmate of the infirmary at Newcastle-upon-Tyne, where she had one of her toe-nails taken off. After she left the infirmary she returned to her father's, but her toes still continued bad. Mr. Meggison, surgeon, of Whickham, was called in to attend her, and it was considered advisable to remove the nail from the great toe of her right foot. Mr. Meggison and his assistant attended about one o'clock on Friday afternoon last, to perform that operation. No one was present when the operation was performed but Mr. Meggison, his assistant, and myself. She moaned after the nail was off; on which Mr. Meggison dashed water in her face, when her eye moved. He afterwards put some brandy into her mouth, and she rattled in her throat. He also bled her in the arm and neck, but very little blood flowed. She never recovered.

*   *   *   *

"The CORONER then addressed the jury, briefly explaining the law of the case. The JURY then retired, and, after a few minutes' absence, returned with the following verdict:—"We are unanimously of opinion that the deceasd, Hannah Greener, died from congestion of the lungs, from the effect of chloroform, and that no blame can be attached to Mr. Meggison, surgeon, or to his assistant, Mr. Lloyd."

"The inquisition was then made out in the usual form, and the jury dismissed."

1849

Published February, 1960

"It has been said that America's greatest contribution to medical science was the introduction of anesthesia into surgical procedures. If this is true, then the controversy that followed the Morton demonstration of October 16th, 1846 is, by way of contrast, the sorriest contribution America has ever made to medical science. Nowhere in the annals of medicine can there be found a story more filled with greed, sordidness, chauvinism, and selfishness than this one."

So runs a recent appraisal of the Great Ether Controversy, and there must be few who have delved into the details of that dismal saga who would disagree. Indeed, a mere two years after the discovery became generally known, the public was wearied to death of the controversy, which continues even today, more than a century later. Each of the participants recognized the importance of the truly historic event, and each entered vigorously into the struggle for the honors and the expected great wealth. The claims and countercharges that were made, the petty letters and repulsive tracts that were written, the bitter enmities that grew, all but dimmed the luster of the greatness of the fact. But, perhaps not unreasonably, each claim was valid in its own way.

Certainly the magnitude of Morton's contribution can never be held in serious doubt (Classical File, *Survey of Anesthesiology*, February, 1957). The Boston dentist did in fact administer the ether at the first public demonstration of surgical anesthesia; and if he was not the actual discoverer of anesthesia, he was, at the very least, mainly responsible for its introduction into surgical practice. There is little question that Morton "borrowed" some of his ideas from others. Morton had been Horace Wells' student in Hartford, and from him Morton had learned all about nitrous oxide, its effects, and its preparation; it was this knowledge that put Morton upon the trail of anesthesia. Morton had also been a student of Charles Thomas Jackson, chem-

ist and geologist, and it was from him that Morton learned of sulfuric ether. Yet in spite of these indebtednesses, the fact remains that Morton was the man who gave surgical anesthesia to the world.

Wells' contribution was also of undoubted magnitude. The Hartford dentist had witnessed the public entertainment during which Colton amused the audience with the antics of volunteers who inhaled "laughing gas," and he perceived instantly the significance of the fact that one of the volunteers sustained a severe skin bruise without feeling pain and even without apparent knowledge of the injury. He was quick to apply the concept of anesthesia, first to himself and then to his dental patients; and, indeed, he was applying nitrous oxide anesthesia almost as a routine in his dental practice nearly two years before Morton's triumph at the Massachusetts General Hospital (Classical File, *Survey of Anesthesiology*, February, 1958). It was only the robustness of the patient and the failure to attain a sufficient depth of anesthesia during Wells' own abortive demonstration at Boston that kept Wells from achieving the public acclaim that Morton won the following year.

Jackson, the chemist, was led to press his claim because of a fierce and driving envy, but his was perhaps a lesser contribution than that of any of the others. It is true that Jackson suggested the use of ether to Morton—a fact which Morton never denied—but he did so with tongue in cheek, secretly believing that its usefulness would prove to be of little value. It was only *post facto* that Jackson, poisoned with maniacal envy, went to the Academy of Arts and Sciences, to the newspapers, and finally to Congress itself, either to obtain recognition for himself or to prevent it for Morton. These endeavors were as fruitless as had been his previous energies to gain the credit for William Beaumont's remarkable researches on the progress of digestion through the famous gunshot accident to Alexis St. Martin, which left a "window" in the young French-Canadian's stomach; or his even earlier attempts to gain the credit for Morse's invention of the telegraph.

All three of these men—Morton, Wells and Jackson—were to a certain extent essential to the introduction of anesthesia. In retrospect, it seems a shame that the bitter controversy arose, for there was surely credit enough in the presentation of anesthesia to mankind for all to share. But, in fact, the controversy was only just beginning, for Crawford Williamson Long, of Jefferson County, Georgia, had, in many respects, the best claim of all. He was familiar with ether, had made observations of its analgesic effects that were strikingly similar to those made by Wells on nitrous oxide, and had administered ether as a surgical anesthetic as early as 1842. Indeed, he was to all intents and purposes the discoverer of anesthesia, except for one fatal mistake—his failure to present his discovery to the world. This failure he rectified belatedly, seven years too late, in the *Southern Medical and Surgical Journal 5:* 705–713, December, 1849, under the title of "An Account of the First Use of Sulphuric Ether by Inhalation as an Anaesthetic in Surgical Operations."

AN ACCOUNT OF THE FIRST USE OF SULPHURIC ETHER BY INHALATION AS AN ANAESTHETIC IN SURGICAL OPERATIONS

C. W. LONG, M.D.

Jefferson, Jackson Co., Georgia

South. Med. Surg. J., 5: 705–713, 1849

"For nearly three years, the various medical journals have contained numerous articles on the employment of Sulphuric Ether by Inhalation, for the purpose of rendering patients insensible to pain during surgical operations.

*   *   *   *

"In the month of December, 1841, or January, 1842, the subject of the inhalation of nitrous oxide gas was introduced in a company of young men assembled at night in this village, (Jefferson,) and several persons present desired me to prepare some for their use. I informed them that I had no apparatus for preparing or preserving the gas, but that I had a medicine (sulphuric ether) which would produce equally exhilerating effects; that I had inhaled it myself, and considered it as safe as the nitrous oxide gas. One of the company stated, that he had inhaled ether while at school, and was then willing to inhale it. The company were all anxious to witness its effects. The ether was introduced: I gave it first to the gentleman who had previously inhaled it, then inhaled it myself, and afterwards gave it to all persons present. They were so much pleased with the exhilerating effects of ether, that they afterwards inhaled it frequently, and induced others to do so, and its inhalation soon became quite fashionable in this county, and in fact extended from this place through several counties in this part of Georgia.

"The first patient to whom I administered ether in a surgical operation, was Mr. James M. Venable, who then resided within two miles of Jefferson, and at present lives in Cobb county, Ga. Mr. Venable consulted me on several occasions in regard to the propriety of removing two small tumours situated on the back part of his neck, but would postpone from time to time having the operations performed, from dread of pain. At length I mentioned to him the fact of my receiving bruises while under the influence of the vapour of ether, without suffering, and as I knew him to be fond of, and accustomed to inhale ether, I suggested to him the probability that the operations might be performed without pain, and proposed operating on him while under its influence. He consented to have one tumour removed, and the operation was performed the same evening. The ether was given to Mr. Venable on a towel; and when fully under its influence I extirpated the tumour. It was encysted, and about half an inch in diameter. The patient continued to inhale ether during the time of the operation; and when informed it was over, seemed incredulous, until the tumour was shown him. He gave no evidence of suffering during the operation, and assured me, after it was over, that he did not experience the slightest degree of pain from its performance. *This operation was performed on the 30th March, 1842.*

"The second operation I performed upon a patient etherized was on the 6th June, 1842, and was on the same person, for the removal of another small tumour. This operation required more time than the first, from the cyst of the tumour having formed adhesions to the surrounding parts. The patient was insensible to pain during the operation, until the last attachment of the cyst was separated, when he exhibited signs of slight suffering, but asserted, after the operation was over, that the sensation of pain was so slight as scarcely to be perceived. In this operation, the inhalation of ether ceased before the first incision was made: since that time I have invariably desired patients, when practicable, to continue its inhalation during the time of the operation."

1853

Published April, 1975

Over the course of the last 19 years, *Classical File* has, at one time or another, and in one form or another, republished writings by all of the participants in the Great Ether Controversy, except one. We have heard from William Thomas Green Morton (twice!), in Henry Jacob Bigelow's initial paper on "Insensibility during Surgical Operations Produced by Inhalation" in the November 18, 1846 issue of "Boston Medical and Surgical Journal," and in a paper written by Morton but published posthumously by his son William J. Morton, "The First Use of Ether as an Anesthetic. At the Battle of the Wilderness in the Civil War," in the April 23, 1904 issue of the "Journal of the American Medical Association." We have heard from Horace Wells in his pamphlet, "A History of the Discovery of the Application of Nitrous Oxide Gas, Ether, and Other Vapors, to Surgical Operations," which was published in 1847 by J. Gaylord Wells, corner of Main and Asylum Streets in Hartford (right across from Wells' dental office!). We have heard from Crawford Williamson Long in his paper on, "An Account of the First Use of Sulphuric Ether by Inhalation as an Anaesthetic in Surgical Operations," in the December, 1849 issue of the "Southern Medical and Surgical Journal." But we have never heard from Charles Thomas Jackson. It is time to rectify that omission.

Jackson was Professor of Chemistry at Harvard and one of the greatest chemists of his time; he was also the most insufferable figure in the Great Ether Controversy. He had an ego as big as a mountain, and he could not live without prestige. There are 3 uncharming incidents illustrative of this.

The first of these occurred on the transoceanic packet-ship *Sully* in 1832. The *Sully* sailed from Le Havre headed for New York and, because of constant headwinds, did not arrive there until 40 days later. Jackson was a passenger, returning to Boston to establish a practice of medicine after more than 2 years of postgraduate study of medicine at the Sorbonne and continuing researches in geology (he was, in addition to being a doctor and a chemist, a thoroughly competent geologist) at the *Ecole des Mines*. Another passenger aboard the *Sully* was Samuel F. B. Morse, a brilliantly versatile man who, after studying physics at Yale, had pursued a thoroughly successful career in portraiture.

The voyage, as noted above, was extended; and since Jackson had purchased a number of pieces of equipment for his research laboratory while in Paris, he used an electromagnet (which was among these items) in a series of demonstrations of electricity to amuse his fellow passengers— and, of course, to make himself the center of attention. Following one of these shows, Morse remarked to Jackson at the dinner table that, if the presence of electricity could be made visible in any part of the circuit, there was no reason why intelligence could not be transmitted instantaneously by electricity. The idea gripped Morse and served as the seed for the invention of the telegraph, which he and his collaborators perfected and patented in 1837. His shipboard notes, following the chance conversation with Jackson, involved a sending apparatus to transmit signals by the closing and opening of an electric circuit; an instrument for receiving, to record these signals on a strip of paper fed by clock movements; and the "Morse code" for enciphering letters and numbers into dots and dashes.

Morse's success, and patent, devoured the envy-driven Jackson, who promptly asserted a claim for the invention. In May of 1839, the following item appeared in "The Boston Post": "We are informed that the invention of the electromagnetic telegraph, which has been claimed by Mr. S. F. B. Morse of New York, is entirely due to our fellow citizen, Dr. Charles T. Jackson, who first conceived the idea of such an instrument during his return voyage from Europe on the packet-ship *Sully* in October 1832." Jackson pressed his claims again in 1846, and once again in 1849; but he had become so thoroughly discredited by then that nobody took him very seriously. Morse wrote of the legal deposition made by Jackson on the subject, "There was never a more finished specimen of wholesale lying than is contained in it. He is certainly a monomaniac, no other conclusion could save him from an indictment for perjury."

The second uncharming incident involved the military surgeon Beaumont who, because of the famous gunshot accident to Alexis St. Martin which left a "window" in the young French-Canadian's stomach, made the first important researches into the physiology of digestion. These were epochal studies, not to be surpassed for almost two-thirds of a century

with the brilliant work in Russia by Pavlov and his pupils.

The incident started innocently enough when Beaumont, who toured with St. Martin, exhibiting him before various medical societies, left some gastric juice with Jackson in Boston to make a chemical analysis of its properties. The supply was small and soon Jackson sought more, when he learned to his dismay that Beaumont had been ordered to a new post in the West and that therefore St. Martin would no longer be available for Jackson's experiments. This prompted the incredible Jackson to petition the Secretary of War, with the signatures of more than 200 members of Congress, to change the military orders which had been issued to Beaumont:

"Being informed that Dr. Charles T. Jackson, an eminent chemist of Boston, is successfully prosecuting an analysis of the gastric fluid of Alexis St. Martin, the Canadian boy attached to Dr. Beaumont, surgeon of the United States Army, and that the analysis cannot be satisfactorily accomplished without the presence of Dr. Beaumont and Saint Martin; and regarding the case as furnishing a rare and fortunate opportunity of demonstrating important principles in physiology, by which credit may be conferred on the medical science of our country and important benefits accrue to humanity; also, understanding that several scientific bodies are anxious to draw Saint Martin from this country for the purpose of prosecuting the investigations now making by one of our countrymen, who is in every way competent to the work; and persuaded that the opportunity now afforded, if neglected, will be lost to our country forever, we request that the Honorable Secretary of War WILL STATION DR. BEAUMONT AT BOSTON, OR IN THE VICINITY, FOR THE TERM OF FOUR MONTHS, OR LONGER IF NECESSARY FOR THE OBJECT."

Only the bureaucracy of Army orders— which already had the good doctor headed West—saved the credit for his famous discoveries in physiology to Beaumont, discoveries which Jackson would surely have claimed!

The third uncharming incident concerned the discovery of anesthesia.

The alleged facts concerning this incident vary; but certain it is that Jackson—by conversation, by chance remark, or by lecture—turned Morton's attention from nitrous oxide to ether as a possible form of anesthesia (the word had not even been introduced at the time!). One version, very possibly apocryphal, is that Morton actually boarded at Jackson's house following his departure from Hartford to go to Boston, and that Jackson told him of the anesthetic effects of ether when applied to the skin (undoubtedly a form of refrigeration anesthesia from the evaporation). Morton used the method on the tooth of a young woman, Miss Parrot, in July of 1844, for a painful filling, and, noting that the surrounding parts of the face were numbed, wondered if the entire system could not be brought under the influence of the drug.

Another version, probably equally apocryphal, was that Morton chanced upon the effect of ether by an accident:

"In the winter of 1841–1842, I was employed in giving a few lectures before the Mechanics Charitable Association in Boston, and in my last lecture, which I think was in the month of February, I had occasion to show a number of experiments in illustration of the theory of volcanic eruptions, and for these experiments I prepared a large quantity of chlorine gas, collecting it in gallon glass jars over boiling water. Just as one of these large glass jars was filled with pure chlorine, it overturned and broke, and in my endeavors to save the vessel, I accidentally got my lungs full of chlorine gas, which nearly suffocated me, so that my life was in imminent danger. I immediately had ether and ammonia brought, and alternately inhaled them with great relief . . . . I determined, therefore, to make a more thorough trial of the ether vapor . . . . I continued the inhalation of the ether vapor, and soon fell into a dreamy state, and then became unconscious of all surrounding things . . . . Reflecting on these phenomena, the idea flashed into my mind that I had made the discovery I had for so long a time been in quest of—a means of rendering the nerves of sensation temporarily insensible, so as to admit of the performance of a surgical operation on an individual without his suffering pain therefrom."

Yet a third version has Morton going to Jackson's laboratory to obtain a new bag to contain his nitrous oxide, and being told in an off-hand manner by Jackson that ether had the same effect on the central nervous system as nitrous oxide, and was a good bit easier to handle.

Whatever the truth, there is no question that Jackson got into the act when it became evident that Morton had achieved an overnight triumph with ether anesthesia. Jackson sent letters to a friend in the French Academy of Sciences which, without so much as mentioning the name of Morton, proclaimed himself as the discoverer of anesthesia. He read a paper to the American Academy of Arts and Sciences in which he publicly announced himself as the discoverer of ether. He petitioned Congress for a "reward" of 100,000 dollars for his contribution to America. He even wrote of his use of ether to cure mental disease. He was, in short, in the very midst of the Great Ether Controversy.

Outside of his claims to the discovery, Jackson wrote very little about anesthesia—which was reasonable, since he knew so little about clinical anesthesia. He did write one piece discussing anesthesia in 11 different animals; and then the following letter, which was published in the January, 1853 issue of the "Southern Medical and Surgical Journal" (*South. Med. Surg. J., 9:* 5–20), addressed to "Prof. L. A. Dugas."

LETTER TO THE EDITOR

BOSTON, October 23d, 1852.

PROF. L. A. DUGAS:

My Dear Sir—I comply most cheerfully with your request, that I should prepare a short account of the use of Anesthetic Agents in Surgery and Midwifery for publication in your valuable medical journal. I have for some time had it in contemplation to prepare for the press a volume, containing all the information that I possess on the subject, with a digest of the numerous works that have been published upon it by distinguished scientific and medical gentlemen of Europe, but my professional and offical duties have occupied my time so completely as to have prevented my accomplishing this task; and I should desire to visit Europe, in order to collect all the best observations, before publishing a work of so important a character. I have decided, however, to begin here, and to work up such materials as are in my hands; after which, I hope to have the pleasure of consulting with my generous friends in Europe, and to collect all the scattered information of a practical character that may be needed to complete a work worthy of the subject, and sufficient to meet the wants of the medical world. This, the public may expect from my hands.

I have now before me a number of books and pamphlets, on the use of anesthetic agents, which have emanated from the presses of Europe—twenty-one of them are in the German language, one in Latin, three in French, and one in Italian, while only two or three pamphlets have been published in England, on Chloroform, and only one regular work on the use of Ether and Chloroform in Child-birth, and a pamphlet on Ether, have, thus far, appeared in America. Unfortunately, the public mind has been more occupied with the disputes which have taken place here as to the origin of the discovery, than with the rational investigation of the principles and practice of Etherization. This, I trust, will cease to agitate us much longer; for the question of discovery has been passed upon by the highest of scientific tribunals—the Institute of France—and it is no longer open for discussion, excepting so far as concerns the appropriation of some reward for the discovery by the Congress of the United States, and even that I have not sought, prefering that the act should emanate spontaneously from the councils of the nation. France and Sweden have already shewn, by liberal acts, their approbation of this discovery, and it is hoped that our own country will not long delay that justice which is expected from her hands.

* * * *

It is well known, that the use of ether vapor for the production of insensibility to pain in surgical operations was made by me, and that the Institute of France so decided, after a full examination of the claims of numerous contestants for the honor of this discovery.

1856

Published August, 1977

There probably is no more pathetic, disheartening—and, yes, even terrifying—sight in medicine today than to watch the average pediatric resident or medical student attempting to resuscitate a depressed newborn infant.

Her, or his, Chairperson of Pediatrics has argued long and loud that the resuscitation of the newborn infant is the bailiwick of the pediatrician and, after much vituperative declamation, has made the point at numerous Faculty meetings, Dean's Office conferences, or gatherings of the Curriculum Committee: the Department of Pediatrics will assume responsibility for the resuscitation of the newborn!

But who is going to teach these poor, benighted pediatric residents and medical student clerks *how* to resuscitate the newborn infant? Not the Professor and Chairperson of the Department of Pediatrics, because there are no Professors and Chairpersons of the Department of Pediatrics in the delivery room at 2:00 A.M. when the depressed infant is born. Not the Associate Professor of Pediatrics, because there are no Associate Professors of Pediatrics in the delivery room at 2:00 A.M. Not the Assistant Professor of Pediatrics, because there are no Assistant Professors of Pediatrics in the delivery room at 2:00 A.M. Not the Instructor of Pediatrics, because there are no Instructors of Pediatrics in the delivery room at 2:00 A.M.—just the pediatric resident and/or medical student clerk assigned to Pediatrics.

It is an awe-inspiring scene.

A large cart is wheeled in which contains all the necessary, or even conceivable, equipment.

There is a mask, a bag, and an oxygen tank—which is empty; but this really is not important, since the pediatric resident or medical student clerk does not know how to open an oxygen tank, let alone get a flow of oxygen out of it.

There is a laryngoscope with an infant blade—which is not checked to see whether the bulb will light, that the batteries are not dead, or, in other words, whether it is functional.

There is a collection of various sizes of infant endotracheal tubes, ranging in size from 00, through 0, to 1, but no one looks through the lumens of these tubes to be sure that they are patent (and history records that there are a number of ways in which endotracheal tubes can become plugged).

There are ampules of bicarbonate, epinephrine, glucose, nalorphine, levallorphan, naloxone, sodium chloride, *et cetera, et cetera.*

Then the charade begins.

The wee bairn is about to be born, but first the pediatric resident and/or medical student clerk must draw up: (1) a syringeful of sodium bicarbonate; (2) a syringeful of glucose; (3) a syringeful of epinephrine; (4) a syringeful of nalorphine, or a syringeful of levallorphan, or a syringeful of naloxone; *et cetera, et cetera.*

Meanwhile, back on the delivery table, the wee bairn is indeed born, and the bairn is in a depressed state.

The first thing to be done, obviously, is to fill out the elaborate form which will provide information about every conceivable factor which might bear on the development of fetal depression.

When the form has been properly filled out, the ECG electrodes must be applied to the chest.

Then, immediately, the trachea must be intubated.

Well, there really is no point in going on with the sorry tale—by now the reader has a mental picture of the dreadful nightmare.

In point of fact, some years ago Shnider laid out a very structured, reasonable, and all-inclusive procedure for the resuscitation of the newborn:

I. Establishment and maintenance of an airway
   A. Position
      1. Keep head lower than trunk from birth
      2. Hold by feet, with mouth lowermost, for best drainage
      3. In bassinet, keep head down, neck extended, body at lateral tilt
   B. Suction of pharynx
      1. Perform very briefly and gently
      2. Avoid prolonged suction; laryngospasm or bradycardia may result
II. Laryngoscopy and endotracheal suction, if:
   A. Meconium is present
   B. Rales and rhonchi are heard in lungs
   C. Blood or other debris is present in mouth
III. Evaluation of infant
   A. Determine Apgar score
IV. Administration of oxygen (if baby is depressed—score of 7 or less)
   A. Mild depression (score 5 to 7)
      1. Blow oxygen over face
      2. Stimulate feet
      3. Avoid anal dilation
      4. Avoid back slapping
   B. Moderate to severe depression (score 1 to 5)
      1. Administer oxygen by intermittent positive pressure via mask or endotracheal tube
   C. Proper ventilation
      1. See chest expand
      2. Hear bilateral breath sounds; listen over both lung bases and stomach
      3. Observe improvement in con-

dition of newborn, *e.g.*, increasing heart rate
4. Avoid excessive pressure (above 25 cm. H$_2$O for more than 2 seconds)
V. Administration of sodium bicarbonate (if Apgar score is under 5 at 5 minutes, despite adequate ventilation with oxygen)
   A. Insert catheter into umbilical artery (under sterile precautions)
   B. Administer slowly sodium bicarbonate, 2 to 8 mEq. per kg.
VI. Administration of drugs (Nalline, Lorfan, or analeptics are rarely necessary and must be used with caution)

More than a century before the preparation of this lucid, step-by-step list of instructions for the resuscitation of the newborn by Shnider, Marshall Hall had made his own list of what he termed "RULES," which he presented in a paper that he read before the Harveian Society on Thursday, November 20th, 1856. This was published under the title of "The Asphyxia of Stillborn Infants, and its Treatment" in the November 29th, 1856, *Lancet* (pp. 601–602), and is reprinted below.

THE ASPHYXIA OF STILL-BORN INFANTS, AND ITS TREATMENT

MARSHALL HALL

Lancet, 2: 601–602, 1856.

We must remember that the newly-born infant is a creature of high irritability and low stimulus, and that the foramen ovale and ductus arteriosus are open—both events calculated to protract life and hope in the case of apnea; and we must long, very long, *persevere* in our efforts to save the still-born.

Resuscitative efforts are directed at 1) measures to induce efficient respiration, and 2) measures to maintain the circulation.

Treatment may be summarized in the form of *Rules*:
1) Place the fetus on the face.
2) Sprinkle the general surface briskly with *cold* water.
3) Make gentle pressure on the back; remove it, and turn the infant on the side; and again place it prone with pressure.
4) Rub the limbs, with gentle pressure, *upwards*.
5) Repeat the sprinkling only now, with cold and hot water (of the temperatures of 60° and 100°F.) alternately.
6) Continue these measures, or renew them, from time to time, even for hours. The embers of life may not be entirely extinct.

1857

Published August, October, December, 1961

"But if you are an Indian, and believe the things an Indian does and think the way an Indian thinks, then the making of a batch of curare is a difficult and an awesome task. To begin with, it takes four or five hard days in the jungle to gather your materials and prepare them. Certain roots are gathered; and certain of the long trailing lianas, or tree vines, are sought for with patience and cunning instinct, so that they may be pulled down from the trees and cut into sections short enough for the curare pots. Certain plants are hunted and their bark removed, since only that part of them is used.

"Meanwhile, you have a selected spot for making the flying death far out in the jungle, hidden away from the rest of your people, for that is custom. It is there you store your ingredients as you find them, and it is there you put the especially made clay pots and lay in a supply of firewood which will keep your curare boiling continuously for several days. You must do all that away from your clanhouse and your people. You know that if you made the curare under your own roof all your household would be weakened and made ill by its magic, just as you know that the people of your household would have a weakening effect on the drug.

"At last everything is ready in your jungle retreat so that, undisturbed, you can go through the ritual of making flying death . . . and steep yourself in the ultimate jungle magic.

"You have built a lean-to, for you will continue your vigil as a poison maker alone and away from the world for several days. During that time you cannot be with or even—it is better—see your wife; and in your retreat you are happy in the knowledge that the one thing in all the jungle which would most weaken your poison cannot happen: no pregnant woman will come within sight of your pots of boiling poison. If that should happen, you might as well throw the stuff away, for you know, as your fathers before you have known, that it would be weak and useless and would not harm the smallest bird that flies in the jungle.

"Also, for a day or so before you are actually ready to make curare, you have taken no salt or chicha or any *aji*, the violently hot little pepper of which you are so fond at other times. Sometimes you have not even taken anything containing sugar during that period, though usually—in this region—during the actual making of the poison you are permitted to chew sugar cane for nourishment.

"On the very last day before you actually begin to make the deadly stuff you eat nothing at all. All that—the fasting and the keeping away from your woman and your household you call the 'sacrifice,' and you are proud of having made it. After it is all over, you tell your friends that you have been a man . . . and that you make very good poison indeed.

"Early in the morning of the day you fast, you make the final preparations. The one or more large clay jars with the pointed bottoms—the ones you use only for curare making and which gather strength the more times they are used—are carefully balanced on the unlit fires made only from three large sticks. The smaller, traditionally bowl-shaped pot for the final thickening of the curare is carefully inspected. It is very old, and has thickened many batches of curare for you. You feel it is full of magic, and that it is part of all the other jungle magic.

"After that, you check over the large vine-tied bundles of the mysterious ingredients with which you are about to work: the roots and bark scrapings, and the long twisted sections of tree vines. You name them over to yourself carefully, to see if you have missed anything. The names given them in the ancient lore slip easily through your mind, as you look at them: the stick-which-catches-fire; the toucan-tongue; the thick-gold-stick; the vine-which-is-like-a-frog; the magic-stick-that-grows-beside-big-waters; the black-poison-stick; and the stick-which-is-like-a-boa. Sometimes there are other ingredients— roots from the plant-which-talks-in-the-wind, for example. Usually there are not. But always, since you are of this region, you use at least these which you now have before you.

"Patiently you work with the magic plants. After they have been thoroughly cleaned, they must all be shredded as fine as possible, so that in their cooking you may extract the last particle of their magic strength and power. To do this, you beat them for hours, over and over again, a bit at a time, on a large flat rock, and are careful to use only a wooden cudgel so that you will not lose a single splinter or a single drop of their potent juices.

"When you are sure that everything is ready, you may take a long bitter swallow of the juice of the soul-vine. Then you go into your lean-to to sleep with your hunger, and dream strange dreams about the magic of curare, and the mighty hunting you will do with this that you are about to make.

"Early the next morning, while the mists are still on the jungle and before Inti has made you warm, you quickly rinse your hunger-tasting mouth with the acrid *gua-yusa* and swallow a mouthful of some food which has no salt and chew a bit of sugar cane. By then you are ready for the actual making.

"While your fires are burning up bravely against the dampness of the dawn mists, you turn your attention to your shaped-by-magic ollas, or, as you would probably call them, your *jambi-mangacuna*, your huge clay pots with the pointed bottoms, in which your deadly brew will simmer for the next two days. By that time you will be ready to bring it to its final state in the small open casserole-sort of cooking vessel. This, until you need it, you keep carefully covered with a piece of bark cloth so that its magic will not escape.

"Your brittle clay ollas are very old, and have been used—fragile and unwieldy as they are—many times before in the making of curare. They are veterans, and being veterans, are better able to resist the spirits of the foaming black magic which will shortly be in them. When they are new and untried, you know they are weak in spirit, and are likely, mysteriously as those things happen, to break without warning when they are on the fire, and let the result of your hard-worked witchcraft run out on the jungle floor in a thick, dark-brown pool. You handle them carefully, for you respect them as you would respect any jungle comrade. . . .

"When you are ready, you rub them quickly and thoroughly with handfuls of *cuilin* leaf, which gives them a smooth watertight coating on the inside. The cuilin leaf itself is not a magic plant. At other times, your woman has used it to line the inside of her cooking and chicha pots.

"Then immediately, while the black juices of the cuilin are still wet on the inside of your ollas, you place the great pots (you are probably starting off with three) on the fires. When they are hot enough, the coating of cuilin juices will be as hard and shiny as thin black lacquer. After they have been on the fires awhile, you spit carefully into the hollow cone of their bottoms. If the slight crackle you hear above the sound of the fire seems right to your sensitive ears, you hastily throw about a quart of water into each pot to hold them at just that heat.

"Quickly, then, you go from fire to fire and distribute arm-loads of your pounded ingredients—the roots, the bark, the long gnarled liana sections—among your ollas until you have no more left to put in them.

"You have been careful, in the filling of your pots, to wave certain bits of the flying death plants three times around your head before you put them in with the rest. Just why you do that you have never known. It is part of the ancient lore, and even your father, the aged twisted Old One, could not tell you why it was necessary. It is just that you must do it, and you know that it is better that way.

"Now that you have arranged your dry ingredients, as you have always been taught, you put five or more gallons of the water in each great, open-mouthed pot so that it is completely filled.

"Then for two long days and nights you tend your fires so that the stuff you are cooking will simmer correctly. When it is not raining, and your fires are not covered with their individual canopies of great leaves, you lie beside them—constantly awake and watchful—and think of the things a man should: the meat you will kill with the poison you are making; the stealthy walking along hidden game trails; the poisoned dart in the blowgun; your lean, root-hard body held in patient readiness for the shot; the eating of much food again . . . and your woman to prepare it for you . . . and then your woman . . .

"And when it *is* raining, you squat in sodden stolidness under your lean-to, with the water streaming out of your ash-streaked matted hair and over your suddenly shivering body, and hope that soon Inti will return and help you with your fires. Ane even as you hope for Inti, the good sun, you hope that Supay, who is evil, will not take it into his mind to make your poison weak and like a woman-thing. You hope that for your days of labor and your sacrifice you will get a pound of fine strong curare out of the many gallons which are boiling in front of you.

"By late afternoon of the second day, when the shadows—dark as the brown-black stuff you have been boiling for so long—fall slanting across your ollas and across your hands, which have become tired from fanning fires with a feather fan, you see that it is time for another step. By now the good jungle strength has been extracted from your ingredients. So, being very careful not to inhale their magic, you fish them, hot and steaming, out of the pots and throw them away in the bush, covering them well with leaves so that others will not see them. After that, the amount of liquid remaining is so small that, strained two or three times through a piece of hand-beaten bark cloth, it can all be put in one pot.

"Arranging the single, pointed-bottomed olla on a fresh fire directly in front of your lean-to, for another night you squat sleepless beside it, fanning it and tending it. And as you chew your bit of sugar cane and wolf down a meager handful of unsalted yucca, you look out past the small fire into the greatness of the night. The loneliness of your vigil and the emptiness of your hunger bring before you the spirits of the Beings of the ancient lore which you have heard at so many night-fires. Somehow you confuse them with the sounds the jungle makes at night.

"When the mist-broken light of the third day filters down to where you are squatting on the floor of the jungle, you see that the amount of liquid in the olla is now about one syrupy, foam-covered gallon. The foam is a dirty amber in color, and as thick as beaten white of egg. When you see it, you say 'Yah . . . !' to yourself with satisfaction, for it is a sign that the poison will be good. Also, it is important to you at the moment, for with it you make the first real test of your jambi.

"Carefully you skim it off with half of a sun-hardened gourd which has holes in its bottom so that the liquid will run out and the foam will remain. When you have collected the foam and placed it in another small gourd, you dip half a dozen blowgun darts in it, and then hastily dry their poisoned points before the fire.

"After that, and after you have arranged your fire so it will burn evenly for at least an hour, you take your blowgun, and the freshly-coated darts, and slip off into the jungle to see if the magic of your jambi will be good, or if it will be a weak thing and shame you when you return to the house of your family.

"In all the ancient lore which has come down to you by word of mouth from so many fathers of fathers, there has never been anything about white-tiled laboratories, and undeviatingly-accurate toxicity tests, and the careful computation of animal protocols resulting from those tests. You have your own jungle-rigid means of proving that your poison is strong and deadly, that, when it is made and you have coated many arrows with it, it will kill for you with a sureness which may save your own life.

"The lore of the poison tells you there are only three animals on which you may try it . . . that you may try only its foam before the jambi itself is completed . . . and that the trial must be made on the first of three animals you see during your hour's walk away from the fire.

"Possibly you may see, and succeed in catching, a large water toad. That is one of the animals. If you do, you will hold him in one hand, and force deeply into the delicate white underskin of a hind leg the poisoned tip of one of your darts. Then you will put him on the ground and prod him so that he will jump, and your eyes will glitter with the hope that your work has been good. The toad must collapse, completely paralyzed, within six to eight jumps. You count them carefully, "Shuc . . . ishcai . . . quimsa . . . chuscu . . . pichca . . . sucta! YAH! YAH! . . .!'

"Or—and you would rather have it happen this way—when you walk through the bush you suddenly see, high up in the branches ahead of you, a large toucan or, darting behind the long extended roots of a tree, you see a *pavo del monte* (a grouselike bird). In either event, you and your long tapering blowgun are suddenly no more than a noiseless jungle shadow, as you glide as close as possible to the bird you have seen. Then in complete silence, you blow your dart and watch again to see if your magic has been good. If the bird, feeling the prick of the small dart, flies at once a few feet to the branch of another tree, and—even as it is alighting on the branch—quivers and falls, your curare is strong and is a man-poison.

"You return to your fire contented with the flying death you are making, and refreshed with having hunted and killed. Before night comes again you will have finished and, carrying your jambi-mangacuna and your new curare, you will return to your house and to your woman.

"When there is no more foam and the thick molasses like liquid has been reduced to less than two quarts, you transfer it to the small olla, which you have unwrapped and prepared. All through the middle of the day you sit beside the small cooking pot, impatient and restless, but more careful with your fire than you have been at any time before.

"While the hot black stuff is simmering down to about the volume of a pint, it must not be allowed to scorch. Guarding your hand with a thick green leaf, you anxiously remove individual embers from the fire or, if you think best, shove them closer to the pot and blow gently on them. It is your only means of temperature control in the most delicate and nerve-racking procedure in all the jungle . . . and the most exacting work which you, a jungle man, will ever have to do.

"But you have been careful and precise, and your magic has been good. As the afternoon wears on, and the poison in the jar looks more than ever like melted pitch, you commence to touch its surface with the tip of a blowgun arrow. Suddenly, one of the times you touch it, a long, sticky black thread rises up behind the arrow's tip. It has come to its 'point.'

"Quickly you lift the little jar from the fire and, before it has time to cool and harden, you pour the thick black syrup into a gourd or a long thin tube of bamboo. If you intend to trade it with others who do not know the secret of making it, you may divide it among several small clay pots, each of which holds about three ounces. As soon as it has congealed, you carefully cover the mouth of the container with a bit of leaf which you size down with a thread of *pita* fiber.

"You have finished. The sacrifice has been good, and the jambi is good. It is the flying death, and it will kill much meat for you and your family or, if you trade—it is valuable among those Indians who do not make it—it will bring you much flake gold or animal skins or whatever it is you feel at the time you and your people most need. You carry it home with pride through the bush to the place where your yucca is planted, and where your house is, and where your woman is waiting for you . . ."

Thus runs the description of curare making in Richard Gill's fascinating volume, *White Water and Black Magic* (New York: Henry Holt and Company, 1940). Gill's account retains all the mystery and voodoo that Gill himself has done so much to dispel by his arduous journeys into the jungle and his procurement of botanical specimens which permitted "the medical civilizing of curare."

Almost a century earlier, the genius of Claude Bernard had done equally as much to dispel the mystery surrounding the mechanism of action of the flying death in a series of elegantly-conceived and meticulously-executed experiments, which he reported in his lectures at the College of France, where he held the chair of medicine. *Survey* and its readers are indebted to the Williams & Wilkins Company—the publishers of *Survey*—for the translation into English of lectures seventeen through twenty-six from Bernard's book, *Leçons Sur Les Effects Des Substances Toxiques Et Médicamenteuses* (Paris: J. B. Balliere et Fils, 1857). These lectures will be published in this and the succeeding two issues of the Journal.

LEÇONS SUR LES EFFECTS DES SUBSTANCES TOXIQUES ET MÉDICAMENTEUSES

CLAUDE BERNARD

J. B. Bailliere et Fils, Paris, 1857

LESSON SEVENTEEN

May 9, 1856

Summary: Physical and chemical properties of curare. . . . Extraction of its active principle. . . . Boussingault and Roulin, Pelletier and Petroz, etc. . . . Chemical characteristics of curarine. . . . Chemical antidotes to curare.

LESSON EIGHTEEN
May 16, 1856

Summary: Physiological action of cu-rare. . . . Facts reported by authors (Brodie, Watterton). . . . Our first experiments (1844). . . . Conclusions. . . . Differences in absorption of curare by the various mucosal surfaces. . . . Its quite special effect on the nervous system.

LESSON NINETEEN
May 21, 1856

Summary: Experiments on the absorption of curare.—Curare is not changed by the gastric juice.—It is not absorbed by the mucous mem-branes, gastric, vesical, or conjunctival.—It is absorbed by the rectal mucosa, but especially by the respiratory mucosal surfaces and by glandular surfaces.—The intestinal mucous membrane of birds and reptiles absorbs cu-rare.—The lack of absorption by the gastric mucous membrane of mammals is not an ab-solute fact.—The skin of mammals and of birds does not absorb curare.—That of frogs absorbs it under certain conditions.

*   *   *   *

LESSON TWENTY-ONE
May 28, 1856

Summary: Curare is without effect on the active organs of the circulation, and it does not take away from the blood its physiological properties.—Effect of curare on the nervous system: it abolishes the manifestations of the nervous system and leaves the muscular system intact.—By this, it can be proved that muscu-lar contractility and the excitability of the mo-tor nerves are two distinct properties.—Exper-iments relating to this subject.

LESSON TWENTY-TWO
May 30, 1856

Summary: Curare acts on the nervous sys-tem.—It must not be thought that it acts, si-multaneously and in the same way, on the sensory and the motor properties.—Its transi-tory action excludes the idea of an anatomical lesion.—Difference between its effects and an-esthetic effects.—On the dosage of curare and of medicaments in general.

LESSON TWENTY-THREE
June 4, 1856

Summary: Curare acts exclusively on the motor nerves. . . . Experiments. . . . It leaves intact the sensory nerves, the muscles, and all the other tissues of the body. . . . Experiments on muscular respiration. . . . Special indepen-dence of the movements of the heart; their relations with the nervous system. . . . An anal-ogous phenomenon seems to be produced in other muscular movements.

LESSON TWENTY-FIVE
June 11, 1856

Summary: Galvanization of the pneumogas-tric nerve arrests the movements of the heart: experiments with the cardiometer. . . . It no longer stops them in an animal poisoned with curare. . . . The near mechanism of death by curare is asphyxia through cessation of the respiratory movements. . . . Curare considered as a medicament. . . . It cannot be regarded as the antidote to strychnine.

1858

Published August, October and December, 1969

This fall—December tenth, to be pre-cise—marks the one hundred and twenty-fifth anniversary of the discovery of anesthe-sia.

It was in the evening of that day that Horace Wells and his wife, Betsy, went to Union Hall in Hartford (Connecticut) to hear the itinerant showman, "Professor"

Gardner Quincy Colton, lecture on the marvels of the new science, chemistry. And it was during the course of that lecture and demonstration that the shrewd Yankee mind of Horace Wells deduced the concept of general anesthesia. This fact has not been popularly acknowledged by all men in all places. It is not acknowleged in Jefferson, Georgia. It is not acknowledged in upper New York state. It is not acknowledged in certain parts of the United Kingdom. And it is most ceratinly not acknowledged in Boston. But facts are facts; and the facts on the matter are that the evidence in support of Wells' claim as the discoverer of anesthesia is overwhelming.

The Honorable Truman Smith, United States Senator from Connecticut in the thirty-second Congress of the United States, was the most vigorous advocate of Wells' rightful claim, just as History has been the most effective. Smith collected and collated all of the pertinent information concerning this claim, and drew attention to his brief in an address to a distinguished group of Hartford women which was published in 1858.

"Ladies: I venture to address you on a subject in which I have been led to take a deep interest, and which can hardly fail, on being properly presented, to arrest your attention. Are you aware that the city of Hartford was a few years since the theatre of one of the most wonderful discoveries of modern times? In the month of December, 1844, the late Horace Wells, of your city, a dentist of great intelligence and respectability, conceived the idea of throwing the human system, by the use of certain means, into a state of insensibility to pain, under the most severe dental or surgical operations.This, by a bold experiment which he caused to be tried on himself, he soon ascertained could be done; and thus originated, on the banks of your beautiful river, the modern art of Anaesthesia, which early attracted the attention of learned men everywhere, and was ere long introduced into practice throughout the civilized world.

"But notwithstanding the facts alluded to were notorious in your city, and a whole cloud of witnesses can be, and, indeed, have been called to establish their truth, a pre-

tender ere long appeared in the person of W. T. G. Morton, who has been, and is, seeking to arrogate the fame of this great discovery, and to appropriate all the rewards which public gratitude should doubtless accord to it. This he attempted both at the first and second sessions of the Thirty-second Congress; and being then a member of the U. S. Senate, and conversant with all the facts, I felt it to be my duty to oppose to his claims an uncompromising, as I did a successful, resistance.

"This put an end to the efforts of Morton, so far as Congress is concerned; but within a few weeks, he has made his appearance in this city, and has been addressing appeals to the municipal authorities for grants of public moneys, on the ground that he alone should be recognized as the author of Anaesthesia. Having finished the work here, it is understood he is then to carry his appeal elsewhere, and thus obtain, if possible, universal recognition and a great national reward.

"Under the influence of precisely the same motives which prompted my course at Washington, I have felt it my duty to stand up again in opposition to pretensions which I verily believe to be founded on imposture, and the result is a 're-presentation' of the case of Dr. Wells in the accompanying publication, to which I respectfully invite attention.

"But up to this date the contest has been an unequal one. Morton has been sustained by the most ample pecuniary resources, obtained from one Tuckerman, now justly incarcerated at Wethersfield for robbing the U. S. mail. The case of Dr. Wells has had little other support than my humble advocacy, much indebted, I admit, for its intelligence to Dr. Ellsworth, of your city, and for publicity to Mr. Joseph Wales, a near relative of Dr. Wells.

"But that publicity has been, and must continue to be, very limited without some assistance. Ought not the facts to be known? Should not imposture and fraud be put down, and truth and justice vindicated? It has occurred to me that an appeal could be addressed to you, ladies of Hartford, with propriety and success; to you who can so readily ascertain the facts, and who, indeed, know them already; to you whose hands are ever prompt and ready for every work of beneficence, and whose hearts never fail to beat in unison with the promptings of humanity and the suggestions of rectitude. I venture, therefore, to make to you that appeal, but ask no higher appreciation of the case than is consistent with other obligations and other claims. For wise purposes, God has apportioned to your sex the larger share of the pain and anguish incident to our common humanity. It seems to me, therefore, that you may well feel that something is due to the memory of the man who discovered the means not merely of alleviating but obliterating both the one and the other."

The *re-presentation* to which the Senator referred was published in book form by John A. Gray, Printer, 16 & 18 Jacob Street (Fire-proof Buildings), New York, in 1858, under the title, "An Examination of the Question of Anaesthesia, arising on the Memorial of Charles Thomas Wells." It was directed "to the United States Senate, Second Session, Thirty-second Congress, and Referred to a Select Committee, of Which The Hon. Isaac P. Walker is Chairman." Because of its length, parts of it only will be reproduced here and in the subsequent 2 issues of *Survey of Anesthesiology.*

*   *   *   *

These excerpts established—from the depositions made by Dr. Linus T. Brockett, David Clarke, Elizabeth Wales, Dr. John M. Riggs, and Gardner Q. Colton—that Horace Wells, as early as 1840, had envisioned some substance which might be employed to allay pain in dentistry; that during the moment in which he perceived that the young pharmacy clerk, Cooley, had injured himself without knowing of it while

under the influence of nitrous oxide, the thought flashed to his mind that nitrous oxide might be such a substance; that he then immediately arranged an experiment upon himself to prove his point; and that the successful result of the experiment was not just a fortuitous coincidence, but that—as indicated in the further extracts of the depositions from Dr. Riggs and Mrs. Elizabeth Wells, and the depositions of Dr. E. E. Marcy, Dr. P. W. Ellsworth, Dr. John B. Terry, John Braddock, the Honorable James Dixon, Edward W. Parsons, Francis C. Goodrich, John Gaylord Wells, William H. Burleigh, Norman A. Goodrich, Horace E. Havens, Thomas Martin, and Franklin R. Slocum—nitrous oxide was indeed an effective pain reliever in dental surgery.

The final set of excerpts, indicate that the new pain-relieving substance, nitrous oxide, was as effective during surgery as during dentistry.

AN EXAMINATION OF THE QUESTION OF ANAESTHESIA, ARISING ON THE MEMORIAL OF CHARLES THOMAS WELLS

Hon. Truman Smith

DIRECTED TO A SELECT COMMITTEE OF THE UNITED STATES SENATE, 32ND CONGRESS.

John A. Gray

Printer,
16 & 18 Jacob St, N.Y., 1858

Published February, 1973

European countries are generally far in advance of the United States in the matter of the development and design of ambulances that are equipped to provide immediate and comprehensive treatment for patients who are being transported to hospital. Indeed, less than a generation ago it was not uncommon in this country for the local hearse to also double as the ambulance

for the community, a tacit admission, perhaps, that no one regarded the one form of transportation as being really very different from the other.

In Europe, on the other hand, the ambulance has become a highly sophisticated vehicle which contains all of the life-support systems that would be available in a well equipped and efficient Emergency

Room or Accident Ward. In some instances, they are virtually operating rooms on wheels, complete with a stretcher capable of acting as an operating table and the facilities (lights, suction, instruments, and the like) to cope with life-threatening situations during the trip from the site of the accident to the hospital.

These ambulances also, of course, have all of the necessary equipment and facilities for both respiratory and cardiac resuscitation—oxygen cylinders, oxygen inhalers, portable hand-operated self-inflating bag and mask units with connections for oxygen, various sizes of Guedel airways, orotubes for mouth-to-mouth resuscitation, emergency intubation sets, emergency tracheostomy sets, a hard flat surface for the thoracic portion of the stretcher to permit closed cardiac compression, cardiac stimulants, cardiac puncture cannulae, defibrillators, and in some instances an electrocardiograph.

In addition, there is a vast amount of miscellaneous equipment, including special sets of instruments for venous cutdown, emergency amputation, puncture of a major cavity (pneumothorax needles, etc.), and a complete array of drugs and intravenous infusions.

These vehicles have proven their worth in terms of saving lives and lowering morbidity. A recent review of 200 emergency calls responded to by the ambulances of the University Hospital of Mainz is quite revealing when broken down according to the admitting service at the hospital: 32.2 per cent were surgical, 37.5 per cent were medical, 5.7 per cent were obstetrical, 3.1 per cent were psychiatric, 3.5 per cent were pediatric, 12.2 per cent were poisoned, and the rest were in miscellaneous categories. Oxygen therapy was employed 63 times, intubation performed 57 times, artificial ventilation was necessary 46 times, external cardiac compression was applied 29 times, endobronchial suction was used 28 times, artificial airways were inserted 23 times, 4 pneumothoraces were decompressed, and 2 obstetrical procedures were performed. Also of interest was the variety of drugs administered: intravenous solutions, 82 (dextran 6 per cent, 46; glucose 5 per cent, 14; sodium bicarbonate, 13; plasma, 5; and

hypertonic solution, 4); isoproterenol, 9; meperidine, 8; muscle relaxants, 8; epinephrine, 5; phenothiazines, 5; cortisone, 2; and atropine, 2 (*Can. Anaesth. Soc. J.,* 15: 15, 1968).

Now the British have gone one step further and are advocating the use of Entonox in the ambulance service. Entonox is the trade name for a mixture of 50 per cent nitrous oxide and 50 per cent oxygen, available premixed in cylinders, which is widely used in England for obstetrics (*Lancet,* 2: 964, 1961; *Br. Med. J.,* 1: 732, 1964; *Lancet,* 1: 1229, 1965) and postoperative analgesia. The concept of premixed gases is not new, having been suggested by Barach and Rovenstine as early as 1945 as a means of obviating the hazards of anoxia during nitrous oxide anesthesia (*Anesthesiology,* 6: 449, 1945), and has the great advantage of having the nitrous oxide used for analgesia made inseparable from a safe proportion of oxygen by a process which depends neither on a mixing device nor on two cylinders with different rates of emptying. There are still dangers, of course, since at low temperatures there may be partial liquefaction of the cylinder contents (*Br. Med. J.,* 2: 915, 1963, *ibid,* 1: 732, 1964) and as the cylinder is emptied the oxygen concentration falls until in severe cases the final portion of the cylinder contents may consist of an hypoxic mixture. This hazard can be prevented by storage in a horizontal position, and the British Oxygen Company (B.O.C.) provides Entonox in cylinders with rounded bottoms, so that they cannot be stored vertically; the B.O.C. also advocates that all cylinders which are delivered in cold weather should be kept in a room in which the temperature will not fall below 5°C. for 24 hours before use (*Br. Med. J.,* 2: 715, 1968).

The use of this nitrous oxide mixture for pain relief during the ambulance trip was the subject of a pilot trial in South Gloucestershire in 1969, starting with 9 ambulances and being expanded to the whole county (26 ambulances) the following year. Strict precautions were necessary and observed. An absolute essential was that the men be fully trained; no one was allowed to supervise the administration of the gas until he had received full instruction, including lectures and practical demonstrations on the basic properties, pharmacology and action of Entonox. The principle of self-administration was particularly emphasized, since with this technique it becomes highly unlikely that the patient will become unconscious and lose his protective laryngeal reflexes, or become disoriented and uncooperative by entering the second stage of anesthesia. Similarly, the possibility of carbon dioxide retention and narcosis occurring due to the administration of a high concentration of oxygen to a chronic bronchitic is avoided by self-administration. Careful contraindications were also observed, and no Entonox inhalations were offered to patients with head injuries if there was impairment of consciousness or disorientation, patients with maxillofacial injuries, or in cases of drunkenness (*Proc. Roy. Soc. Med.*, 65: 7, 1972).

The results were excellent. Marked pain relief was obtained in 195 cases (64 per cent); partial relief in 99 (33 per cent); and no relief in only 11 (3.5 per cent). Not only was the pain relief convincing, but both the ambulance men and the receiving casualty officers remarked on the improvement in peripheral circulation in many of the shocked cases, no doubt due to the combination of good analgesia and oxygen therapy. Furthermore, the shortcomings of what must be considered the mainstay analgesics, the opiates, were avoided. These include the respiratory and cardiovascular depression and the unreliable absorption and excretion which are associated with these drugs and which are accentuated in the accident and emergency situation.

In this country, however, the opiates, despite their shortcomings, remain the principal analgesics for accident victims and emergency situations. Morphine and meperidine are the standards, administered either intramuscularly or intravenously. In fact, these drugs, administered by these routes, are so common that it is hard to conceive of treating the accident patient without them, and we sometimes forget that such therapy was not possible until the invention of the hypodermic syringe by Pravaz in 1853 and the invention of the hollow needle by Alexander Wood

in 1855. Wood made his discovery known first in a short notation under the proceedings of Medico-Chirurgical Society of Edinburgh in the *Monthly Journal of Medicine* in January, 1855, and then published a lengthier version under the title, "Treatment of Neuralgic Pains by Narcotic Injections," in the August 28, 1858 issue of the *British Medical Journal*. The latter paper is republished below with the kind permission of the publishers.

TREATMENT OF NEURALGIC PAINS BY NARCOTIC INJECTIONS

ALEXANDER WOOD, M.D.

Edinburgh
Br. Med. J., 2: Aug. 28, 1858

*   *   *   *   *

"A lady, troubled with neuralgic pains, had been punctured upwards of one hundred times, always in different places; but no sooner had the pain been driven from one spot, than it took up its seat in another. At last, I had expelled it from every part of the body, except a corner of the head, and there I was puzzled how to deal with it. The fact was, I could detect no painful point in the scalp. I would impress upon you that the instrument is not to be put into the place where the patient complains of the pain, but into the spot where you find you can awaken the pain upon pressure. Well, I could find no pain by pressing upon any part. The lady's husband, a medical man, took her to the German baths, in the hope that they might furnish what was wanting to the cure. She resided there for several months, but without the slightest benefit; and at length her husband brought her back to me, saying, he was satisfied unless I could cure her, nobody else could. I twice examined the part of her head affected; once more, the second time, I succeeded in finding out the point where the needle should be inserted; introduced the instrument; and from that day she has never had a touch of neuralgia again, though she has suffered from rheumatic gout.

"Another lady, also the wife of a medical man (and I take these cases, because on that account I am better able to get at the symptoms), was suffering from very intense neuralgia in the forehead, which had lasted, at irregular intervals, for ten days. The pain was so severe that it rendered her completely useless. I at once inserted the needle; the pain became instantly relieved, and soon left entirely. Since then it has never returned.

*   *   *   *

"I believe the remedy I have been speaking of acts in two ways. First, the injection into the cellular tissue in the neighborhood of the nerve, the needle being charged with narcotic solution, affects the nerve. In the second place, I believe it acts by being passed into a part which rapidly absorbs the medicine and sends it through the system, thus producing an almost instantaneous effect. In this little instrument we possess the means of bringing the patient almost directly under the influence of opium. It is truly astonishing to see how rapidly it affects the system. If you throw in a large quantity, you will see the eyes immediately injected, and the patient narcotised; and, in a few minutes afterwards, you will see him in a profound sleep.

*   *   *   *

"The instrument is of the simplest construction, and is a modification of Mr. Ferguson's already alluded to. It consists of a small glass syringe graduated like a drop measure, and to this is attached a small needle, hollow, and having an aperture near the point like the sting of a wasp. The painful point being ascertained, the syringe, being charged, is pressed firmly in to such a depth as to reach the nerve, when the piston being shoved home, the charge is delivered. No haemorrhage follows; and, in the many cases in which I have operated, I have never seen any disagreeable local effects, except a slight blush of urticaria round the wound".

1868

Published February, 1963

Dr. Edmund W. Andrews was a man of many parts, but without question his most important accomplishment was his epochal work in anesthesia.

He was born in Putney, Vermont, on April 22, 1824, to a family that was theologically inclined on the paternal side and medically inclined on the maternal side. His boyhood was a nomadic one, since his family moved successively westward from Vermont to West Bloomfield, to Mendon and to Pittsford, New York; and to Armada, Michigan. He matriculated at the University of Michigan and was graduated (A.B.) in 1849. He proceeded on into medicine and graduated from the medical Department of the University of Michigan in 1852. He then served his alma mater as a demonstrator in anatomy until 1855, when he was appointed professor of anatomy at Rush Medical College. The state of medical education at Rush was at a low ebb at that time, however, and the "diploma mill" environment disgusted Andrews so much that, in company with a number of others, he founded the Chicago Medical College, which ultimately became the Northwestern Medical School. During the Civil War, he served the North in the campaigns against Shiloh, Corinth, and Vicksburg, and was in the personal service of both General Sherman and General Grant. Following the

War, he resumed practice in Chicago, where he spent almost 50 years of professional activity before dying in 1904 at the ripe old age of 80.

So much for the biographical facts; they tell little of the catholicity of interest and profound accomplishments in diverse fields that characterized the man. He was an excellent sholar, an effective speaker and a succinct writer. He was a talented artist who illustrated his own scientific articles, painted ornithologic pictures and, while with General Sherman, painted numerous scenes around Memphis and Vicksburg. He designed his own book plate and a church organ, and even built the latter. He was an all around naturalist, well grounded in botany and zoology, but particularly interested in geology. He was one of the founders of the Chicago Academy of Sciences and it was before that body that he first proposed a scientific explanation of the intermittent eruption of geysers. He wrote a book and a number of geologic papers on glaciers and the sequelae of their action, based in part on observations made in the Georgian Bay region of the Great Lakes, where for many years he camped during the summer. He read Latin, Greek, and Hebrew fluently; and not only translated Latin and Greek Poems into English, but even wrote his own poems in these languages.

All of this he accomplished while pursuing his profession as a physician and surgeon. He developed increasing interests in both genito-urinary and orthopedic surgery, and invented a number of useful surgical instruments, important implements of traction and several types of urethral dilators. His operative work was done at Mercy Hospital in Chicago or in the homes of his patients, as was customary at that time. In the absence of either chemical or pathologic laboratories in the hospitals of those days, he performed diagnostic urinalyses and surgical pathology in his own home. While serving with the Army of the North, he introduced a system of case records of military surgery and wrote the first monograph on the mortality of military surgical diseases. He acquired an extensive knowledge of anal and rectal diseases at a time when most doctors were unwilling to contaminate their hands by even touching these parts, and wrote a scientific treatise on rectal diseases. He made a monumental contribution to medical education when, with N. S. Davis, father of the American Medical Association, he helped to establish the first graded curriculum in the United States.

His interest in nitrous oxide anesthesia arose from his observation of the painless extraction of teeth under the influence of undiluted nitrous oxide gas as administered by dentists; and that interest was whetted further by a statistical study which indicated that the mortality from chloroform was about eight and a half times greater than by ether, and that nitrous oxide was the safest of the three agents. He felt that the availability of nitrous oxide anesthesia in the field of general surgery would be a great step of progress, but he was well aware of the asphyxial nature of the undiluted gas. This led him to experimentation and clinical trial of the addition of oxygen to the inhaled anesthetic mixture, a milestone of incalculable importance in the history of anesthesia. These investigations were published under the title, "The oxygen mixture, a new anaesthetic combination," in *The Chicago Medical Examiner* (9: 656–661, November, 1868) and are reprinted below.

THE OXYGEN MIXTURE, A NEW ANAESTHETIC COMBINATION

E. ANDREWS, M.D.

Prof. of Principles and Practice of Surgery, Chicago Medical College Chicago, Illinois

The Chicago Medical Examiner, 9: 656–661, November, 1868

*　　*　　*　　*

"I have for some time been experimenting, to see whether by the addition of free oxygen to the nitrous oxide, a mixture would not be obtained, by which a patient might be anaesthetized for an indefinite period without danger of asphyxia, and thus render gas available for the most prolonged operations of surgery. These experiments are not yet finished, but they have advanced far enough to show that the preparation, which I have named the Oxygen Mixture, is certainly available for a large part of our operations, and that for pleasantness, and probable safety, it is infinitely superior to chloroform, ether, or unmixed nitrous oxide".

* * * *

Published December, 1971

Aristotle, the Greek philosopher, is not usually associated with respiratory physiology, and yet he made perhaps the first recorded scientific experiment on the ventilatory aspects of respiration.

Aristotle was a man of prodigious talents. His work covered all of the branches of human knowledge extant in his times, and estimates of the number of books which he wrote range from an astounding 400 up to an incredible 1000. The scope of his concerns was equally incredible and included not only the field of logic, for which, of course, he is best known, but also natural science, basic metaphysics, ethics and politics, and rhetoric and poetry.

Aristotle was born in Stagira, on the Aegean seacoast, in 384 B.C. His father, Nichomachus, was court physician to Amyntas II, the grandfather of Alexander the Great. Aristotle's childhood included a thorough-going education in the natural sciences at the hands of his father, and then at the age of 17 he went to Athens, where for 20 years he studied philosophy with Plato. Inevitably, he acquired many of the thought processes of his famous teacher; but although he respected Plato's theories, he was also allowed to disagree with them.

Aristotle's philosophy differs from Plato's in that it is far more systematic and more reconciled with the material world as it exists. He delved at length into the philosophy of logic, and he examined in detail the form of reasoning known now as syllogism, or deductive logic; *e.g.*, all animals which produce milk to feed their young are mammals, the whale produces milk to feed its young, therefore the whale is a mammal. H. G. Wells, writing in *The Outline of History*, said, "He (Aristotle) anticipates Bacon and the modern scientific movement in his realization of the importance of ordered knowledge. He was the first natural historian. Other men before him had speculated about the nature of things, but he, with every young man he could win over to the task, set himself to classify and compare things. Plato says in effect: 'Let us take hold of life and remodel it'; this soberer successor: 'Let us first know more of life, and meanwhile serve the king.'"

It is ironic that Aristotle's logic led him to the wrong interpretation of the results of his major experiment in respiratory physiology. He made the correct observation that animals in airtight boxes soon died, but he incorrectly ascribed their deaths to the inability of the animals to cool themselves. This was not, on the basis of the state of knowledge in the fourth century B.C., an entirely illogical conclusion, since up until the time of Harvey's announcement of the discovery of the circulation in 1615, respiration was considered a mechanism for keeping the body cool.

Knowlege of respiratory physiology has developed slowly over the course of the 23 centuries since Aristotle's time, and much of that knowledge has only come in the past few hundred years. Leonardo da Vinci (1452–1519), another intellectual giant, recognized that fire consumed something in air and that animals could not live in an atmosphere which could not support a flame, but it was more than another 250 years before Priestly discovered oxygen, and even then he did not grasp its true relationship to respiration.

Knowledge of the control of respiration has been even more recent and in fact is still developing. A major milestone in this area was the identification of the mechanism of the Hering-Breuer reflex. This work was reported in detail by Breuer to the Academy of Sciences in Vienna on November 5, 1868, but a preliminary report was published earlier that year in the Proceedings of the Imperial Academy of Sciences by Hering under the title, "The Self-

Regulation of Respiration Mediated by the Vagal Nerve" (S. B. Akad. Wiss. Wien., 57: 672–677, 1868). *Survey* and its readers are greatly indebted to Dr. Ernest O. Henschel, Chairman of the Department of Anesthesiology at The Medical College of Wisconsin (formerly Marquette University School of Medicine) for the translation which is published below.

THE SELF-REGULATION OF RESPIRATION MEDIATED BY THE VAGAL NERVE: REPORT OF AN INVESTIGATION CARRIED OUT BY DR. JOSEPH BREUER IN THE INSTITUTE FOR PHYSIOLOGY OF THE IMPERIAL AND ROYAL JOSEPH'S ACADEMY

HERING, E.

S. B. Akad Wiss. Wien., 57: 672–677, 1868.

Hering states that most of the confusion regarding the role of the vagus in regulation of respiration arises from experiments which stimulate the central end of the cut vagus.

He then notes the differences in the respiratory pattern of patients suffering dyspnea from pneumonia contrasted with dyspnea of tracheal stenosis. He cites the observations on the respiratory effort of animals with tracheotomy when the trachea is occluded at end-expiration contrasted to occlusion at the end of inspiration, and compares both of these with the respiratory effort of the animal when breathing an oxygen free gas mixture.

He postulates: "These remarkable phenomena have found their explanation in the fact that the neural center for respiratory movement, by way of the vagal fibers ending in the pulmonary parenchyma, is in a continous dependency on the state of distension of the lung: In other words, that the respiratory movements are influenced by the degree of distension of the lung."

1876

Published February, 1964

The advent of thiopental, and its ardent support in such influential journals as *McCall's* and *Good Housekeeping*, have made the rigors of a good old-fashioned inhalation induction merely a memory from a bygone era. Induction today is as pleasant for the patient as a single pin-prick, and as simple for the anesthetist as the performance of venipuncture. But even before the introduction of thiopental, the sport was going out of induction. An agent such as nitrous oxide, or ethylene, or cyclopropane, would usually produce a comparatively rapid and pleasant induction for the patient, and one which was relatively simple

and carefree for the anesthetist to accomplish.

It was not always thus. There was a time when the induction of general anesthesia was a suffocating, fiendish nightmare for the patient, and a perspiring ordeal of combatting secretions, coughing, breath-holding, cyanosis, and laryngospasm in a thrashing patient, for the anesthetist. Untold numbers of patients suffered the tortures of the damned during induction, and countless anesthetists grayed prematurely from the tribulations of the second stage. The man who changed all of this was Joseph Thomas Clover.

Clover was born on February 28, 1825, in the town of Aylesham, Norfolk County, England. The Clover family was descended from sound Yeoman stock and had long been established in Norfolk. Clover's great uncle had been a distinguished veterinarian surgeon there in the city of Norwich, and had devoted his life to veterinarian science: he invented an apparatus for the cure of broken tendons and bones in horses, and was the discoverer of the manner in which larvae of bots (a disease caused by the botfly in horses, cattle and sheep) are conveyed from the coat of a horse into its stomach. These qualities of creator, inventor, and investigator, appeared again in the same family in the person of Clover himself.

Clover was the third of the six children (two sons and four daughters) born to John Wright Clover, who had married Miss E. M. A. Peterson. He was educated at the Gray Friars Priory School at Norwich. He then was apprenticed to Mr. Gibson of Norwich and in 1842 became a dresser at the Norfolk and Norwich Hospital. Two years later, at the age of nineteen, he proceeded to University College, London, and University College Hospital.

These were momentous times in medicine, and Clover was in the midst of the inception of great happenings. Joseph Lister was a fellow student, the renowned Robert Liston and the equally renowned James Syme were among his teachers, and he was present at the advent of anesthesia in Europe when Liston performed his first surgical operation upon a patient under ether on Monday, December 21, 1846: "I was a junior student at University College when Ether was first used there and saw Liston amputate a man's thigh under its influence. I was also present when the same surgeon brought some chloroform and gave it by means of a glass breast pump. The chloroform took the place of ether immediately, and until the fatal case occurred in the practice of Sir John Fife of Newcastle we were unanimous in preferring chloroform."

Clover showed great aptitude for clinical work as a student, and he became house surgeon to Morton and then in 1848 to Syme. He next was appointed Resident Medical Officer, a post which he held for five years, during which he administered many anesthetics and showed that interest in anesthesia which was to shape his future career. John Snow, in his classic work *On Chloroform and Other Anaesthetics*, mentions Clover's ability as an anesthetist in the discussion of a fatal case which had occurred at University College Hospital: "this plan of administering chloroform with the head and shoulders of the patient covered with a towel, was introduced by Mr. Clover, who was for several years a resident officer of the institution; and it is right to state that it led to no accident in his hands; in those of his successors it was, however, less successful; three accidents having occurred in a little more than a year and a half."

Clover passed his final F.R.C.S. examinations in 1850, and began private practice in 1853, at the age of 28 years. He practiced as a general practitioner, but continued interest in, and the administration of, anesthesia. The sudden death of John Snow in 1858 was one of the factors which led Clover to specialize almost entirely in anesthesia, and he was in due course appointed Lecturer in Anaesthetics to University College Hospital, Chloroformist to the Westminster Hospital, and Administrator of Anaesthetics to the London Dental Hospital.

Among Clover's great contributions to anesthesia were his inventions for improved techniques of administration, and he had a workroom in his residence, completely equipped with benches, tools and lathes, where he spent a great deal of his spare time inventing and perfecting original apparatus to improve anesthetic administration. He developed a chloroform bag inhaler, which enabled the administrator to provide a mixture of air containing a definite proportion of chloroform—similar in principle to the present-day method of injecting a measured amount of halothane from a calibrated syringe into a closed rebreathing system to produce a precise concentration of halothane. He also developed an ingenious portable bellows which enabled him to charge the bag of the inhaler with a measured dose of chloroform. By 1868, Clover could report to the Odontological Society of Great Britain that he had used his apparatus in 1,802 cases, "not only without any fatal results, but with uniform success, in the induction of complete anesthesia", including an administration of anesthesia to Her Majesty Queen Alexandra, when Princess of Wales, for an operation on the knee.

Despite Clover's personal record of safety, by 1863 the number of cases in which death could be positively assigned to the inhalation of chloroform had reached the formidable total of 123, and many of these occurred during the performance of trivial or minor surgical operations. The medical profession was becoming increasingly disturbed, and this led the Royal Medical and Chirurgical Society to appoint a committee in 1864 "to give their anxious attention to devise means for obviating such accidents." The findings of the committee were unequivocal in stating that ether was a much safer and quite as efficient an anesthetic as chloroform but, "it's odor is disagreeable, it is slow in operation, and gives rise to greater excitement than chloroform." The committee went on to advise the use of chloroform mixtures, such as A.C.E. mixture which contained one part alcohol, two parts chloroform, and three parts ether. It was at this point that Clover, who was not favorably impressed by either the safety or the value of the chloroform mixtures, began his long but successful search for a method by which ether could be used efficiently.

After the tragic failure of the demonstration by Horace Wells of nitrous oxide at the Massachusetts General Hospital in 1845, this agent fell into disrepute and was not employed for many years. However, its use was revived by Colton, and with great success, in 1862. Colton had amassed an experience of 24,000 cases at the Colton Dental Association in New York City, which was established as an institution devoted exclusively to the extracting of teeth with nitrous oxide anesthesia. It was at this time that Colton visited Paris to attend the International Exhibition and the First International Medical Congress. While in Paris he met Dr. T. W. Evans, a fellow

countryman who had practiced in the French capital as a dental surgeon for some years, and instructed Evans how to prepare and administer nitrous oxide gas. Evans was an apt and enthusiastic pupil, and used the agent for the extraction of teeth with great success. In March, 1868, Evans went to London and gave several demonstrations at the National Dental Hospital. Evan's demonstrations were attended by the leading metropolitan anesthetists and dentists of the day and were described by Clover: "the results of his cases were on the whole in favor of the gas but the appearance of the patients, their lividity and convulsive movements, were regarded as alarming, and a few of his patients were insufficiently narcotized. . . . Dr. Evans brought the gas in a large India rubber bag which was placed on the floor, a tube of several feet led from this to the mouthpiece—a flat piece of ebonite which was placed between the patient's teeth." It was while attending Evan's demonstrations that Clover's genius foresaw the possibility of modifying his own chloroform apparatus to permit the patient the pleasantness of induction with nitrous oxide and the potency of anesthesia with ether—and "gas-ether" was born. It was the major contribution of a career which had, in the words of the *British Medical Journal*, "during the past twenty or thirty years done more for the benefit of the world's suffering millions than almost anyone of his generation." Clover's paper was published in the July 15, 1878, issue of that journal under the title of, "On an apparatus for administering nitrous oxide gas and ether, singly or combined" (Clover, J. T.: *Br. Med. J.*, 2: 75–77, July 15, 1876), and is reprinted below.

ON AN APPARATUS FOR ADMINISTERING NITROUS OXIDE GAS AND ETHER, SINGLY OR COMBINED

J. T. CLOVER, F.R.C.S.

Br. Med. J., 2: 75–77, 1876

"For several years, my attention has been directed to the improvement of the way of administering ether. At first, I spared the patient the unpleasant choking sensation of ether by first getting him asleep with chloroform. My next plan was to dilute the ether-vapour with a known proportion of air, the supply of ether-vapour being rendered more uniform by attention to its temperature, which was kept within limits by causing the expired air to pass through the ether-vessel in a kind of worm. I called this the double-current apparatus, and showed it at the meeting of the British Medical Association in London, in 1873. At the same time, I explained the two methods I had used for giving gas preparatory to ether. By the first plan, I simply exchanged the gas-inhaler for the ether-inhaler as soon as the patient was unconscious. By the second, I caused the current of gas to pass through a vessel of ether, after the first three or four respirations of pure gas had made the patient indifferent about its taste. This plan answered very well for cases not requiring more than three or four minutes' anaesthesia; but I found it difficult to supply sufficient air to prevent muscular twitching, without admitting enough to cause a return to partial consciousness".

1878

Published August, October, December, 1963

Oxygen is transported in the blood by the hemoglobin of the red cells, and only negligible amounts are carried as physically dissolved oxygen in the plasma. In a patient with a normal hemoglobin level, breathing air at atmospheric pressure, arterial blood contains about 19.5 volumes of oxyhemoglobin per 100 ml. of blood, while only approximately 0.25 volumes per cent of oxygen is carried in the blood in simple physical solution in the plasma. The latter is of special importance, however, because it is in physical solution, and its level can be raised simply by raising the ambient pressure. If the patient is placed in a pressure chamber and administered oxygen under 2 atmospheres of pressure, the amount of oxygen in solution in the plasma is raised from 0.25 to 4.2 volumes per cent, or more than 16 times the normal level, and the oxygen content of the blood is therefore raised from less than 20 volumes per cent almost up to 25 volumes per cent—a quite considerable increase. However, in addition to this there is a further potential benefit, for by increasing the tension of oxygen in the blood stream the rate of oxygen diffusion into poorly perfused and anoxic tissues is enhanced. For while the red cells act as floating storehouses for oxygen, the rate at which oxygen will diffuse from the blood through the capillary wall to the tissue fluids, and hence to the cells of the part, depends upon the partial pressures between the plasma and the tissue cells.

These facts have allowed Boerema and his colleagues to dilute the circulating blood of the pig, using plasma and macrodex to replace the removed whole blood, until only 0.4 per cent of the original hemoglobin remained. The blood at this dilution was a clear liquid and the animals were a startlingly pale color, but in oxygen under 3 atmospheres of pressure they maintained normal electrocardiograms throughout the experiment. On the contrary, breathing 100 per cent oxygen but at normal atmospheric pressure, the hemoglobin could be reduced only to 11 or 12 per cent in the animals before abnormalities were observed on the electrocardiogram.

This ability of hyperbaric oxygenation to

saturate the whole body, the blood plasma, the intercellular fluid, and the cells themselves with a very high level of physically dissolved oxygen has been under intense study as a therapeutic tool by Boerema and his associates in Amsterdam and Illingworth and Smith in Glasgow for much of the past decade, and enthusiastic interest spread to this country about 2 years ago. The original investigations were of use as an aid to open-heart surgery, but they soon proved to be of value in a number of other areas.

As might be anticipated, drenching the body with oxygen has been particularly beneficial in the treatment of anaerobic infections. In the therapy of *Clostridium welchii* infections, hyperbaric oxygenation has resulted in detoxication within 24 hours, and has permitted postponement of radical amputations and the subsequent sparing of many extremities. Antibiotics have been administered against secondary infection, but the use of anti-gas-gangrene serum has not been necessary. Of 26 such patients treated in Surgical University Clinic in Amsterdam, in only one patient was death clearly due to gas-gangrene, and in one other patient the cause of death was indirectly related to the infection.

One of the most obviously logical applications of oxygen under high pressure (OHP) has been the treatment of carbon monoxide poisoning. Hyperbaric oxygenation at 2 atmospheres of pressure has been shown to be far more effective than either 5 per cent or 7 per cent carbogen mixtures or 100 per cent oxygen at ambient pressure. This form of treatment has rapidly corrected the anoxia and increased the speed at which carbon monoxide was removed from the blood and tissues. Of 22 patients with severe carbon monoxide intoxication admitted directly to the Western Infirmary, Glasgow, during a 12-month period, all recovered completely, despite the fact that the carboxyhemoglobin content averaged 40 per cent and ranged as high as 69 per cent on admission.

Hyperbaric oxygenation has been employed rather extensively in the treatment of peripheral vascular insufficiencies. Acute arterial insufficiency, caused by injury to the main vessels to a limb, has been treated in the hyperbaric chamber with promising results, the immediate danger of gangrene being averted until sufficient collateral circulation could develop to maintain the vitality of all or most of the part. Chronic arterial insufficiency and soft tissue necrosis have been treated with hyperbaric oxygenation and have shown improvement in the healing ability of soft tissues in patients with chronic arterial insufficiency not correctible by surgery. Patients with chronic obliterative disease of the lower extremity, such as atherosclerosis and thromboangiitis obliterans, do not, of course, show improvement of the gross organic vascular changes, but in many such patients the severe rest-pain—often severe enough to prevent sleep—was relieved.

The initial research studies and clinical experiences from the group in Glasgow indicate a possible potential in the treatment of extensive myocardial infarction. They ligated the main left coronary circumflex artery in the dog, and were able to reduce the mortality rate from 50 to 60 per cent in unprotected dogs to 10 per cent in the animals breathing oxygen at 2 atmospheres pressure. The therapy has been applied to human beings for periods up to 3½ days with complete recovery and with no evidence of subsequent hemodynamic failure.

The Glasgow group also has investigated the effect of hyperbaric oxygenation on cerebral vascular occlusion in the dog by occluding both carotid and both vertebral arteries low in the neck. When this was done at atmospheric pressure, signs of cerebral anoxia developed rapidly, the electroencephalogram showing deterioration within 15 seconds, and a complete loss of cortical rhythm within 1 minute. By contrast, when the clamps were reapplied during full oxygenation at 2 atmospheres of pressure, the electroencephalographic record remained normal throughout the experimental period of about 30 minutes. These observations could have important clinical implications in relation to cerebral disease and in relation to operations on the brain.

The potential value in open-heart procedures, as already mentioned, underlies much of the recent interest in hyperbaric oxygenation. As an adjunct in major surgery for patients with increased cardiac risk, it is of proven value, for the patient's state of oxygenation can be improved immensely before surgery. Reduction of cardiac irritability and the prevention of ventricular fibrillation has been demonstrated by Boerema's group, and they have been operating on deeply cyanotic children with congenital heart disease who would have been inoperable otherwise.

The most longstanding of the newer applications of hyperbaric oxygenation has been its use as an adjunct to radiation in the treatment of malignant tumors. Hypoxia reduces the sensitivity of tumor cells to radiation and many viable tumor cells are probably rendered hypoxic because of inadequate blood supply. In the past, attempts have been made to return anoxic tumor cells to full radiosensitivity by the inhalation of oxygen at atmospheric pressure. Hyperbaric chambers are now being utilized as a means of increasing the oxygen tension in tumors and thus increasing the radiosensitivity of the tumors.

In view of these many possible uses of oxygen under pressure, it is interesting to recall the statement made by Sir Michael Foster that science travels in circles: the concept followed yesterday may be dropped today and rediscovered tomorrow. This suggestion has certainly been true of hyperbaric therapy as a clinical tool in medicine. More than a century ago, a number of health spas in Europe offered hyperbaric therapy for a variety of ills; Paul Bert's classic volume on the physiologic effects of barometric pressure which was published in 1878 describes a number of these facilities and their therapeutic endeavors. During World War II, it became of first importance to the Allies that this great classic on pressure physiology should be made available in the English language to the flying personnel of our armed forces. Accordingly, it was translated by Dr. Fred A. Hitchcock, Associate Professor of Physiology at the Ohio State University, and his wife, Mary Alice Hitchcock, formerly Professor of Romance Languages at the University of Akron, and published by the College Book Company, Columbus, Ohio, in 1943. Three sections of "Title II. Increased Pressures" in Bert's book (Bert, P.: *La Pression Barometrique, Recherches de Physiologie Experimentale*, pp. 1168, G. Masson, Paris, 1878.)—Chapter II, "Low Pressures" (under 2 atmospheres), Chapter III, "Theoretical Explanations and Experiments," and Chapter IV, "Summary and Conclusions"— will be published in this and the succeeding 2 issues of *Survey of Anesthesiology*.

LA PRESSION BAROMETRIQUE, RECHERCHES DE PHYSIOLOGIE EXPERIMENTALE

Paul Bert

G. Masson, Paris, 1878

In the three chapters from Title II, Increased Pressures, originally published in Survey, Bert reviews the existing literature thoroughly and draws numerous apt conclusions.

In the summary and comments, attention is drawn to the phenomena due to compression: pains in the ears; the rise in pitch of the voice; the enlargement of the thorax and slowing of the respiratory rate; the decrease in pulse rate; and the changes in the central nervous system.

During decompression, the necessity to be slow is emphasized. Up to 2 atmospheres no symptoms are evident, but beyond that cutaneous itching, painful swelling of the muscles, and periarticular pains appear. Above 3 atmospheres, symptoms appearing after decompression include sensory disturbances, blindness, deafness, paralysis of the lower limbs, cerebral disturbances, loss of consciousness, and even death.

The cause of the severe disturbances were not known at that time. But conjectured were visceral congestions of blood and the escape of free gases from the blood.

1879

Published February, 1978

The first written reference to curare—a word for the arrow poison which has endured such indiscriminate variations as urari, uirari, ururara, uirary, urali, ourari, wourari, wourali, woorari, woorara, curara, curari, and others, depending upon the region, the date, and mere quirk—is probably contained in the great book on the New World, *De Orbe Novo*, written by the Italian monk, Peter Martyr d'Anghera, in 1516:

"They like to use bows and poisoned arrows. They poison their arrows with the stings of scorpions, the heads of certain ants, poisons which they manufacture, and those little plums I have mentioned, as well also as the juice they distil from certain trees in which they dip their arrows. But everybody is not permitted to make this mixture. There are certain old women skilled in the art, who are shut in at certain times and furnished with the necessary materials; during two days these women watch and distil the ointment. As soon as it is finished the house is opened, and if the women are well and not found lying on the ground half dead from the fumes of the poison, they are severely punished, and the ointment is thrown away as being valueless; for the strength of the poison is such, that the mere odor of it, while compounding almost kills its makers.

"Whoever is wounded by one of these poisoned arrows dies, but not instantly, and no Spaniard has yet found a remedy for such wounds. The natives know some, but the remainder of one's life, after being cured, is sufficiently disagreeable; for it is necessary to abstain from many things one likes. First of all from sexual pleasure for two years, and afterwards, during a lifetime, from liquors, excessive pleasures of the table, and all exertion. Otherwise death quickly follows. Our monks have seen many wounded Indians, for they live in a state of perpetual war, but they assisted at the death of only one woman, who was unwilling to undergo the cure; the women fight by their husbands' sides. Nobody has been able to extort from them the secret of this antidote."

Some 80 years later, Sir Walter Raleigh—who was both a soldier and sailor (General and Admiral, respectively), a treasure hunter and a pirate, a courtier, a poet, a historian, and who introduced potatoes and tobacco to the Western World—wrote in 1595:

"There was nothing whereof I was more curious, than to finde out the true remedies of these poisoned arrowes, for besides the mortalitie of the wound they make, the partie shot indureth the most insufferable torment in the world, and abideth a most vgly and lamentable death, sometimes dying starke mad, sometimes their bowels breaking out of their bellies, and are presently discolored, as black as pitch, and so vnsauery, as no man can endure to cure, or to attend them; And it is more strange to know, that in all this time there was never Spaniard, either by gift or torment that could attaine to the true knowledge of the cure, although they have martyred and put to inuented torture I know not how many of them. But euery one of these Indians know it not, no not one among thousands, but their soothsaiers and priests, who do conceale it, and only teach it but from the father to the sonne.

"Those medicines which are vulgar, and serue for the ordinarie poison, are made of the iuce of a roote called Tupara: the same also quencheth maruellously the heate of burning feauers, and healeth inward wounds, and broken veines, that bleed within the body. But I was more beholding to the Guianians than any other, for Antonio de Berreo told me that he could neuer attaine to the knowledge thereof, and yet they taught me the best way of healing as wel thereof, as of al other poisons. Some of the Spaniards have been cured in ordinary wounds, of the common poisoned arrowes with the iuce of garlike: but this is a generall rule for all men that shall hereafter trauell the Indies where poisoned arrowes are vsed, that they must abstain from drinke, for if they take any licor into their body, I say, if they drink before the wound be dressed, or soone upon it, there is no way with them but present death."

Within 24 years of the discovery of America, the potency of the Indian arrow poison had made such a fearsome impression upon the early explorers of the New World that they were convinced of the following: (1) that there were several varieties of arrow poisons—which was true; (2) that one variety was obtained by distillations of certain trees—which was also true; (3) that the arrow points broke off on hitting the target—which was sometimes true, depending upon the marksman, the quality of the arrow, and the target; (4) that the darts were made of palm wood—which was certainly not necessarily true, but rather concerned the availability of types of wood in the geographical area under discussion; (5) that the natives knew an antidote—which was almost certainly not true; and (6) that cauterization of the wound caused by a poison arrow was practiced by the Indian—which was sometimes true and sometimes untrue, depending, again upon the place from which the statement emanated.

Many of these so-called established facts were, therefore, myths and legends, reshaped and misshaped in the telling and retelling of the tales. The way that the apocryphal tale of the "old women" became gospel, for instance, was a feat in the "hard sell" which modern day Madison Avenue could envy.

The man who did much to separate these facts and unfacts from fancy, myth, and legend was Charles Waterton, the Squire of Walton Hall. "He was at one and the same time a charming Victorian and a thorough-going eccentric. He was an expert ornithologist, a taxidermist, and a naturalist who created one of the first bird sanctuaries by surrounding Walton Hall's 300 acres by a three-mile wall, six feet high, to keep out the poachers and foxes. He was totally without fear of animals, including reptiles: it is recounted that he once captured a cayman (crocodile) by jumping on its back and riding it to captivity. On another occasion, he is said to have 'climbed into a cage with a not-too-well-schooled orangutan, and inspected its hands and teeth, whereupon the ape did the same for him, and added greatly to the amusement of the spectators by commencing a careful and critical study of the Squire's hair!"

"Waterton's family owned estates in what is now British Guiana, and from 1804 to 1812 Waterton himself aided in the administration of these interests. During this time he made expeditions into the interior from which he gained firsthand knowledge of wourali poison, its use in hunting, and something of its concoction; and he collected specimens of it which he brought back to England upon his return."

Waterton's account of his adventures, told with charm and lucidity, were contained in his book, *Wanderings In South America*, published by MacMillan & Company, London, in 1879, of which pages 126–144 are reprinted below without the permission of either the author or the publisher.

WANDERINGS IN SOUTH AMERICA

CHARLES WATERTON

Chapters II and III, pp. 126–144

MacMillan and Company, London, 1879.

"Grammatici certant, et adhuc sub judice lis est."

The Macoushi Indians—Poison vendors—Apparent failure of poison—Collecting materials for wourali-poison—Preparing the poison—Superstitions—The blowpipe gun—The Ourah—The Samourah—Silkgrass—Acuero fruit—Coucourite palm—Wild Cotton—Arrows—Quivers—Jaw of

Pirai—Packing the arrows—Cotton basket—Gun sight made of Acouri teeth—Poisoned fowl—Suspending the guns— The bow—Ingenious arrows—Small quivers—A wild hog shot—Utilization of indigenous products.

*   *   *   *

1880

Published February, 1969

Several years ago, Noel Gillespie's classic volume on *Endotracheal Anesthesia* (Madison, Wisc., University of Wisconsin Press, 1941), only one of a number of significant contributions to the specialty to emanate from the Department of Anesthesia at the University of Wisconsin, was beautifully updated and revised by Karl Siebecker and Betty Bamforth. They managed to retain the style and flavor of the original text, while at the same time making the many changes and additions which had become necessary since the publication of the first edition in 1941. One need only read Gillespie's original section on the advantages of endotracheal anesthesia to realize how far the technique has progressed in the mere span of a generation or so:

"It is evident from the literature that many of the objections expressed in the past have been directed, not at endotracheal anaesthesia itself, but at some particular route or technique of which a given author disapproved. It must therefore be stressed at the outset that this consideration of its advantages and disadvantages applies to any form of endotracheal anaesthesia, provided that it is competently administered.

"The arguments in favor of endotracheal anaesthesia fall into three main groups: freedom of airway, the control of intrapulmonic pressure, and artificial ventilation.

"Endotracheal anaesthesia procures an absolute freedom of the patient's airway which is mechanically assured. All authorities are agreed that the most frequent cause of difficulty or danger in the administration of an anaesthetic is obstruction of respiration. Intubation removes this cause, and the following advantages result:

"With a tube in place in the trachea, spasm of the larynx, should it occur, cannot interfere with the efficacy of respiratory exchange. Laryngeal spasm may be the result of direct irritation of the glottis by too sudden a concentration of a pungent vapor, by a drop of mucus, or by an ill-fitting pharyngeal airway. If its onset is recognized it can usually be abolished by finding the cause and removing it. Once spasm is established, however, intubation is usually the only effective treatment. Reflex glottic spasm is often initiated by surgical stimulus in light anaesthesia, and therefore safety demands either a degree of anaesthesia sufficiently profound to abolish the glottic reflex, or else intubation as a means of maintaining a plane of anaesthesia which is both light and safe. Although any intense surgical stimulus may cause reflex glottic spasm, it occurs most frequently during abdominal operations. Unless the plane of anaesthesia is sufficiently deep to cause paralysis of the glottis, reflex spasm usually results from the stimulus of traction on the peritoneum or of palpation of the structures adjacent to the diaphragm. This spasm, in turn, causes a lack of oxygen which enhances the tension of the unrelaxed muscles, and makes the surgeon's task difficult if not impossible. Until the spasm is relieved and respiratory exchange is re-established it is impossible to deepen the anaesthesia. This vicious circle is familiar to all surgeons as well as to anaesthetists. As long ago as 1903 Kühn pointed out that in abdominal operations intubation promoted smoother anaesthesia, and urged this argument in its favor. Cotton and Boothby were inclined to favor intubation for sub-diaphragmatic operations. Their surmise was confirmed a generation later by Boyle and Hewer. This has in recent years been the common experience of almost all anaesthetists.

"If a free airway for the patient is assured, it becomes superfluous for the anaesthetist or his apparatus to remain in close juxtaposition to the patient's head; and he can safely withdraw to a distance without losing anything of his accurate control of the administration, provided that he uses a stethoscope and blood-pressure cuff fitted with sufficient lengths of tubing to permit of close and constant observation of the behaviour of the patient's cardio-vascular system. The movements of the breathing bag will naturally provide him with the necessary information as to the character of the patient's respiration. So long as the anaesthetist's hands and apparatus, neither of which could be kept sterile, perforce encroached on the surgical field at intervals, no true asepsis was possible in any operation upon the head. A tube, once in place, can be treated as part of the surgical field, and remains undisturbed during the operation. In this way endotracheal anaesthesia has made a definite contribution to the recent advances in plastic and cerebral surgery.

"In almost all the operations of otorhino-laryngology, if anaesthesia by inhalation is employed, a conflict of access to the operative field takes place between the anaesthetist and the surgeon, because the upper air passages are themselves the site of the operation. This very difficulty was the stimulus which excited the work of Kühn, and he solved it by using intubation, as he says, 'for the purpose of bringing the air in the trachea into direct contact with the outside air.' This 'exteriorization of the larynx' enables the surgeon to work unfettered by the necessity either of maintaining a free airway himself or of being interrupted periodically by the anaesthetist's efforts to do so. In certain operations inside the thorax or upon the stomach it is sometimes a help to the surgeon if an oesophageal bougie or stomach tube can be passed.

If the patient has been intubated, this can be done without any interruption of the administration of the anaesthetic.

"Closely allied to the foregoing advantage is the ability to prevent the aspiration of vomitus, blood, mucus, or pus into the lower respiratory tract. 'Aspiration pneumonia' was a fairly frequent sequela of any operation upon the upper air passages in days before intubation was currently used. The aspiration of foreign fluids can always be prevented during operation by the skilful use of endotracheal methods. This fact is of importance not only in operations upon the upper respiratory tract but also in any condition liable to cause the patient to vomit during anaesthesia.

"Intubation of the trachea enables the anaesthetist to remove fluids easily, and at any time, from the bronchial tree by suction through or alongside the endotracheal tube. This applies not only to an excess of mucus secreted by the trachea and bronchi, but also to blood or pus. The latter are usually seen only during pulmonary operations, but unless they can be rapidly removed they are a grave menace to the patient. Certain precautions, however, are expedient when applying either negative or positive pressure deep in the respiratory tree.

"It has long been recognized that certain positions of the patient upon the operating table, although necessary to the operation, greatly impede the mechanics of normal respiration. The chief offenders in this respect are the prone position, the steep 'Trendelenburg' position, and any arrangement of the patient which involves raising of a 'bridge' beneath the lower ribs. Not only is respiratory movement hindered, but in these positions it is often difficult if not impossible to prevent upper respiratory obstruction, especially in anatomically 'difficult' subjects. Several early workers with endotracheal anaesthesia reported that the incidence of 'operative shock' was lower when this technique was in use and suggested that this more favorable condition was due to an absence of exertion during respiration in the intubated patient. Even the very experienced anaesthetist occasionally encounters patients so anatomically abnormal that he is unable to maintain unobstructed respiration with the aid of an artificial airway in the pharynx. In these rare cases intubation will remove the obstruction to respiration where all other measures fail.

"Finally endotracheal methods are of great value in those rare cases in which a mechanical obstruction to respiration is either present or anticipated. The least uncommon of these is probably thyroidectomy undertaken for the relief of obstructive symptoms. Naturally intubation must then be accomplished with a tube certain to remain patent under any pressure to which it may be subjected, and of sufficient length to reach beyond the point of constriction of the air passages.

"If the pleural cavity is opened, the lung which it contains collapses. This collapse can be prevented or remedied by raising the pressure inside the lung. The simplest way to do this is to apply positive pressure to the anaesthetic vapor. The mechanical means of doing this are discussed on pages 112–115 and 153–154. The application of positive pressure can often be achieved by the use of an accurately fitting facepiece. If, however, glottic spasm occurs, or the patient vomits during anaesthesia, it will be impossible to control the intrabronchial pressure. If the glottis is intubated, on the other hand, spasm cannot occur, and vomiting, with suitable precautions, need not disturb the control of the intrapulmonic pressure.

"Atelectasis may occur during anaesthesia. If it is diagnosed, the presence of a tube in the trachea renders its immediate treatment possible, by suction drainage of the tracheo-bronchial tree and gentle manual reinflation of the lungs.

"The complete collapse of one lung is occasionally desirable during the performance of certain modern operations upon the lung itself. This condition can be secured by the intubation of a main bronchus with a tube carrying a cuff which, when inflated, occludes the bronchus of the diseased side. Respiration is then carried on by the sound lung only.

"The complicated positive and negative pressure cabinets designed for the purpose of preventing pneumothorax during thoracic operations, which enjoyed a considerable vogue at the beginning of this century, have disappeared from use. Increasing experience has thus clearly shown that an appropriate form of endotracheal anaesthesia is both the simplest and the most efficient method of avoiding the difficulties and dangers inherent in the condition of pneumothorax.

"Centuries before the discovery of anaesthesia the resuscitative value of mechanical ventilation was demonstrated ... and the ability instantly to transmute the maintenance of anaesthesia into the process of resuscitation is a great safeguard to the patient. To such an extent is this true that within the space of a few years the 'apnoea' which but recently was the terror of the anaesthetist has under certain circumstances become an accepted technique of anaesthesia. Intubation is no more essential to controlled respiration than to control of intrapulmonic pressure, for adequate respiratory exchange can usually be effected with a bag and a facepiece. Yet when the maintenance of this exchange is essential to life, and obstruction of the air passages may at any moment interrupt it, intubation offers too valuable a safeguard to be neglected.

"Operations in the course of which respiratory failure may occur were formerly embarked upon with trepidation. If intubation is resorted to in such cases, the surgeon can proceed secure in the knowledge that, should respiratory failure occur, the anaesthetist is in a position to substitute effective manual exchange of gases for spontaneous respiration.

"Writing at a time when specialist anaesthetists were all but unknown, Kühn said that intubation enabled the surgeon 'Herr der Lage zu sein and zu bleiben' (to become and remain master of the field). This is indeed the only possible concise statement of the advantages of intubation: that it makes the anaesthetist master of every mechanical aspect of respiratory exchange, under any circumstances of functional disturbance, and for any period of time."

The technique of endotracheal intubation, as we know it today, was introduced in Glasgow in 1880. In that year, William

MacEwen, a Scottish surgeon, published his epochal paper, "Clinical Observations on the Introduction of Tracheal Tubes by the Mouth Instead of Performing Tracheotomy or Laryngotomy" (*Br. Med. J.*, 2: 122–124, 163–165, 1880), which is republished below.

CLINICAL OBSERVATIONS ON THE INTRODUCTION OF TRACHEAL TUBES BY THE MOUTH INSTEAD OF PERFORMING TRACHEOTOMY OR LARYNGOTOMY

MacEwen, W.

Br. Med. J., 2:122–124, 163–165, 1880

Prior to this, attempts at orotracheal and nasotracheal intubation of the larynx to treat respiratory obstruction of recent onset had been largely unsuccessful, although mechanical dilation of chronic tracheal stenosis had been successfully performed. MacEwen reports on successful orotracheal intubation of four patients using his finger as a guide. Two patients suffered from tumor of the pharynx, one of burn and one of infection, all with recent onset of partial respiratory obstruction. His last of ten deductions states, "Such tubes may be introduced in operations on the face and mouth, in order to prevent blood from gaining access to the trachea, and for the purpose of administering an anaesthetic; and they answer this purpose admirably."

1881

Published August, 1964

During the past decade, a considerable interest has been generated in the use of hyperventilation as a technique in anesthesia. There have been two main applications of this technique in clinical practice: first, the use of hyperventilation as a means of reducing brain volume during neurosurgical procecures, particularly craniotomies; and, second, the use of hyperventilation to produce a quieter operative field and to decrease the quantities of anesthetic and muscle relaxant drugs required during other types of surgery, particularly intra-abdominal operations.

One of the first reports concerning the use of hyperventilation in neurosurgery to decrease brain volume was that by Furness, which appeared in the British literature in 1957. She reported her empirical experiences in 100 neurosurgical procedures, employing a combination of thiopental-nitrous oxide-curare and hyperventilation produced with a mechanical ventilator of the positive-negative type, set to deliver a minute volume exchange of 10 liters per minute. She believed that the use of a negative phase during expiration was an essential part of the technique, and that it significantly aided in reducing venous bleeding, since it favored the maintenance of negative pressure in the thorax, which otherwise would tend to become positive and lead to an increase in venous pressure, which in turn would be transmitted to the brain. Slocum and his colleagues, at the Walter Reed Hospital in this country, have employed a similar technique to relieve brain swelling during neurosurgery, but have not included a negative phase of respiration, believing that venous pressure could be controlled by gravity through the use of the headup or sitting position during surgery. It has been the opinion of these groups on both sides of the Atlantic that hyperventilation is superior to induced hypotension, hypothermia, or chemical dehydration as a technique to produce a "relaxed" brain and good operating conditions with a minimum of physiologic morbidity. Rosomoff, however, has recently reported studies which challenge whether hyperventilation in fact does reduce brain volume. His data indicate a decrease in intracranial blood volume and a compensatory increase in cerebrospinal fluid volume; no change was seen in either brain water or brain solids, nor was there a decline in cerebrospinal fluid pressure. He concluded that observations to the effect that the brain is smaller because it "appears to be slack" during hyperventilation are illusions of the human eye, and that in fact a reduction of intracranial tension is produced by hyperventilation only if hypercarbia due to underventilation was present before the onset of artificial ventilation.

The use of hyperventilation during other types of surgery has been championed by the Liverpool school of anesthetists, under the leadership of Professor T. Cecil Gray, as a technique which will decrease the need for both general anesthetic and muscle relaxant drugs. Gray has pointed out that, when relaxant drugs have been administered, the degree of abdominal relaxation will be influenced by the efficiency of pulmonary ventilation: if this is inadequate, the hypercarbia which results will stimulate the respiratory center, more frequent impulses of greater intensity will pass down the motor nerves to the muscles, and a larger dose of relaxant will be required to produce a given degree of paralysis or relaxation. Others have suggested that hyperventilation achieves its relaxing effect not by hypocarbia, but by inhibition of abdominal muscle reflexes. Still other workers have implicated hypoxia as the reason for deepening of anesthesia and the decrease in the requirement for anesthetic drugs: hyperventilation is known to produce cerebral vasoconstriction and increased cerebrovascular resistance; and in one study, cerebral oxygen tension, as measured by an oxygen electrode, dropped markedly during hyperventilation. Caution must be exercised in the interpretation of results obtained from the use of oxygen tension electrodes on the surface of, or within, the brain, however, as artifact may be present from either compression of capillaries at the tip of the electrode, or actual disruption and damage of the tissue.

It is rather intriguing to realize that the present widespread interest in hyperventilation was preceded by a similar period of interest when hyperventilation was introduced as an anesthetic technique by a Philadelphia dentist more than 80 years ago. *Survey* and its readers are indebted to Dr. J. Alfred Lee, of Southend-on-Sea, Essex, England, and Dr. David A. Davis, of Chapel Hill, North Carolina, for bringing the writings of Dr. W. G. A. Bonwill to the attention of "Classical File." Two of Dr. Bonwill's contributions to the literature are reprinted below. The first, "The air as an anaesthetic", was published in the *Philadelphia Journal of Dental Science*, volume 3, pages 57–61, in 1876; the second, "Rapid breathing as a pain obtunder in minor surgery, obstetrics, the general practice of medicine and of dentistry", appeared in *Scientific American Supplement*, No. 275, pages 4386–4389, April 9, 1881.

RAPID BREATHING AS A PAIN OBTUNDER IN MINOR SURGERY, OBSTETRICS, THE GENERAL PRACTICE OF MEDICINE AND OF DENTISTRY

W. G. A. BONWILL, D.D.S.

Scientific American Supp., No. 275, 4386–4389, 1881

"Through the kind invitation of your directors, I am present to give you the history of "rapid breathing" as an analgesic agent as well as my experience therein since I first discovered it.

*   *   *   *

"I think we are now prepared to show clearly the causes which effect the phenomena in rapid breathing.

"The first thing enlisted is the *diversion of the will force* in the act of forced respiration at a moment when the heart and lungs have been in normal reciprocal action (20 respirations to 80 pulsations), which act could not be made and carried up to 100 respirations per minute without such concentrated effort that ordinary pain could make no impression upon the brain while this abstraction is kept up.

"Second. There is a specific effect resulting from enforced respiration of 100 to the minute, due to the *excess of carbonic acid gas set free from the tissues,* generated by this enforced normal act of throwing into the lungs five times the normal amount of oxygen in one minute demanded, when the heart has not been aroused to exalted action, which comes from violent exercise in running or where one is suddenly startled, which excess of carbonic acid cannot escape in the same ratio from the lungs, since the heart does not respond to the proportionate overaction of the lungs.

"Third.—Hyperaemia is the last in this chain of effects, which is due to the excessive amount of air passing into the lungs preventing but little more than the normal quantity of blood from passing from the heart into the arterial circulation, but draws it up in the brain with its excess of carbonic acid gas to act also directly upon the brain as well as throughout the capillary and venous system, and as well upon the heart, the same as if it were suspended in that gas outside the body".

1884

Published June, 1965

Cocaine hydrochloride is a white crystalline powder that is freely soluble in water and is fairly stable, decomposing only slightly except on prolonged boiling. It is the benzoic acid ester of the base ecgonine, which in turn is esterified with methyl alcohol. It is obtained from the leaves of the Erythroxylon coca, a small shrub with vivid green leaves which is indigenous to the Andes mountains of Chile, Bolivia and Peru, where for centuries the native Indians have chewed coca leaves to increase their physical strength and endurance.

Cocaine stimulates the central nervous system from above downward. In animals, the cortical action is manifested mainly by increased motor activity, which is coordinated at first, but is characterized by tremors and convulsive movements as the dose is increased, and eventually leads to clonic and tonic convulsions. In man, the first action on the cortex appears as garrulity, restlessness, and euphoric excitement.

The action of cocaine on the medulla results in rapid, shallow breathing, and the vasomotor and vomiting centers share in the stimulation. Depression then replaces the central stimulation, and unconsciousness ensues; eventually the depression includes the vital medullary centers, and death results from respiratory failure.

Cocaine also has effects upon the sympathetic nervous system activity, but not direct effects on sympathetically innervated structures. It does, however, have the property of potentiating both excitatory and inhibitory responses of muscles and glands to epinephrine or adrenergic nerve impulses, perhaps by preventing the destruction of epinephrine since it inhibits amine oxidase, the enzyme concerned with the oxidation of epinephrine.

Cocaine is a marked pyretic, and hyperthermia is often a striking feature of cocaine poisoning. Pyrexia probably results from increased heat production as a result of the muscular activity attending central stimulation, from decreased heat elimination due to vasoconstriction produced by central vasomotor stimulation, and perhaps from a direct effect on the heat regulating centers.

The effects of cocaine upon the cardiovascular system vary with the dosage. Bradycardia may result from small doses due to central vagal stimulation, but as the dose is increased a definite tachycardia is produced. This tachycardia, coupled with vasoconstriction due to central vasomotor stimulation, causes a pronounced increase in blood pressure. In addition to this vasoconstriction of central origin, the application of cocaine to blood vessel walls will produce direct vasoconstriction. The administration of a large intravenous dose of cocaine may result in immediate death from cardiac failure due to a direct toxic action on heart muscle.

The effect of cocaine on skeletal muscle has been the subject of considerable investigation because of its well known reputation for relieving or delaying fatigue from physical exertion. There is no evidence, however, that cocaine increases the strength of muscular contraction, and it has been concluded that central stimulation and euphoria simply mask the sensations of fatigue.

By far the most important action of cocaine is its ability to block nerve conduction when brought into direct contact with nerve tissue. It was this property from which the entire field of regional, nerve block, and conduction anesthesia grew. The development and use of cocaine as a local anesthetic was chiefly the work of Karl Koller, who reported his investigations to the Ophthalmological Congress held in Heidelberg on September 14 and 15, 1884. His studies were published under the title of "Ueber die Verwendung des Cocaïn zur Anästhesirung am Auge." *Wiener Medizinische Wochenschrift 34:* 1276–1278, 1309–1311, 1884. *Survey* and its readers are indebted to Dr. Carl S. Hellijas of the Department of Anesthesiology, Hartford Hospital, for the English translation of this article which is reprinted below.

CONCERNING THE USE OF COCAINE FOR ANESTHESIA OF THE EYE

DR. KARL KOLLER
Assistant Physician of the
Royal Imperial General Hospital,
Vienna

Wiener Medizinische Wochenschrift, 34:
1276–1278, 1309–1311, 1884

*   *   *   *

"At the outset, I considered using cocaine therapeutically in two ways: first, as a *narcotic for painful eye ailments* and second, as an *anesthetic for operations on the eye.*

"As to the first usage, I expected to gain much from its effect, especially on *corneal and conjunctival ailments associated with pain and photophobia.* I used cocaine (in 2% solution) in a large number of patients with conjunctivitis lymphatica with eruptions and ulcerations on the cornea and on one patient with vascular banding. All of the patients so treated stated that they felt far better a few minutes after the instillation: the pain subsided and the photophobia decreased considerably. Correspondingly, however, the patients complained that 2 to 3 hours after the instillation pain and photophobia returned.

*   *   *   *

"I now come to the second way of using cocaine, that is as an *anesthetic for operations on the eye.* Cocaine is first rate for *removal of foreign bodies from and out of the cornea,* often difficult because of the patient's restlessness. I have set about establishing anesthesia in a goodly number of these patients (about 30 cases) by having the patient, who was sitting or standing, look at the floor while I put 2 drops of a 2% solution on the cornea; the instillation was repeated once again in 3 to 5 minutes. All of the patients stated that they had lost the feeling of a foreign body; at removal of the fragment from the cornea with a needle, all patients kept the globe motionless and on questioning about what they felt, all answered that they felt nothing at all".

Published June, 1959

The history of anesthesia abounds with proof that great discoveries and events do not usually occur unexpectedly as the result of sudden inspiration in the mind of one man, but rather proceed logically and almost inevitably from preceding events and discoveries. It is therefore perhaps also inevitable that the thought which kindled a great discovery often occurred in more than one man's mind at almost the same instant in time. The introduction of direct nerve block anesthesia is a cogent example.

The pertinent preceding events in this instance were, of course, the development of the syringe and hollow needle, and the discovery of the local anesthetic properties of cocaine. The former occurred in 1853 when the Scotsman, Alexander Wood, devised the modern type of metallic hollow needle at the same time that the Frenchman, Charles Gabriel Pravaz, attached an improved hollow needle to a specially constructed syringe, called, on the continent of Europe, the "Pravaz syringe," in honor of its inventor.

The discovery of the local anesthetic properties of cocaine was made in 1884 by Carl Koller, but might well have been attributed rather to the great psychoanalyst, Sigmund Freud, had not Freud's romantic interest taken him away on a holiday to meet his fiancee at that time—perhaps lending support to Freud's later thesis that sex is the dominant force in man's activities. As it was, Koller's discovery that the application of a few drops of cocaine solution to an animal's eye would render that eye insensitive to mechanical, chemical, thermal and faradic stimulation, was demonstrated in a human patient at a congress of ophthalmology which met at Heidelburg on September 15, 1884. The news traveled like wildfire and the use of cocaine for eye surgery was so enthusiastically accepted and extolled that one medical editor was constrained to write: "The loneliest doctor in the world is the ophthalmologist who hasn't written an article on cocaine." Nor was the use of the drug confined to eye surgery, for the drug was employed extensively also in laryngology and rhinology, and for operations in the male urethra.

Very obviously, the thought of applying cocaine directly to a nerve trunk by injection was the next logical and inevitable step, and on November 22, 1884, within ten weeks of the public demonstration of the local anesthetic properties of cocaine at Heidelburg, Dr. W. C. Burke, Jr., of South Norwalk, Connecticut, wrote to the Editor of the New York Medical Journal:

"A.B., a phlegmatic German, about 40 years of age, on Friday, the 14th instant, while cleaning a revolver, accidentally shot himself in the right hand. The ball (.22 caliber) entered the palm of the hand opposite the third carpophalangeal articulation, and, passing outward under the flexor tendons of the hand, lodged against the first phalanx (inner surface) of the little finger, about half an inch in front of the articulation with the corresponding bone. Twenty-four hours after the accident the man came to my office to have the wound dressed. At that time the hand, which naturally was very large and thick, was considerably swollen and inflamed; there was also considerable pain. I gave him a hypodermic injection of 5 minims of a 2-per-cent solution of the hydrochlorate of cocaine on the back of the hand, at the inner side of the last metacarpal bone—deeply injected, so as to bring the drug as near as possible to that branch of the ulnar nerve supplying the inner side of the little finger. Five minutes later another hypodermic of the same amount was given along the back of the first phalanx of the little finger, the solution being thrown in as the needle was withdrawn. He said that the introduction of the needle the second time gave not the slightest pain, the first one having hurt him and been followed by smarting (probably due to the alcohol). After waiting five minutes longer, I made the necessary incision, an inch or an inch and a half long and quite deep, owing to the size of his finger and its swollen condition. Neither the cut or the subsequent manipulation in the removal of the ball, nor the dressing, gave him *any pain whatever.* He described his sensations in the hand as being 'numb or asleep.'"

Four days later, on the 26th of November, Dr. R. J. Hall of the Roosevelt Hospital in New York City, also wrote to the Editor of the New York Medical Journal to describe the experiments and clinical trials which he had been carrying out in conjunction with Dr. William S. Halsted on the injection of cocaine for direct nerve block. Rightfully or wrongfully, the names of Burke and Hall have been relegated to lower-case type in the histories of local anesthesia, and the name of William Stewart Halsted has been placed in capital letters as the man who introduced nerve block anesthesia with cocaine. Nevertheless, Hall's letter to the Editor must stand as one of the published landmarks of regional anesthesia: entitled "Hydrochlorate of Cocaine," it was published in the December 6, 1884, issue of the *New York Medical Journal* and is reproduced below, together with the Editorial entitled, "The New Local Anaesthetic," which appeared in the same issue.

LETTERS TO THE EDITOR

"HYDROCHLORATE OF COCAINE"

HALL, R.J.

New York Medical Journal, 40: 343–349 (Dec. 6) 1884

Dr. Hall described a number of experiments made by Dr. Halsted and himself injecting a four percent solution of cocaine subcutaneously and noting the resulting sensory anesthesia. In addition to the area of anesthesia, "marked constitutional symptoms appeared", including giddiness, nausea, and cold perspiration. Hall reported on the successful administration in a number of cases in the outpatient department, and in addition had persuaded his dentist to use it on himself.

In addition, the lead article in the journal reviewed the introduction of this new technique for inducing anesthesia. In conclusion, it stated, "no doubt much yet remains to be done in the way of experiment and observation before the precise sphere of the new anesthetic can be defined, and it would be prudent for those who may undertake to furnish us with these data not to count too much upon the innocuousness of the drug, for it should be noted that Dr. Hall experienced marked consitutional symptoms from an injection of 32 minims of a four percent solution of the hydrochlorate."

1885

Published June, 1960

The claim for the introduction of a new technique in medicine frequently is subject to revision following more arduous search by medical historians into the dusty archives of the past. This situation most certainly has been true in the field of anesthesia, the most celebrated example being, of course, the notorious Ether Controversy involving Morton, Jackson, Wells and Crawford Long (*Survey of Anesthesiology,*

February, 1960). The history of the development of conduction anesthesia contains no such celebrated disputation as that Great Ether Controversy, but a number of differing interpretations of historical facts have been developed as unbiased (or perhaps more biased) historians have unearthed older and older records.

One prime prerequisite to the development of conduction anesthesia, for instance, was the hollow needle, and this invention is generally credited to the Scotsman, Alexander Wood, in 1853; however, the first hollow needles were quills, of the type used by Sir Christopher Wren around 1656 for his intravenous injections of opium, and probably also by Sigismund Elsheltz in 1665 for his injections of opiates. A second prerequisite for the development of conduction anesthesia was certainly the discovery of a local anesthetic agent, which is generally credited to Karl Koller following his demonstration of the anesthetic properties of cocaine before the Ophthalmologic Congress held in Heidelburg on September 15, 1884; however, as early as 1860, Albert Niemann, who obtained the alkaloid of cocoa leaves in crystalline form and named it "cocaine," reported the numbing effect of this drug on the tongue; and in 1873, Alexander Bennett demonstrated the anesthetic properties of cocaine. Even the penultimate step in the development of conduction anesthesia, the actual injection of a local anesthetic agent to produce anesthesia, generally credited to William S. Halsted in 1884, had been taken by Vasili Konstantinovich von Anrep as early as 1878, when he injected a weak solution of cocaine under the skin of his own arm, experienced a sense of warmness which was followed by anesthesia that lasted for about half an hour, and suggested the possibility of the employment of cocaine as a local anesthetic agent.

But perhaps the chief disagreement in the interpretation of historical facts relative to the development of conduction anesthesia concerns the introduction of spinal anesthesia. August Bier is generally considered to have performed the first spinal anesthesia in man in 1898. There is little doubt that it is to Bier that credit must be given for endowing surgery with the method of spinal anesthesia, but in point of fact it was James Leonard Corning who performed the first injections of cocaine into the human spine in 1885. Whether Corning had obtained true spinal anesthesia at this time, or merely had produced epidural anesthesia, remains a debated question. Certain it is that Corning's experiment was based on faulty physiologic and anatomic premises, since he believed that cocaine injected into the region between two spinous processes would be absorbed by the circulation and "transferred to the substance of the cord, and give rise to anesthesia of the sensory and perhaps motor tracks of the same." He did, however, clearly suggest the possibilities of the utility of a form of spinal anesthesia for surgery, whether or not he realized the importance of the subarachnoid space in the production of spinal anesthesia as it is defined today. His original observations were published under the title, "Spinal Anaesthesia and Local Medication of the Cord," in the October 31, 1885, issue of the New York Medical Journal.

SPINAL ANAESTHESIA AND LOCAL MEDICATION OF THE CORD

J. Leonard Corning, M.D.

New York Med. J., 43: October 31, 1885

*   *   *   *

"*Experiment I*. This was performed on a young dog. At ten o'clock, a. m., I injected twenty minims of a two-per-cent solution of the hydrochlorate of cocaine into the space situated between the spinous processes of two of the inferior dorsal vertebrae. Five minutes after the injection there was evidence of marked inco-ordination in the posterior extremities; the dog threw his hindlegs about aimlessly, holding them far apart, much after the manner of some ataxic patients. A few minutes later there was marked evidence of weakness in the hind-legs, but there were no signs whatever of feebleness in the anterior extremities. I now tested the condition of sensibility by means of a powerful faradaic battery, one of the conducting cords of which was attached to a fine wire brush. When the wire brush was applied to the hind-legs, there was no reflex action whatever on the part of the latter, at least such was the case except when the most powerful currents were employed. But, on the other hand, when I applied the wire brush to either of the anterior extremities, the limb was drawn away violently, and the animal set up the most dismal howls. Similar effects were observed on pinching and pricking the limbs.

"These phenomena persisted for a considerable length of time, and traces of inco-ordination were observed two hours after the injection had been made. After the lapse of about four hours, however, the dog seemed to have recovered his usual health, and walked about without difficulty.

"During the duration of the experiment nothing of an abnormal nature was observed in the fore-legs. I infer from this fact that the action of the anaesthetic was practically local, being confined, for the most part, to that portion of the cord situated immediately beneath the point of injection. It is conceivable, however, that, had the quantity of anaesthetic fluid injected been greater, the anterior limbs might also have been affected. An *absolute* localization of the anaesthesia is indeed hardly within the range of possibilities, on account of the numerous blood-vessels. It is true, nevertheless, as we have seen, that the local action of the drug is greatly favored, at least, so far as the inferior segment of the cord is concerned, by reason of the lethargy of the circulation at this point".

1894

Published August, 1962

Chloroform has so many admirable features as an anesthetic drug that it has stayed around considerably longer than would seem justifiable on the basis of its clinical record for mortality. It has a sweet, not unpleasant odor, and is only mildly irritating on inhalation. It is a fully potent drug, and provides a rapid and usually smooth induction which does not require the use of a preliminary induction drug such as nitrous oxide or ethylene. One needs only the simplest of equipment for its administration—a piece of lint and a dropper bottle. It can provide magnificent muscular relaxation: certain Canadian anesthetists refer to it as "The Great Softener" because of its ability to render the most robust Cape Breton coalminer as limp as a rag in a matter of breaths. It is totally nonflammable, permitting the use of electrocoagulation and electronic equipment without fear of fire or explosion. Very low concentrations are required for even the most profound anesthesia, so that extremely high concentrations of oxygen are possible in the inhaled mixture. It is chemically stable and easily preserved. It is so inexpensive that a total anesthesia may cost only a matter of cents. In fact, on a number of counts it comes close to the ideal inhalation anesthetic—except for the mortalities.

The mortalities from chloroform began to occur soon after the introduction of the drug into clinical anesthetic practice by Simpson in 1847. Hannah Greener was the first, a brief 10 weeks after Simpson's initial report on the use of chloroform for anesthesia; but she was only the beginning. The redoubtable John Snow, at the time of his death in 1856, had collected 50 deaths from chloroform; and in view of the small number of operations at the time, this was no mean mortality rate. A quarter of a century later, in 1882, Henry M. Lyman devoted 50 pages of his book on anesthesia to case reports of 393 chloroform deaths collected from a variety of sources: a small number had died at the beginning of the inhalation, a large number before complete insensibility, another large number during maintenance, and a goodly number post-operatively. On this side of the ocean, Edmund Andrews of Chicago reported 43 deaths in 117,078 chloroform anesthesias, or a mortality rate of 1 : 2723. The mortalities continued down through the years: during one very black week in 1899, no fewer than 9 deaths under chloroform were reported in a single issue of the *Lancet*—2 from Liverpool, 4 in various London hospitals, 2 in military hospitals, and one at the county borough of Dudley. Even as recently as 1956, Siebecker and Orth at the University of Wisconsin reported 2 deaths from 7 chloroform anesthesias for thoracic surgery, both from fatal hepatic damage, and 2 other patients also had severe hepatic damage which, however, was not fatal.

The role of hepatic damage in the production of death following chloroform anesthesia went unrecognized for many years. In fact, it was not recognized until chloroform had been in use as an anesthetic in England for 47 years, and chloroform was used in almost every patient during that time. Leonard George Guthrie was the man who put Delayed Chloroform Poisoning on the map. (He was, incidentally, no relation to Samuel Guthrie, of Sackett's Harbor, Long Island, who shares the credit for the chemical manufacture of chloroform with the German, von Liebig, and the Frenchman, Soubeiran, all 3 men having discovered the drug independently in 1831). Leonard Guthrie was born in 1858, qualified at Oxford in 1888, and died on Christmas Eve, 1919, aged 61. He was physician and pathologist, and formerly chloroformist, to the Paddington-Green Chil-dren's Hospital, so he was particularly well situated to bring to light this obscure condition, which mostly affected children. This he did in 2 articles entitled, "On Some Fatal After-Effects of Chloroform on Children," which were published in the January 27 and February 3, 1894, issues of *Lancet* (Guthrie, L. G.: *Lancet, 1:* 193–197, January 27, and 257–261, February 3, 1894), and which are reprinted below.

ON SOME FATAL AFTER-EFFECTS OF CHLOROFORM ON CHILDREN

LEONARD G. GUTHRIE, M.A., M.D. OXON., M.R.C.P. LOND.,

Assistant Physician and Pathologist (Late Chloroformist), Paddington-Green Children's Hospital; Assistant Physician, Northwest London Hospital; Physician; Regent's Park Hospital for Epilepsy and Paralysis

Lancet, 1: 193–197 and 257–261, 1894

Ten children are described in whom the administration of chloroform for operation was followed in all but one with death. After a thorough analysis, including autopsy in those who succumbed, it was concluded that: the deaths were primarily due to autointoxication; a fatty condition of the liver existed before the operation; and chloroform and operative shock combined to aggravate the condition already present.

1899

Published June, 1962

August Bier was one of the last of the great German Geheimrat Professors of Surgery, but when he died in his 88th year on March 14, 1949, it was his contribution to anesthesia that was most prominently featured in his obituaries.

Bier was the son of a surveyor, Thedor Bier, and was born in 1861 at Helsen, a small town on the Wesser between Westphalia and Hesse-Nassau. He attended the local village school and continued his education at the Gymnasium in Korbach, the chief city of the former principality of Waldek. He then faced the perplexing problem of choosing a career. His great love of wood and field made it difficult to decide whether to become a forester or a doctor, but he finally chose medicine. He studied in Berlin, Leipzig, and Kiel, and came under the influence of both Karl Friedrich Wilhelm Ludwig, one of the most important physiologists of the last century, and Professor Friedrich von Esmarch, who had won his fame with the elastic rubber bandage for "bloodless" operations. Bier completed his studies in Kiel with distinction in 1886, took his doctoral examination in 1888, became an assistant of Esmarch's, and qualified as an instructor in 1889.

From then on, Bier's career in medicine became one of increasing distinction. He was a man of intuition, quick decision, had the courage of his convictions, and became a surgeon of towering stature. He was a bold and rapid operator, with a quick recognition and evaluation of the pathologic problem at hand. He was an inspiring teacher. On the podium he was a magnet— kept his listeners fascinated, enlivening even the dryest subject. He had the great gift of simplication, his epigrammatic sentences often humorously revealing the core of things.

Shortly after the discovery of general anesthesia, Diffenbach, one of Bier's predecessors in the Chair of the Department of Surgery at the University of Berlin, had extolled the new miracle: "A dream has come true. Pain has been conquered!" Some fifty years later, Bier gave this truth a new impetus through the introduction of spinal anesthesia. In 1891, Quincke had described the technique of lumbar puncture and demonstrated its usefulness as a diagnostic procedure. Quincke had apparently been unaware of the possibilities of spinal anesthesia, but he had shown that the introduction of a needle through the dura was feasible; and this revelation in itself was enough to fire the imagination of August Bier. The report of Bier's earliest studies is fascinating, not only as the milestone marking the clinical introduction of spinal anesthesia, but also because it contained a clear and precise description of postspinal headache, including even the probable etiology and treatment! *Survey of Anesthesiology* and its readers are indebted to Associate Editor, Dr. Gertie Marx, for the translation into English of Bier's paper, "Versuche über Cocainisirung des Rückenmarkes," which was published in the *Deutsche Zietschrift fur Chirurgie, 51:* 361–369, 1899, and which is reprinted below.

EXPERIMENTS REGARDING THE COCAINIZATION OF THE SPINAL CORD

Professor Dr. August Bier

The Royal Surgical Clinic of Kiel
Zeitschrift fur Chirurgie, 51: 361–369,
April, 1899

*   *   *   *

"I have attempted to render large areas of the body insensible to pain by introducing cocaine into the spinal cord. This was carried out in the following way: with the patient lying on his side, lumbar puncture is performed according to the familiar method of Quincke. The needle should be very fine. After the subarachnoid space is entered, the stilet of the needle is removed; the opening is immediately covered by the finger so that very little cerebrospinal fluid can escape. The desired amount of cocaine is then injected with the help of a "Pravaz" syringe, which fits the needle tightly. Of course, one has to add the volume of cocaine held by the injecting needle (with our needles, this equals 1½ lines on the "Pravaz" syringe). To prevent absorption of cocaine by adjacent tissues, the needle with the syringe is left *in situ* for two minutes, after which it is removed. The puncture is sealed off with collodion.

* * * *

"The cocaine spreads in the cerebrospinal fluid and comes in contact not only with the surface of the spinal cord, but also with the non-myelinated nerves passing through the subarachnoid space and with the ganglia. I believe that paralysis of pain sensation following intrathecal injection of a small quantity of cocaine is due to the action of the drug on these sheathless nerves

and probably on the ganglia as well. I would like to use the words, "cocainization of the spinal cord" with this meaning in mind; I chose these words because of their brevity.

* * * *

"These experiments proved to us that an exceedingly small quantity of cocaine (0.005 gm.) injected into the intrathecal space can narcotize two-thirds of the body to such a degree that major surgery can be performed painlessly. Loss of sensation develops in the legs 5 to 8 minutes after injection. Most likely, the effect of cocaine is on the sheathless nerves, the nerve-roots and the ganglia, rather than on the spinal cord itself. The area of numbness gradually increases; with a small dose and in a large person numbness results as far as the nipples (Case 1, 2, 5, and Dr. Hildebrandt). A dose which is greater in relation to the size of the body causes anesthesia of the entire body with the exception of the head (Case 4: 0.005 gm. cocaine given to an 11-year-old boy). With smaller doses (0.005 gm. in adults) anesthesia lasts for about 45 minutes; then sensation returns slowly (Dr. Hildebrandt)".

* * * *

1901

Published August, 1979

Nobody knows for certain whether the "local medication of the spinal cord" which Corning reported in the October 31st, 1885, issue of the *New York Medical Journal* was spinal or epidural analgesia.

Check that. A lot of people know for sure that it was spinal analgesia, and a lot of other people know for sure that it was epidural analgesia. It is just that not everybody can agree.

James Leonard Corning was born in Stamford,Connecticut, in 1855, and received his medical education in Germany,

where he attended the University of Heidelberg and then obtained the degree of doctor of medicine from the University of Wurzburg in 1878. He returned to the United States and specialized in neurology, becoming a member of the New York Neurological Society and practicing in and around New York City—he was a member of the medical staffs of the Hackensack, St. Francis, and St. Mary's Hospitals. As a neurologist, Corning became interested in the effects of cocaine upon the central nervous system, the same interest which led Sigmund Freud to collaborate with Carl Koller in research, which eventually led to the discovery of cocaine as a local anesthetic and thereby opened up the entire field of conduction anesthesia which developed because of that discovery.

Corning's avowed purpose when he undertook "local medication of the spinal cord" was to determine whether or not anesthetization of the spinal cord, using the hydrochlorate of cocaine, "was within the range of practical achievement;" and he established that clearly it was. The experiment which he performed on a young dog consisted of the injection of 20 minims of a 2.0 per cent solution of the hydrochlorate of cocaine into the space between the spinous processes of 2 of the inferior dorsal vertebrae. Within 5 minutes there were evidences of marked incoordination in the posterior extremities; and within 10 minutes there was no response to electrical stimulation of the hindlegs, whereas when the wire brush was applied to the anterior limbs the leg was withdrawn violently and "the animal set up the most dismal howls." The incoordination was still present at the end of 2 hours, but by 4 hours the dog appeared to have recovered completely and walked about without difficulty.

Corning next performed the experiment on a patient by injecting 30 minims of a 3.0 per cent solution of the hydrochlorate of cocaine into the space between the spinous processes of the 11th and 12th dorsal vertebrae. At the end of about 8 minutes, there was no numbness, tingling, or other evidence of modified sensibility, so Corning injected another 30 minims of the solution in the same place and in the same manner. This time he was rewarded, after about 10 minutes, by the patient stating that his legs "felt sleepy" and by discovering that the sensibility to both pinprick and electrical stimulation was greatly impaired in the lower extremities, whereas full sensation and muscle activity were present in the upper extremities. The patient subsequently experienced some vertigo and headache, but otherwise there were no constitutional symptoms. The passage of a sound to treat the patient's seminal incontinence, "although usually accompanied by considerable pain, remained almost unperceived, and an urethral electrode caused no inconvenience, even when strong currents were used." Corning concluded that, "whether the method will ever find an application as a substitute for etherization in genitourinary or other branches of surgery, further experience alone can show."

Some authorities state quite unequivocably that, whatever the result, it clearly was not Corning's intention to deposit a local anesthetic agent in the subarachnoid space. He deposited approximately 120 mg. of cocaine, dissolved in 4 ml. in 2 doses, within slightly more than 10 minutes, near the lower thoracic region of the spinal canal. Had this drug been deposited in the subarachnoid space, it seems more than likely that he would have observed the rapid onset of analgesia which should have included the upper extremities, which it did not.

Other observers, however, believe just as strongly that Corning did indeed produce true spinal analgesia, and point out that, in the dog experiment, only about 40 mg. of cocaine dissolved in about 2 ml. was injected and this was both an insufficient dose and an insufficient volume of solution to produce such widespread analgesia of the hindquarters of the animal had the drug been deposited in the epidural space. In further support of their contention that Corning's injections were in fact spinal (intrathecal), they stress the occurrence of headache as a sure sign that there must have been a subarachnoid puncture.

In any event, 2 French physicians, Jean-Althanase Sicard and Fernand Cathelin, reported experiments within 1 week of each other which clearly identified the extradural space and the feasibility of performing injections into it via the caudal canal. Sicard's paper, "Les injections médicamenteuses extradurales par voie sacro-coccygiene", was published in *Comptes rendus hebdomadaires des séances et mémoires de la Société de biologie, 53:* 396–398, Apr. 20, 1901; and Cathelin's report, "Une nouvelle voie d'injection rachidienne. Méthode des injections épidurales par le procédé du canal sacré. Applications a l'homme," was published in the same journal the following week, *53:* 452–453, Apr. 27, 1901. Translations of both are reprinted below.

THE EXTRADURAL INJECTION OF AGENTS BY THE SACROCOCCYGEAL ROUTE

JEAN-ATHANASE SICARD

Laboratory of Professors
Raymond and Brissaud
Salpêtrière Hospital,
Paris, France

*Comptes rendus hebdomadaires
des séances et mémoires de
la Société de biologie, 53: 396, 1901*

"Unfortunately, there is no doubt that the subarachnoid injection of cocaine may present certain difficulties.—Consequently, we have sought another procedure, one which is completely harmless and which allows us to reach, by means of liquid injection, the nerve trunks at the sites of their exit from the spinal cord. The extradural space, located between the dura mater and the bony canal, presents itself for this purpose.

"The trials (in the dog, cadaver and patients) have demonstrated that next to the liquid subarachnoid space there is a cellulo-adipose space, extending between the dura mater and the bony wall, which is readily accessible by the sacrococcygeal route. Solutions injected at this level diffuse easily along the various spinal regions, and bathe, more or less immediately, the nerve trunks traversing the extradural space. The dura mater presents an effective barrier to the passage of such solutions into the subarachnoid space."

1902

Published August, 1978

I was on a troop train heading for the United States Marine Corps base, Camp Pendleton, California, at the precise moment when my college roommate was dying of bulbar poliomyelitis in the Army Hospital at Colorado Springs, just 90 miles north of the railroad tracks over which the troop train was traveling.

I did not know this at the time, of course, but in retrospect it was one of life's bitter ironies. I had introduced Vaughan to his wife, and he had introduced me to mine: because of the exigencies of war, neither of us had been able to attend the other's wedding. But we had planned a real whing-ding reunion and weekend in New York for the 4 of us when the war was over and we had made the World Safe for Democracy by annihilating the Fascist Pigs and the Yellow Hordes. What we had not counted on in planning that reunion weekend was the RNA virus of the picorna group and poliomyelitis.

If I had known then what we know today, and if that troop train had been 90 miles north of where it was, Vaughan need not have died that August night during World War II, and Nancy would not have become a war widow. There are 4 chances out of 5 that my roommate's life could have been saved with today's knowledge and therapies, because he would have been "intubated and placed on a ventilator," a routine procedure which we blithely carry out thousands of times a day in hospitals all over the world, and in all kinds of hospital locations—recovery rooms, intensive care units, coronary care units, emergency rooms, medical wards, surgical wards, pediatric units, even in the obstetric suite, to name but a few. Where there is respiratory distress, be it acute or chronic, the establishment of a secure airway and artificial ventilation of the lungs is the first order of business.

But as short a time as 25 years ago, this type of treatment was infrequent. For one thing, ventilators were rare commodities. Most large hospitals, and some small hospitals too, in this country had one or more Drinker "iron lungs" stored in a basement corridor gathering dust, except during a poliomyelitis epidemic and occasional use for other respiratory situations in certain hospitals. For another thing, intubation of the trachea was seldom undertaken, except in operating rooms or as a rare emergency tracheotomy performed in other parts of the hospital in desperate circumstances. Indeed, aside from the anesthesiologists and the EENT men, there were precious few physicians who knew *how* to intubate a patient—which explains, on an historical basis, why the anesthesiologist became so intimately associated with the first respiratory care wards, the first intensive care units, and became among the first of the pioneers in the emerging specialty of critical care medicine.

There were also the first inklings of today's mandatory approach to respiratory problems by the establishment of a secure airway and the ventilation of the lungs as early as 40 years ago. In England, Lord Nuffield had had the foresight to establish the Nuffield Department of Anaesthetics in the University of Oxford in 1937, and 2 years later he donated a Both type "iron lung" to every Commonwealth hospital requesting one, thereby precipitating the development of specialized units for respiratory care. In this country, the prototypes of such ventilators as the Emerson, the Van Bergen, and the Mörch were being put together and tried out in clinical situations, and the concept of a respiratory care unit was evolving with each poliomyelitis epidemic which occurred. A little later, the Swedish surgeons Bjork and Engström popularized the prophylactic use of prolonged postoperative controlled respiration to combat respiratory insufficiency and chest complications after operation, clearly showing the wider field of usefulness of this therapy. There was still, however, the (possibly) apocryphal story of the eminent surgeon in a major medical center who, on being informed by the nurse anesthetist that the patient had no heart beat or blood pressure, and had stopped breathing, left the operating room, still fully gowned and gloved, to call the Fire Department: after all, the Firemen had the pulmotors and knew how to use them.

It was the magnitude of the catastrophic 1952 poliomyelitis epidemic in Denmark which really changed things around, however, since the experiences in Copenhagen established indisputably that tracheostomy with a cuffed rubber tube and manual ventilation with a bag and a mask was far superior in terms of mortality to the use of the prone position, postural drainage, and tank or cuirass respirator.

The epidemic was overwhelming: between July 24 and December 3, 1952, some 2,722 patients with poliomyelitis were admitted to the Blegdam Hospital in Copenhagen alone: 866 of these patients had paralysis, and 316 of the paralytic patients required special measures, specifically tracheotomy and artificial ventilation. The enormous clinical load is illustrated by the fact that in 4 months the staff of the Blegdam Hospital treated 3 times as many patients with respiratory insufficiency, paralysis of the ninth, tenth, and twelfth cranial nerves, and involvement of the bulbar respiratory and vasomotor centers, as in the preceding 10 years. During the week of August 28 to September 3, the Blegdam Hospital admitted 335 patients, or nearly 50 daily. Lassen, the Professor of Epidemiology in the University of Copenhagen, and the Chief Physician in the Department of Communicable Diseases at Blegdam Hospital, wrote on December 7, 1952: "During these months we have in fact been in a state of war, and at the beginning we were not nearly adequately equipped to meet an emergency of such vast proportions."

Indeed, at times there were as many as 70 patients requiring artificial respiration, and the great number of severely ill patients pouring in made therapeutic improvisations a necessity. At the beginning of the epidemic, one tank respirator (Emerson) and 6 cuirass respirators were available, which proved wholly insufficient when the epidemic progressed into a major catastrophe; and as a result, the mortality rate during the first month was 85 to 90 per cent in patients with respiratory paralysis and/or pharyngeal and laryngeal paralysis. At this point, the Anaesthesia Department instituted what became the treatment of choice: namely, tracheotomy just below the larynx, with insertion of a cuffed rubber tube into the trachea, and manual positive-pressure ventilation with a reservoir bag. (i.e., bag ventilation).

Early tracheostomy was considered to be of decisive importance, because when manifest hypoxia and/or retention of carbon dioxide, in combination with latent or clinical vasomotor shock of even short duration appeared, it led to disastrous effects upon the nerve cells already damaged by virus infection, and to a distinctly worse prognosis. The first step of the operation was tracheal intubation through the mouth, so that tracheotomy could be performed under controlled conditions, allowing effective aspiration of secretions during the surgical procedure and adequate ventilation with oxygen. Cyclopropane was always used, although ether was considered an adequate alternative. Under no circumstances was an intravenous anesthetic or sedative to be used, even in irrational and apprehensive patients, before adequate ventilation was secured. The tube was connected to a soda-lime absorption cannister (Waters to-and-fro) with a reservoir bag, then to a good humidifier (since otherwise incrustation of secretions could occur), and finally to a source of gas mixture consisting of 50 per cent oxygen and 50 per cent nitrous oxide. The final link in the chain leading to adequate manual ventilation was a medical student to squeeze the reservoir bag.

The importance of the medical students in the success of coping with the crisis in Copenhagen during the summer of 1952 was incalculable. The fact of the matter is that the job could not even have been approached without them. During several weeks of the summer and fall there were 40 to 70 patients in Blegdam Hospital requiring continuous or intermittent bag ventilation, and it was necessary to employ about 250 medical students daily, working on 8 hour shifts in relay, to do this. Some of the patients in the epidemic were treated by manual artificial ventilation for up to 3 months, and in all some 1,500 medical students went without formal classes for up to 8 months. It was indeed war.

It was a triumph for the Department of Anaesthesia that so many medical students could be trained in such a short time to maintain adequate ventilation for such long periods by a method in which over-ventilation, under-ventilation, or circulatory disturbances from excessive positive pressure could so easily occur. When the true understanding of the Danish experience sank into the minds of the European medical community at large, and they came to realize that their own countries were as ill-equipped in the event of such catastrophe as Denmark had been, plans for ventilators began flowing off drawing boards like spring freshets. Almost invariably, the ventilator so planned was referred to as the "mechanical student."

The real importance of the experiences of the 1952 poliomyelitis epidemic in Denmark, however, lay in the firm establishment of the fact that the methods employed by the anesthesiologist in the operating room, to establish a secure airway and maintain ventilation by intermittent positive pressure, could be transferred out of the operating room to other parts of the hospital with stupendous benefit.

In retrospect, it is ironical that the basic tenets of "Let's intubate him and put him on a ventilator" had been offered to the medical profession some 75 years ago by a renowned New Orleans surgeon and had lain fallow for the better part of the 50 years preceding the Copenhagen catastrophe. In the January 18, 1902, issue of

American Medicine, Rudolph Matas published his paper titled, "Artificial Respiration by Direct Intralaryngeal Intubation with a Modified O'Dwyer Tube and a New Graduated Air-Pump, in Its Application to Medical and Surgical Practice" (*Am. Med., 3:* 97–103, 1902), which is republished below.

ARTIFICIAL RESPIRATION BY DIRECT INTRALARYNGEAL INTUBATION WITH A MODIFIED O'DWYER TUBE AND A NEW GRADUATED AIR-PUMP, IN ITS APPLICATIONS TO MEDICAL AND SURGICAL PRACTICE

RUDOLPH MATAS

New Orleans, Louisiana

Am. Med., 3:97–103, 1902

*   *   *   *

"In order to investigate with any degree of accuracy the effects of pulmonary inflation by the intralaryngeal method upon the lungs in normal and pathologic conditions, the first requisite was a suitable apparatus which would indicate the positive and negative variations in the intrapulmonary pressure during insufflation (inspiration and expiration), and that would also provide a measure and means of controlling the quantity of air injected into the trachea.—An entirely new apparatus, based on the principle of the pump, would have to be constructed.

*   *   *   *

"When the large duplex pump had been completed it was utilized in our preliminary experiments on dogs and human cadavers to familiarize ourselves not only with the technic of insufflation, but to test the practability of automatic respiration in which the cylinders were used to alternately pump air *into* and *out* of the lungs. But we soon found out that there were many serious obstacles in the way of the successful application of this duplex principle, and the most important of these was the damage done by the suction force exercised by the aspirating cylinder in expiration.—It is fortunate—that the expiratory part of the respiration aid is unnecessary in practice, and that all that is required, so far as the expiration is concerned, is that the apparatus used shall insufflate air into the lungs in sufficient quantity and under proper pressure.

*   *   *   *

"If we now summarize the peculiarities of this apparatus for artificial respiration, we will state—

1. That it is a graduated pump which can be readily adjusted to any quantity of air required, from 1 to 700 cm. (or 1 to 43 cubic inches).
2. That it is provided with a mercurial manometer, which indicates the intrapulmonary pressure and is an index of the peripheral resistance which is overcome by the inflation.
3. That it is provided with an automatic cut-off which effectively prevents any backward leakage of air into the cylinder, and thus puts the inspiratory inflation of the lungs under the control of the operator.—The duration of each inspiratory insufflation will be controlled by the finger of the operator, which closes the outlet in the handle of the canula. So long as the thumb occludes this outlet the insufflated air will be retained in the chest;—when the thumb is lifted from the opening the imprisoned air in the lungs escapes and expiration takes place.
4. It is provided with an air filter interposed between the larynx and the pump, which purifies the air injected through the pump.

"The opportunity has not yet presented itself to apply this pump on the living subject, but our experience with it on the cadaver and dog fully demonstrates its practical working capacity."

Published December, 1962

Time, the weekly newsmagazine, carried the following item in its January 27, 1961 issue:

Relaxed from a tranquilizer, the 65-year-old woman, an abdominal cancer victim, lay quietly on an operating table in the University of Mississippi's Medical Center. Anesthesiologist Leonard Fabian opened her mouth, sprayed a local anesthetic on her throat, inserted an "airway tube" to ensure unobstructed breathing. Under the watchful eye of Surgeon James Hardy, Dr. Fabian attached a tiny electrode to each of the woman's temples. At his signal, a technician turned a control on the face of a small box from which wires trailed out to the electrodes. Within 60 seconds the woman was sound asleep, and the operation began—first ever performed in the United States under electrical anesthesia.

Because sending electric currents through the brain can produce death and convulsions, scientists have long suspected that they could anesthetize surgical patients by some precise combination of voltage, current and frequency. To the U.S. Army, the idea was especially attractive: it was hunting for a safe, simple way to anesthetize battlefield patients without the use of bulky, expensive gas equipment. With Army funds, doctors at the University of Mississippi, experimenting with dogs and monkeys, set out to construct a cheap mobile unit that could be used to shock human patients to sleep.

"Most of the difficulty arises in the fine line that separates anesthesia from convulsions," says Lieut. Colonel John Moncrief, who monitored the project. The Mississippi machine, although still experimental, looks promising: it puts the patient to sleep, keeps him under as long as the current remains constant, permits him to awaken within 60 seconds after the juice is turned off. It uses 22–30 volts, 50 milliamperes, and a frequency that is brought up from 0 to 700 cycles to put the patient under. It causes some spasms, which drugs easily stop, but produces no convulsions, loss of memory or even headache. Its price: $150. Commented the first patient: "I didn't feel a thing."

Time was careful not to state that this was the first electrical anesthesia in the United States, although it was the most spectacularly successful and it did represent a giant step along the trail toward physical, rather than chemical, methods of producing anesthesia. Chemoanesthesia, the dominant approach for over a century now, has inherent drawbacks (physiologic depression, the burden of the metabolism or detoxification or both of the drugs employed, and slow recovery, to mention but a few) and physicians have long been intrigued with the idea of finding a safe and effective nonchemical method of anesthesia. There have been sporadic attempts to produce general anesthesia by the use of an electric current since as early as 1875, but a major problem in this approach has always been the question of the proper combination of voltages, current and frequency. This problem was first seriously studied by the Frenchman, Leduc, and his colleagues, beginning in 1902. *Survey* and its readers are indebted to Miss Harmona Potter, Assistant Librarian at the Hartford Medical Society, for the translation into English of Leduc's articles on "production du sommeil et de l'anesthésie générale et locale par les courants électriques" which were published in Paris in 1902, (Leduc, S.: *Compt. rend. acad. d. sc., 135:* 199, 1902; *135:* 878, 1902) and which are reprinted below.

PRODUCTION OF SLEEP AND OF GENERAL ANESTHESIA BY MEANS OF ELECTRIC CURRENTS

M. Stephane Leduc

Compt. rend. acad. d. sc., 135: 878, 1902

"In a preceding note (*Comptes Rendues,* July 1902), we indicated the manner in which inhibition of the cerebral hemispheres in animals could be achieved, and induction of sleep and general anesthesia brought about by means of 10 to 30 volts and by currents interrupted 150 to 200 times per second. The procedure had the disadvantage of giving rise to clonic contractures or seizures, raising the blood pressure, causing urination and defecation, and bringing about a momentary respiratory arrest.

"These disadvantages are offset by the use in the circuit of a rheostat without self-induction which permits, through a gradual increase, the attaining of the necessary intensity in 3 to 5 minutes. This method requires preliminary placement in the circuit of an electromotive power equivalent, at least, to the maximum power to be achieved; at the same time, the results are all the more successful when the electromotive power used is the lowest possible.

"By the use of a power reducer without self-induction, in such a manner as to increase evenly the electromotive power in 3 to 5 minutes to the required figure, the animals slip smoothly, progressively, without any movements of defense or flight, without a murmur, without any change in respiratory or cardiac movement, from a state of wakefulness into a state of quiet, even sleep, and of complete general anesthesia. The dog's head bows as in drowsiness, then he sits down on his haunches, lies over on his side, and goes off into an apparently restful sleep, without giving the slightest sign of protest or pain."

Published October and December, 1965

In the first 10 years following the introduction of clinical anesthesia, John Snow collected a list of 50 deaths which followed the administration of chloroform. In 5 of these patients, he could unearth no description of the clinical status immediately prior to death; but in all of the patients (*i.e.*, 45) in whom the signs which occurred at the time of death were detailed, there was reason to conclude "that death took place by cardiac syncope, or arrest of the action of the heart."

By 1863, the Royal Medical and Chirurgical Society (the ancestor of the present Royal Society of Medicine) could list 123 deaths attributable to the inhalation of chloroform, and anxiety over these tragedies, many of which occurred "during trivial operations, which, without chloroform, are not attended with risk to life," led to the appointment of a committee "to give their anxious attention to devise means for obviating such accidents." This Chloroform Committee of 1864, as it has come to be known, made a great many experimental observations on dogs, and came to conclusions that were almost identical to those which had already been reached by Snow some 10 years earlier: *i.e.*, that chloroform depresses the action of the heart, and frequently kills by inducing syncope. They also suggested the use of mixtures of chloroform and ether, with or without the addition of ethyl alcohol, as being safer than chloroform alone, since the stimulating effect of ether would offset the sedative actions of chloroform (shades of today's Fluether azeotrope!).

Despite the arduous labors and lengthy report of the Chloroform Committee of 1864, deaths from chloroform anesthesia, and particularly during the induction period, continued to accumulate at a rapid rate. Indeed, by 1882, Henry M. Layman's book, *Artificial Anaesthesia and Anaesthetics*, could devote well over 50 pages to case reports of 393 chloroform deaths and 17 from mixtures or sequences containing chloroform. The majority of these patients died at the beginning of the inhalation, or before complete insensibility was achieved, seemingly bearing out the findings of the Committee relative to the development of cardiac syncope.

Then an extraordinary thing happened. The February 23, 1889, issue of the *Lancet* carried a report of Prize Day at the Hyderabad Medical School, where the prizes had been distributed by their Royal Highnesses the Duke and Duchess of Connaught; and where Surgeon-Major Lawrie, M.D., of the Bengal Army Medical Service and the Principal of the School, had made some brief remarks, "in the course of which he said the male and female students at that institution enjoyed, in many respects, practical advantages of which very few European schools could boast. They had made experiments with reference to the effects of chloroform, which had conclusively decided a question which had been in dispute ever since chloroform was first introduced. They had killed with chloroform 128 full-grown pariah dogs averaging over 20 lb. weight each. What they found was that, no matter in what way it was given, in no case did the heart become dangerously affected in the 40,000 or 50,000 administrations which he had superintended, he had never seen the heart injuriously or dangerously affected by chloroform."

The *Lancet*, of course, was not about to sit still for this type of nonsense, and editorialized in the March 2, 1889 issue: "In a report of the recent prize distribution at the Hyderabad Medical School . . . we learn that a commission had been appointed to investigate the action of chloroform, and the result of the researches made upon pariah dogs was that these animals were killed from respiratory failure, and in no case did cardiac syncope occur directly. (Editor's Note: this commission was appointed in 1888 by the Nizam of Hyderabad's Government at Lawrie's request, and has come to be known as the First Hyderabad Commission.) Unfortunately Mr. Lawrie contents himself with bare statements of results, adding that these results tally with his own experience, which he believes to be uniquely large. . . . All those who are familiar with chloroform are well aware that syncope, when primary, as a rule supervenes in the initial stages of inhalation, while secondary syncope due to respiratory embarrassment is the result of accumulation of chloroform in the blood leading to paralysis of the medullary centres, and occurs in a late stage of the administration. The primary syncope it is rarely, if ever, possible to induce in dogs, although, unfortunately, it is this form of chloroform heart failure which does occur

in human beings, and which it is almost impossible to remedy. While welcoming the attention paid to the subject by the Hyderabad Commission, we cannot but feel that, should the Commission inculcate a disregard of the heart as a factor in chloroform dangers, it will do harm and provoke a slipshod carelessness in the use of that valuable anaesthetic, which must in the long-run do damage to the cause the Commission has espoused."

The acrimonious character of the exchange was stepped up by Lawrie's reply in the May 11, 1889 issue: "In the *Lancet* of March 2nd, 1889, page 438, there is an annotation criticising certain remarks of mine on the subject of chloroform. . . . I have no wish to say anything to give offense to those who hold the same views as the writer of the annotation, but I hold that these views are wrong, and that there is no such thing as chloroform syncope." The *Lancet* came right back: "It is a matter of regret that, instead of complying with our request for fuller information, Mr. Lawrie has contented himself with mere dogmatic assertion and iteration of his former statements. Whatever may be the value of the work done by the Hyderabad Commission—and Mr. Lawrie seems inclined to accept the conclusions arrived at, rather than those of well-known and tried scientists—it is quite impossible for those who have neither seen the experiments to which Mr. Lawrie refers, nor received an authoritative statement as to the methods employed and precautions taken, to accept as evidence the results to which he refers. No mere *ipse dixit* can shake the weight of the large accumulation of facts of which we are now possessed concerning the depressant action of chloroform upon the heart."

The Nizam's supply of diamonds, rubies, and gold was apparently sufficient to the occasion, however (it should have been—20 years ago his worth was estimated at $300,000,000!), for the July 13, 1889 issue of the *Lancet* stated: "We have received a telegram from Surgeon-Major Lawrie to the effect that his Highness the Nizam of Hyderabad offers to place the sum of 1000 pounds from his private purse at our disposal that we may send one or two representatives of the *Lancet* to Hyderabad to repeat the experiments made by the Hyderabad Chloroform Commission . . . and to make any others which we may suggest."

The *Lancet* chose Dr. T. Lauder Brunton, who was a well known pharmacologist with an international reputation, and (perhaps more importantly to the *Lancet*) whose book, *Pharmacology and Therapeutics*, stated that one of the dangers resulting from chloroform was death by stoppage of the heart.

Imagine the shock in London when the *Lancet* received the following telegram from Lauder Brunton in Hyderabad: "Four hundred and ninety dogs, horses, monkeys, goats, cats, and rabbits used. One hundred and twenty with manometer. All records photographed. Numerous observations on every individual animal. Results most instructive. Danger from chloroform is asphyxia or overdose; none whatever heart direct." The *Lancet* was incredulous: "These results apparently indicate such a complete reversal of the view held by Dr. Lauder Brunton at the time he left England . . . that the details of the experiments made by Dr. Brunton, and the reasons for the conclusions he has evidently arrived at, will be awaited with the greatest interest by the profession."

The report of the Second Hyderabad Chloroform Commission was published in sections in the January 18th, February 22nd, March 1st, and June 21st, 1890, issues of the *Lancet*. It supported all of Lawrie's original contentions, for Brunton concluded that failure of the respiration was the only way in which the heart's safety was jeopardized and that the heart never stopped before respiration. He even added a further interesting fillip by stating that the effect of chloroform upon the vagus was beneficial rather than detrimental: "The theory which has hitherto been accepted is that the danger in chloroform administration consists in the slowing or stoppage of the heart by vagus inhibition. This is now shown to be absolutely incorrect. There is no doubt whatever that the controlling influence of the vagus on the heart is a safeguard, and that it is the exhaustion of the nerve which is dangerous."

This Report of the Second Hyderabad

Chloroform Commissions, as might be expected, caused a very considerable commotion. The *Lancet* refused to believe the data produced by its own hand-picked investigator, and promptly appointed another, Dudley Wilmot Buxton. Buxton sent questionnaires to individual doctors and to every hospital of over 10 beds in the United Kingdom, as well as to the larger hospitals on the Continent, in the Colonies, the United States, and India. The tabulations from these questionnaires showed that "the larger proportions of deaths are reported as having resulted from initial heart failure, in opposition to the view to which the physiological researches of the Hyderabad Commission have led." This pronouncement failed to impress the opposition, however, and the beliefs of each of the two schools of clinical thought as to the mechanisms of the danger of chloroform anesthesia remained essentially unshaken.

At this point, the controversy was removed to the physiology laboratory, where it had belonged in the first place. A number of distinguished workers entered into the fray—Gaskell and Shore of the University of Cambridge, J. A. MacWilliams of the Institutes of Medicine of Aberdeen, Leonard Hill of the London Hospital, Augustus D. Waller of St. Mary's Hospital Medical School, and even a new Chloroform Committee appointed in 1901 by the British Medical Association—but perhaps the most important experimental work which served to clear up the state of confusion as to the physiologic action of chloroform was that performed by Edward Henry Embley, Honorary Anaesthetist to the Melbourne Hospital. Indeed, about the only important point that Embley missed was the occurrence of ventricular fibrillation from chloroform anesthesia. His brilliant experimental observations were published in three of the April, 1902, issues of the *British Medical Journal* under the title of "The Causation of Death during the Administration of Chloroform" (Embley, E. H., *Brit. M. J., 1:* 817–821, April 5; 885–893, April 12; and 951–961, April 19, 1902), and they are reprinted below and in the next issue of *Survey of Anesthesiology.*

THE CAUSATION OF DEATH DURING THE ADMINISTRATION OF CHLOROFORM

E. H. EMBLEY, M.D.

Honorary Anaesthetist to the Melbourne Hospital
(From the Physiological Laboratory of the University of Melbourne)

Br. Med. J., 1: 817–821, 855–893 and 951–961, 1902

* * * *

PRESENT INVESTIGATION

"Particular attention was devoted to recording changes in the circulation during the early period of chloroform administration in animals which had not previously received chloroform. This was accomplished in two ways:

1. By performing all operative procedures necessary for studying the circulatory changes under morphine narcosis, either alone or with curare.

2. By inserting the cannulae, etc., under ether anaesthesia, and eight or twelve hours after, when the effects of the anesthetic had passed off, connecting with the recording apparatus. The chloroform was administered off a towel.

"In consequence of the known liability of dogs to die suddenly in the early stage of chloroform anaesthesia, when the chloroform is given by the towel method—a liability to which human beings are also subject in a less degree—these animals were chosen for the experiments.

"In the whole investigation 289 dogs were employed, and 284 graphic records were obtained.

* * * *

CONCLUSIONS REGARDING THE EFFECTS OF CHLOROFORM ON

THE HEART ISOLATED FROM THE CENTRAL NERVOUS SYSTEM.

"1. Chloroform has an immediate and progressively paralytic effect upon the heart muscle. There is no preliminary period of stimulation. There is no abrupt change in the rate or efficiency of the heart.

* * * *

Summary of Conclusions of the Effect of Chloroform upon the Cardiac Inhibitory Mechanism

* * * *

"1. A heart which has been poisoned by inhalations of chloroform of strength 2 per cent, and upwards can always be permanently inhibited by stimulation of the vagi with the faradic current when the blood pressure has fallen to about 40 to 50 mm. of mercury pressure.

2. Chloroform raises the excitability of the vagus mechanism, particularly in the early part of the administration.

3. The increased excitability of the vagus mechanism is due to the action of chloroform on the vagus centres, and the inhibitory action is more intense from being exercised upon a heart whose spontaneous excitability is diminished by the action of the chloroform upon it.

4. Chloroform administered to morphinized dogs in air containing not more than 1.5 per cent. of the vapour, after a period of mild excitation, slowly depresses vagus excitability. The excitability may again be raised with more or less readiness according to the duration of the administration and the endurance of the vagi, by increasing the percentage strength of the chloroform, or by asphyxia.

5. Vagus inhibition is, in dogs, the great factor in the causation of sudden death from chloroform.

6. Dangerous inhibition is liable to occur whenever the strength of chloroform in the air inhaled rises above 2 per cent."

* * * *

Published October, 1975

A few years ago, at the Annual Meeting of the American Society of Anesthesiologists, a self-evaluation program in cardiopulmonary resuscitation was offered which presented a unique opportunity for members, their familes and guests to evaluate their abilities in both cognitive and performance skills in resuscitation. Each examinee was able to demonstrate his or her knowledge, using a confidential self-evaluation examination dealing with basic and advanced measures in resuscitation and emergency cardiac care. They were also able to test their performance skills of basic resuscitation on an automated mannikin. Both examinations were scored on the spot and immediate feedback to the participant was provided by physician experts from the American Society of Anesthesiologists and the American Heart Association.

The standards by which competence was judged were admittedly rigorous, but nonetheless the results were anything but reassuring. In all, 209 people completed both the examination and the mannikin performance test. A majority of the examinees were active members of the ASA, but there were also resident members, wives and guests included in the total number. Of these 209 examinees, 52 (or 25 per cent) passed; 22 (or 10 per cent) passed, but had produced damage (improper ventilation-to-chest-compression ratios, bad hand positions, or poor ventilation) in the conduct of the resuscitation; and 135 (or 65 per cent) failed outright. These are sobering figures for a specialty so intimately involved in CPR. There were 92 examinees who demonstrated inadequate knowledge of how to open up the airway (sic!), while 101 employed improper hand positions as shown by marks or sensors. And among those 135 failing outright were 3 Chairmen of University Departments of Anesthesiology.

Furthermore, as if all this were not bad enough, the anesthesiologist's involvement in teaching CPR did not correlate with his or her ability to pass the overall examination. In reply to the question. "Do you participate in cardiopulmonary resuscitation in your practice?," 9 said "no" and 159 said "yes"—yet 110 of these 159 failed the overall examination. In reply to the question, "Do you teach CPR in your institution?," 86 replied "yes"—yet 56 of these 86

failed the overall test. (On the other hand, 89 answered "no," but 23 of these passed the overall examination with flying colors.) In reply to the question, "Is the Department of Anesthesiology in your institution responsible for CPR, 78 answered yes, 50 answered no, and 43 indicated that they were partially involved.

This showing by those who should be leading the way for the rest of the profession is pretty dismal. If this is the way the anesthesiologists perform in CPR, what about the internist? The surgeon? The dermatologist? The radiologist?

In May, 1973, a National Conference on Standards for Cardiopulmonary Resuscitation (CPR) and Emergency Cardiac Care (ECC) was held and reported in a special supplement of the Journal of the American Medical Association, which was sent to every member of the AMA. Part II of this report is on Basic Life Support and contains sections on Artificial Ventilation, Artificial Circulation (External Cardiac Compression), Precordial Thump, and a special section titled, "Pitfalls in Performance of CPR":

"When CPR is performed improperly or inadequately, artificial ventilation and artificial circulation may be ineffective in providing basic life support. Enumerated below are important points to remember in performing external cardiac compression and artificial ventilation.

"1. Do not interrupt CPR for more than five seconds for any reason, except in the following circumstances.

(a) Under emergency conditions, endotracheal intubation usually cannot be accomplished in five seconds. However, it is an advanced life support measure and should be performed only by those who are well trained and well practiced in the technique and *only* after the victim has been properly positioned and all preparations made. Even under these circumstances, interruptions in CPR for endotracheal intubation should never exceed 15 seconds.

(b) When moving a victim up or down a stairway, it is difficult to continue effective CPR. Under these circumstances, it is best to perform effective CPR at the head or foot of the stairs, then interrupt CPR at a given signal and move quickly to the next level where effective CPR is resumed. Such interruptions usually should not exceed 15 seconds."

"2. Do not move the patient to a more convenient site until he has been stabilized and is ready for transportation or until arrangements have been made for uninterrupted CPR during movement."

"3. Never compress the xiphoid process at the tip of the sternum. The xiphoid extends downward over the abdomen. Pressure on it may cause laceration of the liver, which can lead to severe internal bleeding."

"4. Between compressions, the heel of the hand must completely release its pressure but should remain in constant contact with the chest wall over the lower one half of the sternum."

"5. The rescuer's fingers should not rest on the victim's ribs during compression. Interlocking the fingers of the two hands may help avoid this. Pressure with fingers on the ribs or lateral pressure increases the possibility of rib fractures and costochondral separation."

"6. Sudden or jerking movements should be avoided when compressing the chest. The compression should be smooth, regular and uninterrupted (50% of the cycle should be compression and 50% should be relaxation). Quick jabs increase the possibility of injury and produce quick jets of flow; they do not enhance stroke volume or mean flow and pressure."

"7. Do not maintain continuous pressure on the abdomen to decompress the stomach while performing external cardiac compression. This may trap the liver and could cause it to rupture."

"8. The shoulders of the rescuer should be directly over the victim's sternum. The elbows should be straight. Pressure is applied vertically downward on the lower sternum. This provides maximally effective thrust, minimal fatigue for the rescuer, and reduced hazard of complications for the victim. When the victim is on the ground or floor, the rescuer can kneel or stand at his side. When he is on a bed or a high-wheeled litter, the rescuer must be on a step or chair or kneeling on the bed or litter. With a low-wheeled litter, the rescuer can stand at the victim's side. Problems arise with the use of low-wheeled litters in ambulances. Special arrangements must be made for proper positioning of the rescuer based on the design of the ambulance."

"9. The lower sternum of an adult must be depressed 1½ to 2 inches by external cardiac compression. Lesser amounts of compression are ineffectual since even properly performed cardiac compression provides only about one quarter to one third of the normal blood flow."

"10. While complications may result from improperly performed external cardiac compression and precordial thumps, even properly performed external cardiac compression may cause rib fractures in some patients. Other complications that may occur with properly performed CPR include fracture of the sternum, costochondral separation, pneumothorax, hemothorax, lung contusions, lacerations of the liver, and fat emboli. These complications can be minimized by careful attention to details of performance. It must be remembered, however, that during cardiac arrest, effective cardiopulmonary resuscitation is required even if it results in complications, since the alternative to effective CPR is death."

The above demonstrates that the techniques of CPR have become precise, rational, and, with proper instruction, understandable and performable by almost any group of people. This development is fairly recent, for up until less than a century ago, asystole was thought to be synonymous with death. Indeed, it was almost three-quarters of a century ago that the first successful cardiac massage—at least during anesthesia and surgery—was reported in the literature by Ernest Henry Starling, in an account to the Society of Anaesthetists in the November 22, 1902, issue of *Lancet* (*2:* 1397, 1902). This event is reprinted below with the kind permission of the publishers.

SOCIETY OF ANESTHETISTS

Lancet, 2: 1397, 1902

*   *   *   *

"—Dr. E. A. Starling (Tunbridge Wells) then read the report of his case of Reflex Inhibition of the Heart during the Administration of Ether in which manual compression of the heart was successful in restoring the circulation. The patient was a male, aged 65 years, and the operation was abdominal section for adhesion about the colon. The usual preparations were made and ether was given by a Hewitt's large-bore inhaler preceded by gas. The patient was of the thin, nervous type and had a muffled bruit of the first sound at the apex; otherwise he was healthy. The induction of anaesthesia was easy and normal. The appendix being found unhealthy was removed; then the pulse immediately began to flag; the respiration, which had been shallow, was not affected; more ether was given, but during the trimming of the stump both pulse and respiration stopped together. Artificial respiration by compression of the chest was started at once without any effect; the surgeon (Mr. W. A. Lane) introduced his hand through the abdominal incision and felt the heart through the diaphragm; it was quite motionless; he gave it a squeeze or two and felt it re-start beating, but as the voluntary respirations were still suspended artificial respiration was continued and other restorative measures were adopted; the artificial respiration had to be continued for about 12 minutes when natural respiration re-commenced with a long sighing inspiration. The operation was completed without any more anaesthetic, there being slight movement while the skin sutures were being put in. Except for a little pain about the diaphragm for two days the patient made a good convalescence. Dr. Starling said that he had brought the case before the society, not only because of the successful treatment by direct stimulation of the heart, but because he thought it was somewhat unusual for a patient fairly under the influence of ether to suffer to such an extent from reflex inhibition; and further, though the stimulus to the heart was enough to re-start it, yet the steady persistence with artificial respiration was essential to the recovery."

1903

Published August, 1960

Clinical monitoring of the surgical patient during anesthesia has been part and parcel of the anesthetist's technique of administration since the time of Crawford Long, Horace Wells and Morton; and it goes without saying that an evaluation of the integrity of cardiovascular function has been a major concern of such monitory since those earliest days. The monitoring consisted almost exclusively of the anesthetist's use of his own five senses and powers of observation, and palpation of a peripheral pulse was the anesthetist's main clue to cardiovascular status. Henry Jacob Bige-low, in the first published account of Morton's triumph, drew attention to both the rate and quality of the pulse: "The pulse has been, as far as my observation extends, unaltered in frequency, though somewhat diminished in volume, but the excitement preceding an operation has, in almost every instance, so accelerated the pulse that it has continued rapid for a length of time." Thomas Nathaniel Meggison, whose patient suffered the first recorded death from chloroform anesthesia, pinpointed the role of monitoring the pulse in catastrophe: "I seated her in a chair, and put about a teaspoonful of chloroform into a table-cloth, and held it to her nose. . . . I told her to draw her breath naturally, which she did, and in about half a minute I observed the muscles of the arm become rigid, and her breathing a little quickened, but sterterous. I had my hand on her pulse, which was natural, until the muscles became rigid. It then appeared somewhat weaker—not altered in frequency. I then told my assistant, Mr. Lloyd, to begin the operation, which he did, and took the nail off. When the semicircular incision was made, she gave a struggle or jerk . . . her mouth was open, and her lips and face blanched . . . the last time I felt her pulse was immediately previous to the blanched appearance coming on, and when she gave the jerk."

But for all that, it was obvious that the pulse *per se* was a relatively inadequate sign. The illustrious John Snow, in his classic, *On Chloroform and other Anaesthetics*, published in 1858, wrote: "I have not mentioned the state of the pulse in the above description of the effects of chloroform, for it affords no criterion of the amount of narcotism, and it was better therefore to reserve it for a separate notice. It is nearly always increased both in force and frequency, more especially at the early part of the inhalation. After the patient has become quite insensible, the pulse indeed generally settles down nearly to the natural standard, and in the middle of the most formidable operations, it is often beating with natural volume and force. . . ."

Despite the obvious inadequacy of the pulse as a monitor of cardiovascular function during anesthesia, the clinical anesthetist had little else to rely on for this purpose during the course of the next fifty years. It was at the turn of the century that the incomparable Harvey Cushing, during a period of study in Europe, established the relationship between blood pressure and intracranial pressure in the experimental animal. The importance of blood pressure determination during neurologic surgery was readily apparent to Cushing's genius, but the direct intravascular manometry employed in the physiologic laboratory was obviously an unreasonable routine in the human patient. When, therefore, Cushing chanced upon a practical indirect method of measuring blood pressure, he was quick to apply it to the surgical patient. This major contribution to the monitory of cardiovascular function during anesthesia was published in the *Boston Medical and Surgical Journal, 148:* 250–256, March 5, 1903, under the title, "On Routine Determinations of Arterial Tension in Operating Room and Clinic."

ON ROUTINE DETERMINATIONS OF ARTERIAL TENSION IN OPERATING ROOM AND CLINIC

HARVEY CUSHING, M.D.

Associate in Surgery,
the Johns Hopkins Hospital
Baltimore, Md.

Boston Med. Surg. J., 148: 250–256, 1903

"There has been a long-felt want in the surgical operating room, possibly even more than in the clinic, for some practical form of apparatus which will give with facility numerical equivalents for variations in pulse tension, and by means of which consecutive observations on this quality of the pulse may be diagrammatically charted.

*   *   *   *

"Two years ago, while on a tour among the Italian University towns, I had the good fortune in Pavia to be shown through the medical wards of the old Ospidale de S. Matteo by Dr. Orlandi, a colleague of Riva-Rocci, and to my great interest found that a simple "home-made" adaptation of the latter's blood-pressure apparatus was in routine daily use at the bedside of every patient.

*   *   *   *

"Thanks to Dr. Orlandi, I was given a model of the inflatable armlet which they employed, and practically the same form of apparatus which was in use in Pavia has been utilized at the Johns Hopkins Hospital with increasing satisfaction ever since.

"The instrument, in part, consists of a distensible cylinder or tire of thin rubber covered with a linen jacket. This cylinder, while encircling an extremity, preferably the upper arm, is inflated by means of a double cautery bulb until the pulse-wave, peripheral to its seat of application, becomes no longer palpable. Inserted in the course of the rubber tubing, which connects the bulb and tire, is a simple upright mercury manometer, which records the pressure of the air in the cylinder necessary to obliterate the pulse.

*   *   *   *

"The particular form of the instrument I have to demonstrate is somewhat more carefully constructed than the home-made ones we have heretofore employed, and possesses the advantage, following a suggestion of Dr. H. W. Cook, of having a disjointed manometer tube, enabling it to be enclosed in a smaller compass."

*   *   *   *

1904

Published April, 1962

The Battle of the Wilderness was by no means the most important or famous of the War Between the States, but the true Civil War buff ranks it close to such well-known battles as Gettysburg, Antietam, Bull Run, Fredericksburg, Chancellorsville, Shiloh, Chickamauga and the Siege of Vicksburg.

In 1863, the North adopted a new plan for the war known as the "anaconda policy," after the great snake called the anaconda which squeezes its victims to death: the army in the west was to move eastward from the Mississippi, while the Army of the Potomac was to press down upon Richmond. The Battle of the Wilderness was General Ulysses S. Grant's first important battle as supreme commander of the Union armies, and it marked the opening of his Richmond campaign. Grant's army of 118,000 entered "the wilderness"—the low, tangled underbrush and swampy lands in Virginia to the west of the Chancellorsville battleground of the previous year— on May 4, 1864. They were opposed by the Confederate Army of Northern Virginia, numbering about 62,000, under General Robert E. Lee. The battle began on May 5 and raged for two days without conclusive result, but with 2,246 Union dead, 12,037 wounded and 3,383 missing; the Confederates suffered about 7,750 killed and wounded.

But it was not over: there was more to come. Grant slipped to his left, moving southeasterly off Lee's right toward Spotsylvania Court House. Major General R. H. Anderson with Longstreet's corps got there first and faced the Army of the Potomac. The armies locked in battle, and it became almost like the trench warfare of World War I days. There followed 13 days of assaults, fighting and dying in the woods, small meadows and secondary growth. A stubborn Grant telegraphed Halleck in Washington, "I propose to fight it out along this line if it takes all summer." There were tremendous Federal losses—and Confederate losses, too: only about a third of those of the North, but much harder to replace. In the period from May 5 to May 12, the Union suffered 26,815 killed and wounded and 41,183 missing in action, or 263 casualties out of every thousand effectives, a ratio of one to four.

Literally hundreds of the wounded in these campaigns received anesthesia at the hands of one of the most famous anesthetists of all time, William T. G. Morton, who

18 years earlier, at the classic public demonstration of anesthesia on October 16, 1846, had given the world one of man's greatest triumphs—the triumph over pain.

Morton's desire to minister to the sick and dying was very nearly rebuffed by Grant himself, according to an incident related by Dr. John H. Brinton: "Let me, from personal reminiscence, relate an anecdote in point: in the early summer of 1864, during the fierce contest in the Virginia Wilderness, I was present officially at the headquarters of Lieutenant-General Grant, on whose staff I had previously served. When in conversation with him, an aide approached and said to him that a stranger, a civilian physician, wished to see him for the purpose of obtaining an ambulance for his personal use in visiting the field hospitals. The answer of the General was prompt and decided: "The ambulances are intended only for the sick and wounded, and under no circumstances can be taken for personal use." This response was carried as given to the waiting applicant, a travel-stained man in brownish clothes, whom at the distance I thought I recognized. I went to him and found that he was Dr. W. T. G. Morton. I asked him to wait a minute, and returned to the General. On repeating his request, I received the same answer. 'But, General,' I ventured to say, 'if you knew who that man is I think you would give him what he asks for.' 'No, I will not,' he replied, 'I will not divert an ambulance to-day for any one; they are all required elsewhere.' 'General,' I replied, 'I am sure you will give him the wagon; he has done so much for mankind, so much for the soldier; more than any soldier or civilian has ever done before, and you will say so when you know his name.' The General took his cigar from his mouth, looked curiously at the applicant, and asked, 'Who is he?' 'He is Dr. Morton, the discoverer of ether,' I answered. The General paused a moment, then said: 'You are right, Doctor, he has done more for the soldier than anyone else, soldier or civilian, for he has taught you all to banish pain. Let him have the ambulance and anything else he wants.'"

Possibly the tale is apocryphal: Morton himself relates instant recognition and a hearty welcome by Grant on the basis of a previous introduction in Washington. Morton's own description of his activities during the Battle of the Wilderness was not published during his lifetime, but an abstract from it was furnished by his son, Dr. Wm. J. Morton of New York City, many years later. It was published in the *Journal of the American Medical Association* under the title "The first use of ether as an anesthetic. At the Battle of the Wilderness in the Civil War," (Morton, W. T. G.: *J.A.M.A., 42:* 1068–1073, April 23, 1904) and is reprinted below.

THE FIRST USE OF ETHER AS AN ANESTHETIC AT THE BATTLE OF THE WILDERNESS IN THE CIVIL WAR

W. T. G. MORTON

Boston, Massachusetts

J.A.M.A., 42: 1068–1073, April 23, 1904

"On previous occasions it had been my privilege to visit battlefields, and there to administer the pain-destroying agent which it pleased God to make me the human agent to introduce for the benefit of suffering humanity. How little did I think, however, when originally experimenting with the properties of sulphuric ether on my own person, that I should ever successfully administer it to hundreds in one day, and thus prevent an amount of agony fearful to contemplate.

*   *   *   *

"Having been assigned quarters in a fine old mansion, I commenced going the rounds of the buildings used as hospitals, to administer anesthetics. There was at first a lack of supplies, and many of the wounded, who had been jolted over hard roads some eight and forty hours, were in a bad condition. Several hundred, packed into a church or hall, without change of clothing or washing, made the atmosphere unbearable almost, and gangrene and erysipelas began to make their appearance, but this was soon remedied.

"One of the principal hospitals was the Baptist Church, which was literally packed with wounded. The tank intended for immersion was used as a bathing tub, and the operations were performed in the pastor's small study, back of the pulpit.

*   *   *   *

"On the arrival of a train of ambulances at a field-hospital the wounds were hastily examined, and those who could bear the journey were sent at once to Fredericks-burg. The nature of the operations to be performed on the others was then decided on, and noted on a bit of paper pinned to the pillow or roll of blanket under each patient's head. When this had been done I prepared the patients for the knife, producing perfect anesthesia in an average time of three minutes, and the operators followed, performing their operations with dexterous skill, while the dressers in their turn bound up the stumps. It was surprising to see with what dexterity and rapidity surgical operations were performed by scores in the same time really taken up with one case in peaceful regions."

1908

Published December, 1960

There is the very definite belief in certain quarters that the incidence of surgical cardiac arrest is on the increase. This belief extends beyond the simple statistical fact that the number of surgical operations has increased greatly in the past two decades, and embraces the proposition that the relative frequency of arrest actually has risen enormously in recent years. A number of explanations have been offered: operations are more extensive and difficult today than ever before, and include invasion of the body's most hidden recesses, including the heart, brain and endocrine glands; an increasing geriatric population sends to the operating room more patients with severe intercurrent and degenerative disease processes; more infants and newborns, many with dangerous congenital anomalies, are being operated upon; there is a salutary willingness to undertake the operation that is known to be a calculated risk in the patient who is otherwise doomed; the growing number of anesthetic drugs has led to a malevolent polypharmacy; and so forth.

Without entering into the bitter re-criminations which so often surround the subject, it should be pointed out that, whether or not the actual frequency of cardiac arrest is increasing, certainly the physician's awareness of the problem is on the increase. An almost deafening testimony to this fact may be heard from the speaker's podium of almost any medical meeting; and mute, but equally convincing, testimony is apparent from the veritable flood of papers and even books on the subject which have been published in the past few years. Indeed, it would appear that at least one such contribution is the minimal requisite for advancement of the rising young surgeon, and at least collaboration on one such contribution the requirement for the rising young anesthesiologist. Medical students come to internship prepared to slash a chest at the drop of a systole, and it is a timid house officer indeed who completes his training without ever having at least "almost" resorted to pen knife or razor blade to effect massage in some out-of-the-way corner of the hospital.

This awareness of the problem of cardiac resuscitation is all to the good. Cardiac arrest is not something that permits a leisurely browsing in the library *post facto* to search for the proper course of therapy, except as a preparation for the next case. It is now recognized that severe hemorrhage, by depleting coronary flow, can seriously interfere with the chances of cardiac resuscitation, and should be treated with whole blood transfusions, preferably by the intra-arterial route; or that coronary flow can be maintained by crossclamping the aorta, as is done in some instances of heart surgery, with intra-aortic injection above the site of clamping. It is also recognized that direct massage through a thoracotomy wound is a far more certain method of resuscitation than squeezing the heart through the intact diaphragm via an abdominal incision. It is further recognized that no amount of cardiac massage can prevail unless proper oxygenation of the blood is achieved by the concomitant performance of artificial ventilation. It is recognized, too, that electrical stimulation may be an important adjunct in maintaining cardiac action after stoppage of the heart, and that this can sometimes be effective without opening the chest: *i.e.* with external electrodes. Finally, within the past several months a method of extrathoracic massage (by squeezing the heart between the vertebral column and the sternum with downward pressure of the hands on the latter structure) has been described which may permit cardiac resuscitation without thoracotomy and direct massage.

It is of perhaps more than just passing interest that every one of these points was also recognized and carefully documented more than 50 years ago by Pike, Guthrie and Stewart in the report of their superb investigations entitled, "Studies in Resuscitation: I. The General Conditions Affecting Resuscitation, and The Resuscitation of the Blood and of the Heart", which was published in *The Journal of Experimental Medicine, 10: 371–418*, May, 1908, and is reprinted here.

STUDIES IN RESUSCITATION: I. THE GENERAL CONDITIONS AFFECTING RESUSCITATION, AND THE RESUSCITATION OF THE BLOOD AND OF THE HEART

F. H. PIKE, C. C. GUTHRIE
AND G. N. STEWART

Physiological Laboratories of
Western Reserve University
and the University of Chicago

J. Exper. Med., 10: 371–378, 1908

*   *   *   *

SUMMARY

"Our results may be briefly summarized:

1. Blood, when defibrinated, soon loses its power to maintain the activity of the higher nervous centers, and its nutritive properties for all tissues quickly diminish.

2. Artificial fluids, as a substitute for blood, are not satisfactory.

3. The proper oxygenation of the blood is an indispensable adjunct in the resuscitation of an animal.

4. The heart usually continues to beat for some minutes after it ceases to affect a mercury manometer, and resuscitation of it within this period by extra-thoracic massage and artificial respiration is sometimes successful.

5. Resuscitation of the heart by direct massage is the most certain method at our command.

6. A proper blood-pressure is an indispensable condition for the continued normal activity of the heart.

7. Anaesthetics, hemorrhage and induced currents applied to the heart render resuscitation more difficult than asphyxia alone.

Published June, 1967

The last several years have seen widespread interest in, and extensive use of, intravenous regional analgesia. In fact, the literature for the years 1963 through 1966 includes about 40 papers on the subject. In most instances, these reports have been laudatory; and in some instances they have been downright glowing:

"Regional anaesthesia for surgery of the extremities was produced by intravenous injection of lignocaine into the limb . . . to 514 patients between the ages of 4½ and 86 years, the dose varying from 60 mg. to 800 mg. . . . Of the group receiving 20 cc. of one per cent lignocaine, 92 per cent had good analgesia, while fewer than one per cent had poor analgesia. . . . This method of anaesthesia of the extremities is recommended for the efficient operation of a casualty theatre service."

"The technique of intravenous regional anaesthesia was carried out in 64 patients between the ages 6 and 60 years . . . a new local anaesthetic. . . . Citanest was used . . . in a dosage range of 75 mg. to 800 mg. For this dosage range, 86 per cent had good analgesia, 11 per cent moderate, and 3 per cent poor, providing 97 per cent adequate anaesthesia in the series."

"The effectiveness of this method in the production of anaesthesia cannot be doubted. Only ten patients out of 128 in this series required additional anaesthesia for the completion of a surgical procedure . . . it is probable that the method as described will be completely successful if the following points are remembered: (1) the anaesthetic solution should always be injected into a vein on the back of the hand— if this is not possible, the most distal forearm vein should be chosen; and (2) it is unreliable for procedures in the territories of the intercosto-brachial, lower lateral cutaneous, and posterior cutaneous nerves of the arm."

"Intravenous regional anesthesia for upper extremity surgery is described. In a series of 114 patients, it was characterized by ease of administration, effective anesthesia, and relative absence of complications or side effects observed clinically."

"An experience of 50 intravenous extremity blocks with 46 cases of successful anesthesia (92 per cent) is presented. The procedure has been shown to be simple, rapid, effective, and reliable."

On the other hand, not all of the experiences have been so fortunate:

"Intravenous administration of local anesthetic drugs is not without hazard. In Case 1, the amount of lidocaine hydrochloride introduced into the limb was grossly excessive. Abrupt release of the tourniquet at the end of operation permitted sudden access of this amount into the systemic circulation; convulsions resulted. In Case 2, the dosage was appropriate, but the technic was faulty: with the tip of the plastic catheter lying in the vein proximal to the tourniquet, the lidocaine hydrochloride was injected directly into the general circulation. . . . It is apparent that this technic should only be employed by or in the presence of physicians versed in resuscitative methods and that adequate equipment for resuscitation must always be at hand."

"A clinical trial was made of intravenous regional analgesia using lignocaine in 77 patients undergoing operations on the hand. The average dose of lignocaine administered was 182.5 mg., and the average time between injection and release of the tourniquet was 26½ minutes. . . . Good analgesia was obtained in 85 per cent of patients and good operating conditions in 91 per cent. Neurological side-effects occurred in seven patients, two of whom became unconscious after release of the tourniquet. Cardiovascular side-effects also occurred, a fall in blood pressure and slowing of the pulse rate being frequently noted. Seven patients were found to have arrhythmias or other changes in the ECG and one patient developed cardiac arrest in asystole which was treated successfully with cardiac massage. . . . The previous literature on intravenous regional analgesia is reviewed. In conclusion, we do not feel justified in continuing to use this technique with lignocaine in view of the high incidence of toxic phenomena."

These conflicting experiences and viewpoints were the subject, last September, at a symposium on intravenous regional analgesia which was held in Worcester, Massachusetts, under the sponsorship of Astra Pharmaceutical Products, Incorporated. All of the participants owed their presence at such a meeting to the pioneer work of August Bier, who published the original paper on the subject, "Concerning a New Method of Local Anaesthesia of the Extremities," in 1908 (Bier, A.: Ueber einen neuen weg local anasthesia an den gliedmaasen zu erzeugren. *Archiv fur Klinische Chirurgie, 86:* 1007–1016, 1908). *Survey* and its readers are indebted to Doctor Carl S. Hellijas of the Department of Anesthesiology at Hartford Hospital for his translation of Bier's paper.

CONCERNING A NEW METHOD OF LOCAL ANESTHESIA OF THE EXTREMITIES

Prof. Dr. August Bier

Arch. Klin. Chir. 86: 1908

"Gentlemen:

The allegedly more complicated operations on the extremities, in particular resections of joints, transplantations of tendons and extensive debridements, can be performed under neither infiltration nor conduction anesthesia. I have, therefore, used a new avenue, the blood vessel, to get the anesthetic agent to the end apparatus of the nerves as well as to the nerve trunks. According to my experience, this approach appears to fill the gap I have mentioned. I believe I can best make this very simple procedure understandable by describing to you a selected case of resection of an elbow which I performed with this method, and by pointing out to you on the human arm some of the necessary steps:

* * * *

"The blood was first expressed as much as possible from the extremity from the fingers to above the elbow joint with an Esmarch bandage. Then tourniquets were placed four fingerbreadths above and below the elbow.

"The median vein of the elbow was dissected free, using Schleich's method of infiltration anesthesia, and, as for intravenous infusion, a cannula was introduced distally through a slit in the vein and sutured fast. The vein was ligated proximal to the opening. 100 cc. of an 0.25% solution of novocain were injected into the vein with an ordinary syringe. The solution penetrated easily, without encountering resistance from venous valves, into the section of arm constricted at either end. Directly after the injection was completed, the stiff joint, which previously had been extremely painful on any attempt at motion, could be bent to a right angle with no pain.

"I started the resection immediately. The incisions through skin, muscle and periosteum were wholly without pain, as was the resection itself. At first the patient complained on forceful lifting of periosteum, but after a few minutes she made no further comment during this procedure, during extirpation of the capsule, sawing of ends of bones or scraping and excision of fistulous tracts. It should be noted that the patient was very sensitive, reacting with a loud cry to the needleprick for induction of the Schleich type of anesthesia.

"Sensation below the distal tourniquet was tested at conclusion of the resection (one-quarter hour after the injection of novocain). There was no feeling in this whole section of the arm, but capability of motion was preserved. This anesthesia was then used to make the finger joints mobile once again by forceful flexion and extension, which procedure was rather complete and quite painless."

* * * *

1909

Published June, 1978

It can safely be stated that there are not many anesthesiologists who have not, at one time or another during their professional careers, produced spinal anesthesia to a level that was considerably higher than was either necessary or desirable. These unintentional "high spinals" have often been accompanied by varying degrees of hypotension, respiratory depression, nausea, and other unpleasant and unwanted sequelae; and the memory of these inadvertent administrations would undoubtedly be a source of great personal chagrin if there were not so many of us. However, our numbers are so legion that it is really a matter of "Welcome to the Club."

Consider, then, if you will, those intrepid individuals who have purposefully set out to produce *total* spinal anesthesia. Their aim was to achieve precisely those levels of spinal anesthesia that the rest of us try so desperately to avoid, and to attain levels of hypotension which the rest of us abhor.

The Brooklyn surgeon, Koster, for instance, amassed an astounding experience with intentional high spinal anesthesia which he documented for an incredulous medical audience in 1928 in the American Journal of Surgery under the title of "Spinal Anesthesia. With Special Reference to its Use in Surgery of the Head, Neck and Thorax."

The first paragraph of his report began by stating, "The purpose of this paper is to describe a technique for safely producing spinal anesthesia of the entire body by the injection of an anesthetic solution into the subarachnoid space."

The second paragraph then detailed the technique: "Our method in brief, consisted of a spinal puncture between the second and third lumbar vertebrae, the withdrawal of 4 c.c. of cerebrospinal fluid into an ampule containing 0.1 gm. of neocaine, thorough mixing to produce rapid solution and then reinjection of the cerebrospinal fluid containing the dissolved drug. We found that this procedure gave surgical anesthesia almost up to the level of the nipples and allowed any operative procedure on all structures below the diaphragm."

It was not, however, his ultimate technique.

"Occasionally in doing multiple operations . . . e.g., women in whom it is necessary to do a cholecystectomy and appendectomy and then perhaps some form of suspension and perineal repair. . .the spinal anesthesia did not last long enough to allow for completion of the entire procedure and it was found necessary to finish under gas-oxygen-ether. The addition of the general anesthesia was very unsatisfactory and we began to search for a method of prolonging the spinal anesthesia. We began by gradually increasing the dose of anesthetic substance injected into the subarachnoid space and we found that the anesthesia was prolonged slightly. When the dose was doubled, we prolonged the anesthesia almost 100 per cent."

Koster also found that doubling the dose produced a rather different type of spinal anesthesia than the original technique which he employed: "During the course of the operation the patient asked for some water which he was allowed to drink. A complaint that he could not feel the water passing through his pharynx stimulated us to test out the level of the anesthesia of this particular individual and we found, much to our surprise, that it extended over the entire body, including the scalp. Upon further questioning the information was elicited that although the patient knew that fluid was passing down his gullet, he could not feel it in the pharynx. Repetition of the method in other patients confirmed the original observation that anesthesia of the entire body was produced. Since that time, we have used this method for operating on all parts of the body above the diaphragm, for such conditions as empyema, carcinoma of the breast, diseases of the thyroid, tumor of the tongue, operations on the scalp and skull. We have also used this form of anesthesia experimentally in the last 200 laparotomies for the purpose of testing the efficacy of the method. The level of anesthesia was determined by piercing the forearm, ear lobe and skin of the forehead with a needle. In all of these cases the test demonstrated complete surgical anesthesia. In none of these cases have untoward effects been noted. Contrary to the hitherto generally accepted idea of the effects of anesthetics on the upper portion of the spinal cord and medulla there have been neither respiratory nor cardiac embarrassments."

Koster then went on to describe his final technique in some detail, and in so doing demonstrated his appreciation of the importance of position in the successful performance of lumbar puncture, as well as a knowledge of the fine art of wrestling: "All patients . . . are placed on the operating table in the lateral prone position and an assistant secures flexion of the trunk by approximating the head and knees. Since cooperation of the patient is not always procurable it is wise to be prepared to maintain the trunk flexion while the spinal puncture is being done. It is possible for an individual of average strength to maintain such flexion easily by applying a well-known wrestling principle. With the patient on the left side, the head approximating the knees, and the arms extended overhead, if the assistant stands on the side of the table facing the patient, places his right arm round the neck and his left arm around the knees, both from behind forward so that the hands can be clasped in front of the patient, the latter is rendered helpless."

His list of contraindications was not long ("As yet we have not found any contraindications to its use"), but his list of indications was fairly extensive: "Patients in very early childhood and advanced age tolerate it as well as young adults. Individuals with endocardial and myocardial changes, with renal diseases, respiratory diseases and metabolic disturbances are particularly suited for this type of anesthesia. . . . These are some of the conditions in which spinal anesthesia is particularly valuable. . . . We do not believe that the ordinary cited contraindications should be seriously regarded as such. The best example can perhaps best be found in hypotension cases. Recognition of the 'modus operandi' by which the blood-pressure fall is occasioned in spinal block and the use of Trendelenburg position for gravity drainage to the heart eliminates hypotension as a contraindication to the use of spinal anesthesia."

In evaluating his technique, Koster asks, "Is the anesthesia safe? We have not as yet had a fatality directly attributable to the anesthesia"; but he does describe 4 deaths on the operating table ("He was so dehydrated and so highly toxic that only with reluctance, and because of the minimizing effect of spinal anesthesia on operative trauma, was the operating undertaken") ("During the course of a guillotine operation at the middle third of the thigh, his pulse suddenly became imperceptible and stimulation failed to restore the circulation") ("During the resection her life ebbed out") ("After the dressings were applied, and as the patient was about to be transferred to the stretcher for transportation from the operating room, she ceased to breathe suddenly . . . .") due to the fact that "in each instance the patient was highly toxic and . . . there was marked anhydremia."

The list of advantages was also extensive, but the two clinchers were undoubtedly that, first, "Any one who can do a lumbar puncture can induce spinal anesthesia; the method is reasonably 'fool proof'"; and, second, "Beside the already enumerated advantages it should be remembered that this form of anesthesia can be administered and induced very rapidly, and by its use the surgeon is freed from the vagaries of different anesthetists. This emancipation in itself is a definite advantage."

Some 20 years prior to Koster's paper, another intrepid surgeon, Professor Thomas Jonnesco of Bucharest, had demonstrated how one's enthusiasm for his own technique can often exceed his discretion in a paper entitled, "Remarks on General Spinal Analgesia," which appeared in the November 13th, 1909 issue of the *British*

Medical Journal and which is reprinted below.

REMARKS ON GENERAL SPINAL ANALGESIA

Professor Thomas Jonnesco

Bucharest, Romania

Br. Med. J., 2: November, 1909

"The fundamental principles in spinal analgesia are that puncture of the arachnoid may be performed at all levels, and that to the anesthetic, whether stovaine, tropacocaine, or novocain, strychnine should be added. Puncture of the arachnoid at whatever level is harmless, and the fear of picking the cord unfounded; even if it happens it is not harmful. However, with the patient in the sitting position, superior dorsal puncture between the first and second dorsal vertebrae, and dorsolumbar between the last dorsal and first lumbar vertebrae are easy, and suffice to obtain analgesia of all regions of the body."

A series of 398 operations is reported, performed under spinal analgesia over a period of eight months in 1908–09. Fifteen of these patients were under 10 years of age. High dorsal analgesia was used in 103 patients for operations on the skull (14), operations on the face (45), operations on the throat (23), operations on the thorax (7), and operations on the upper limb (14). Dorsolumbar analgesia was used in 295 patients for intraabdominal, perineal, and lower extremity operations.

"During analgesia patients retain full consciousness, and I am in the habit of speaking to them to divert their attention from the operation, of which the majority are unaware. —A patient may be heard to ask after an operation is finished when it is to be begun."

*   *   *   *

1910

Published June, 1966

The anesthesiologist today speaks often of "balanced anesthesia," and his listeners have no difficulty in understanding his meaning. He is referring to a form of general anesthesia which, with certain individual variations, consists of a short acting barbiturate (usually thiopental), an inhalation mixture (often nitrous oxide-oxygen-halothane), and a muscle relaxant (generally *d*-tubocurare or one of its congeners.) It is safe to say that much of the general anesthesia administered in this country at the present time is composed of this or a rather similar combination of drugs.

The rationale of "balanced anesthesia," of course, is based upon the fact that the anesthetic state must provide a good deal more than mere unconsciousness. It has been recognized for years that unconsciousness, or hypnosis, is only one of several desirable, and indeed necessary, characteristics of full anesthesia. Analgesia, or the obtundation of pain, is an integral component, and can be provided, in the instance of the more superficial surgical ventures, merely by the inhalation of nitrous oxide in combination with oxygen. Deeper probings of the scalpel will require more intense analgesia, either by inhalation of the more potent volatile or gaseous drugs (such as ethylene, cyclopropane, ether, or halothane), or by the intravenous administration of minimal doses of the analgetic drugs, such as morphine, Demerol, Nisentil, Dromoran, Methadon, or other such related compounds. Relaxation of muscles is a third factor in the anesthetic equation, at least for major operations within the abdomen; to achieve it, one requires the use of a muscle relaxant drug, high concentrations of the potent volatile or gaseous drugs, or conduction anesthesia to block the spinal nerves. The final requirement of the anesthetic state is the obtundation of noxious reflex activity; and the latter is also perhaps the most ill-defined of the various components of anesthesia. Noxious impulses of several different kinds—including somatic, sympathetic, and parasympathetic—are recognized but not necessarily distinguished; only on occasion does the anesthesiologist identify the specific reflex that is present and employ a specific blocking drug to prevent further manifestations of such activity. In most instances, the combination of a hypnotic, an analgesic, and a muscle relaxant suffices to provide an anesthetic cover which obtunds noxious reflex activity.

Thus, "balanced anesthesia," in essence, is a form of the practice of clinical pharmacology which employs several drugs to achieve anesthesia, each drug being employed for a specific purpose and in the exact quantity necessary to attain that purpose. This is a far cry from the days when a single, fully potent anesthetic drug was employed to provide all of the several attributes of the anesthetic state, and yet the concept that anesthesia must do more than render the patient unconscious is scarcely a new one. Almost a century and a quarter ago, the ever-astute John Snow wrote, "Ether contributes other benefits besides preventing pain. It keeps patients still, who otherwise would not be. I gave it lately, for this object alone, to a child on whom Mr. George Pollock operated for cataract by drilling. The child was perfectly quiet, and the eye and eyelids were quite passive. It had been operated on before, and without the ether would have made all resistance in its power . . . the relaxing effects of ether are much greater than those of the warm-bath, and emetics. In the case, No. 40 of the list subsequently to be given, Mr. Tatum reduced a dislocation of the shoulder of ten weeks' duration, in a muscular man, under the influence of ether, when it was observed, before the traction was exerted, that the muscles were completely relaxed, and the arm much more moveable than before the inhalation. Other cases of reduction of old dislocations, under the effects of ether, have been related in the medical journals, and also cases in which the surgeon was enabled, by means of it, to reduce strangulated herniae with the taxis, where, otherwise, an operation would have been required. In case 7 of the second list, farther on, the ether superseded one of the most difficult operations in surgery and enabled Mr. Liston to get a catheter into the bladder without using the knife. . . . It is very evident, *a priori*, that an agent which so alters the circumstances of the patient, cannot be without its effects on the ultimate results of capital operations: and since severe pain generally exerts a deleterious influence on the economy, and the use of ether in thousands of trivial operations has shown it, when properly managed, to be attended, either with no danger, or the least conceivable amount of it, it seems to follow that etherization must lessen the danger of serious operations, unless we think (with one or two renowned doubters, who seem to look upon a surgical operation as a natural process, in which pain plays some essential part), that the sufferings of the patient in some way aid his recovery, instead of being deleterious to him."

The bridge between the use of a single drug to provide all of the various attributes of anesthesia and "balanced anesthesia" as we know it today was made of several strong planks. Not the least of these was the concept of Anoci-Association, enunciated by the late George Crile senior and contained in his Ether Day Address, "Phylogenetic Association in Relation to Certain Medical Problems." This paper was published in the December 15, 1910, issue of *The Boston Medical and Surgical Journal*, volume 163, pages 893–904, and is reprinted below.

PHYLOGENETIC ASSOCIATION IN RELATION TO CERTAIN MEDICAL PROBLEMS

G. W. CRILE, M.D.

Cleveland, Ohio

Boston Med. Surg. J., 163: 893–894, 1910

"The discovery of the anesthetic properties of ether and its practical application to surgery must always stand as one of the great achievements of medicine. It is eminently fitting that the anniversary of that notable day, when the possibilities of ether were first made known to the world, should be celebrated within these walls, and whatever the topic of your Ether Day orator, he must fittingly first pause to pay tribute to that great event and to the master surgeons of the Massachusetts General Hospital. On this occasion, on behalf of the dumb animals as well as on behalf of suffering humanity, I express a deep sense of gratitude for the blessings of anesthesia. Two years ago an historical appreciation of the discovery of ether was here presented by Professor Welch, and last year an address on medical research was given by President Eliot. I, therefore, will not attempt a general address, but will present an experimental and clinical research.

*   *   *   *

RECAPITULATION

"The following are the principal points presented: In operations under inhalation anesthesia the nerve impulses from the trauma reach every part of the brain,—the cerebrum that is apparently anesthetized as well as the medulla that is known to remain awake, the proof being the *physiologic* exhaustion of and the *pathologic* change in the nerve cells. Under ether anesthesia the damage is at least four times greater than under nitrous oxide. Inhalation anesthesia is, therefore, but a veneer, a mask that "covers the deep suffering of the patient." The cause of the exhaustion of the brain is the discharge of nervous energy in a futile effort to energize the paralyzed muscles in an effort at escape from the injury just as

if no anesthetic had been given. The exhaustion is, therefore, of the same nature as that from overexertion.

But if the nerve paths connecting the field of operation and the brain be blocked, then there is no discharge of nervous energy from the trauma, and consequently no exhaustion however severe or prolonged the operation.

*   *   *   *

"What is the practical application of this? In operative surgery there is introduced a new principle, which removes from surgery much of the immediate risk from its trauma by establishing *anoci-association*; it places on a physical basis certain of the phenomena of fear; it explains to us the physical basis for the impairment of the entire individual under worry or misfortune; the daily noci-associations of the individual as a social unit; or a noci-influence of a part of the body. On the other hand, it explains the power of therapeutic suggestion and other influences which serve for the time to change the noci-integration, and physical basis for the difference between hope and despair; it explains some of the phenomena of Graves' disease, of sexual neurasthenia, possibly of hay fever and the genesis of the common cold. The principle is probably equally applicable to the acute infections whose chemical noci-association gives rise to many of the phenomena of the disease and explains their cure by natural immunity and by vaccines; it should teach us to view our patients as a whole; and especially should it teach the surgeon gentleness. It should teach us that there is something more in surgery than mechanics; and something more in medicine than physical diagnosis and drugs."

*   *   *   *

1911

Published June, 1963

Man uses his arms and hands constantly. He peels potatoes, slams doors, climbs trees, lights stoves, plays baseball, opens cans, sharpens knives, hammers nails, baits fishhooks, chops kindling, carves meat, sets traps, closes trunks, operates drill presses, shoots guns, whittles sticks, drives tractors, renovates furniture, starts outboard motors, fixes washing machines, splices rope, sets off firecrackers, and seemingly is incapable of resisting signs which say "Danger— High Voltage." As a result he exposes his arms and hands to injury constantly: to burns, cuts, amputations, abrasions, fractures, contusions, dislocations, tears, and half a hundred other results of trauma.

Man also eats constantly. When he is growing up, in a well regulated household at least, he eats three well balanced meals at regular and set intervals three times a day. Or so his mother thinks. She doesn't know about the fireball at recess, the licorice after lunch, the milkshake at the drugstore on the way from school, the ginger ale and cookies on arriving home, the Milky Way when supper is over, the glass of milk before bed, or that candy left over from Halloween for a reassuring bite after the bed is tucked in and the goodnights said. The habit becomes ingrained, and when Man leaves mothers's well-regulated house, with three balanced meals at regular and set intervals three times a day, he goes right on eating. There is breakfast, of course. Then a Danish at coffee-break. Luncheon. A hamburger and frappe in mid-afternoon. Beer and pretzels after a hard day at the plant. Dinner. Popcorn during the movie. A pizza after the show. A quick raid of the icebox before turning in. In point of fact, except between the hours of about 3 and 7 in the morning. Man's stomach is never really empty—proof perhaps, as some nutritionists have claimed, that it never should be, that nature intended frequent small feedings and not three squares a day.

The combination of Man's prehensility and his unflagging appetite keeps a steady flow of patients with injured upper extremities and full stomachs streaming into hospital emergency rooms. This is why the brachial plexus is so frequently the anesthesiologist's favorite group of nerves.

The brachial plexus is formed by the union of the anterior primary divisions of the lower four cervical and first thoracic nerves. It receives contributions from the second and third thoracic nerves, and occasionally from the fourth also. The plexus extends from the lower part of the side of the neck to the axilla. After leaving the intervertebral foramina, the fifth and sixth cervical unite to form a trunk, the upper trunk; the eighth cervical and first thoracic also unite to form one trunk, the lower trunk; and the seventh cervical runs alone as the middle trunk. As these three trunks pass beneath the clavicle, each splits into an anterior and posterior division. The anterior divisions of the upper and middle trunks unite to form the lateral cord, so designated because it is situated on the lateral side of the second part of the axillary artery. The anterior division of the lower trunk passes down on the medial side of the artery as the medial cord. The posterior divisions of all three trunks unite to form the posterior cord which is situated behind the second portion of the axillary artery.

From the anesthesiologist's point of view, the brachial plexus can be divided into two portions: a cervical or supraclavicular, and an axillary or infraclavicular portion. The supraclavicular portion of the plexus has the shape of a triangle, having its base attached to the cervical vertebral column and its apex at the clavicle. The infraclavicular portion consists of the component parts of the plexus forming a close fasces around the axillary artery, lying on the outer side of it. The plexus can therefore be blocked by the paravertebral approach, through the axilla, by the infraclavicular access, or by the supraclavicular route.

And in fact, of course, all four methods have been employed clinically. The paravertebral route was employed by Kappis; the axillary route was used by Hirschel; the infraclavicular route was developed by Louis Bazy; and the supraclavicular route was popularized by Kulenkampff. Kulenkampff described the supraclavicular route in 1912, and in time it became the most widely used method of blocking the brachial plexus. Within the past few years, however, there has been a tremendous resurgence of interest in, and employment of, the axillary route, both because of the simplicity with which the block can be performed by this technique, as well as because the complications are so much less frequent and formidable. It is of some interest, in retrospect, that the axillary technique of blocking the plexus was described by Hirschel a year before Kulenkampff published his supraclavicular technique. *Survey of Anesthesiology* and its readers are indebted to Dr. Aaron Bobrow for the translation into English of Hirschel's article which originally appeared in the July 18, 1911, issue of the Munich Medical Weekly under the title, "Die Anästhesierung des Plexus brachialis bei Operationen an der oberen Extremität" (Hirschel, G.: *Munch. med. Wschr.*, 58: 1555–1556, 1911), and which is printed below.

ANESTHESIA OF THE BRACHIAL PLEXUS FOR

OPERATIONS OF THE UPPER EXTREMITY

PRIVAT DOZENT DR. GEORG HIRSCHEL

Munch. med. Wschr., 58: 1555–1556, 1911

*   *   *   *

"As far as the technique of the injection is concerned, the following remarks should be added:

The arm is placed in marked abduction and a gauze wad is placed in position. This exerts a moderate pressure on the easily palpable blood vessels. This gauze wad must be placed under the pectoral muscles as far upward into the axilla as possible in order to permit enough room for the approach. One fixes the artery with one hand and inserts the needle as far upward as possible under the pectoralis major in the direction of the arm. (Figure 1). As the needle is inserted, Novocain is injected in order to avoid the vessels and to prevent injury to them. In this way one bathes the median nerve above and the ulnar somewhat more anteriorly with a few injections. Another injection under the artery at about the level of the latissimus dorsi is necessary, in order to anesthetize the radial nerve. So the artery is encircled, and with a bit of care injury to it or to the vein will be avoided.

It is important to reach as high as possible in the direction of the first rib with the injection, since otherwise the axillary and the musculocutaneous nerves will be missed."

*   *   *   *

1912

Published October, 1979

Arthur Ernest Guedel was a giant amongst the pioneers of anesthesiology, not only in this country but throughout the world, for he achieved an international reputation which was recognized by the presentation of the Henry Hill Hickman medal by the Royal Society of Medicine of London in 1941—the first outside of the

British Isles to be honored with this prestigious award. In 1951, his own Society, the American Society of Anesthesiologists, presented him with the Distinguished Service Award, the highest tribute the Society can pay an anesthesiologist for his meritorious service and achievement in the course of a career in anesthesia. Over and above his scientific accomplishments and clinical contributions (which have become legendary), however, was Guedel's personality—warm, kindly, full of friendliness and good humor; a man of whom it was said that he had more friends than anybody else in anesthesiology.

Guedel was born in Cambridge City, Indiana* on June 13, 1883, and he was always proud to proclaim that he had one-eighth Cherokee Indian blood, "just like Will Rogers." His early schooling was at the South Side Grade School in Indianapolis, where his father worked for the Atkins Saw Company; and it was while helping his father at the plant at the age of 13 that he lost 3 fingers of his right hand while dusting a machine. This fact did not deter him from later teaching himself to play the piano, and Ralph Waters has written: "An athlete of the first order, he swam with endurance and was adept in the manly art of self-defense, yet no physician I have ever known had the delicate coordination of the smaller muscles that was his. He played the organ and piano with the skill of a natural artist. Many of the pieces of anesthetic apparatus which have come from his hands bear witness to this delicacy of touch."

After graduation from grade school, Guedel went to work for the Atkins Saw

* Ordinarily, the place of a person's birth is of interest only to the person herself/himself, immigration officials, astrologers engaged in the preparation of an individual's horoscope, or those endless bureaucratic governmental questionnaires and forms which the rest of a long-suffering citizenry must fill out promptly and correctly under threat of fine, imprisonment, or both. The fact that Guedel's birthplace was in Indiana, however, brings up an interesting fact about the contribution of the Midwest as a cradle of pioneers and leaders of anesthesia in this country: 9 Midwestern states served as the birthplaces of 14 of the first 42 Presidents of the American Society of Anesthesiologists, and of 15 of the 33 recipients of the Distinguished Service Award.

Company, because there were no funds available for a high school education. Typical of this extraordinary man, he borrowed books, had one of the high school teachers advise him, and gave himself a high school education. His lack of a formal accredited high school education frustrated his ambition to attend medical school only momentarily, because he had the family doctor, one Dr. Brocking, talk to his good friend the Dean of Medical College of Indiana. The result of that little chat was that Arthur Guedel took and passed an entrance examination and matriculated to the medical school in 1903.

He graduated as a first honors student in 1908, took his State Board Examinations the same year, and started a 6 month internship at City Hospital, Indianapolis. This was the start of his career in anesthesia, because he was required to administer ether and chloroform anesthesia, and his feeling of ignorance initiated his studies correlating the eye signs with the depth of anesthesia. The next year, 1909, he started an office for general practice, but his interest in, and facility at, anesthesia soon made this a predominant part of his practice.

When the United States entered World War I, Guedel volunteered but was rejected because of his hand disability. He persisted, however, and eventually was assigned to the Roosevelt Hospital Unit as anesthetist, sailing for Europe in July, 1917.

To quote Ralph Waters, (again and extensively, because he and Guedel were very real and close friends, who exchanged several long letters a month for many years) on the subject of Guedel's career during the war: "Before the first World War the number of true specialists in anesthesia in the U.S.A. could almost be counted on the fingers of one's two hands. In March, 1918, one of these (Leslie Burwell of New Rochelle, New York) reported for duty at the Medical Headquarters of an American unit at Vittel in the Vosges, France. Upon his insistence that he wished to be assigned to work for which he was particularly fitted, the medical officer in command said, 'You will have to see Guedel. He runs the Anesthesia in this region. He blows in here every day or two, like a wild Indian, on a motorcycle. Wait for him.' Sure enough, the next afternoon, with a roar and a put-put the motorcycle arrived in a cloud of dust.

"Burwell's curiosity, as to how an anaesthetist could function on a motor-bike, was soon satisfied. The several hospitals in the neighborhood could be visited frequently only by such means. The scarcity of anaesthetically minded medical officers had made it necessary to assign non-professional, inexperienced persons to duty as anaesthetists. The manner of teaching and directing such personnel under these circumstances is an illustration of the amazing versatility and resourcefulness of Arthur Guedel. He was forced to devise not only simple methods of teaching these willing though inexperienced people but also quick and reliable ways of checking the accuracy and safety of the dosage of ether which they were able, as a result of his teaching, to maintain in the operating rooms of the several hospitals. The difficulties which Guedel surmounted during the first World War were of immense benefit to military surgeons and soldier-patients, it is true, but what greater value were his experiences there to all of us—teachers and pupils alike—all over the world! He insisted that during ether anesthesia movement of the patient's eyeball was a sign which could be checked quickly and which the enlisted-man technician could observe readily and reliably. How often since, have we older teachers found the observation valuable, and even essential, in trying to help medical students and young physicians safely to administer anaesthetics. Guedel's chart of physical signs of ether anaesthesia was born in the military hospitals and while riding army motor-bikes over the rough roads between them. I presume we might even say that the book, later published by Macmillan, as *Inhalation Anesthesia, A Fundamental Guide*, had its foundation built in Guedel's mind in the military hospitals and along the shell-shattered roads of France, during the first war."

Sir Robert Macintosh, the first Nuffield Professor of Anaesthetics at the University of Oxford, must also be quoted extensively on the subject of Guedel's Stages and Signs of Anesthesia. He pointed out that the very first sentence of John Snow's 2 famous books (*On The Inhalation of the Vapour of Ether*, London, 1847; and *On Chloroform And Other Anesthetics*, London, 1858) runs: "The point requiring the most skill and care in the administration of the vapour of ether is, undoubtedly, to determine when it has been carried far enough."

Sir Robert went on to say: "Guedel's chart first appeared in a medical journal in 1920, but its value was appreciated at the time by relatively few. It made a telling impact, however, when it was included in his one and only book written in the easy, chatty style so characteristic of the man himself. The publication of *Inhalation Anesthesia* in 1937 could hardly have been more timely because the second World War was imminent, and it became imperative to train more anaesthetists; and this no doubt accounted in large measure for the demand for twelve reprints in as many years. Since the publication of this popular book, I don't suppose the subject of signs of anaesthesia has been written about or discussed without mention of Guedel's name and chart.

"The name of Guedel is known to anaesthetists throughout the world because of his chart; but to a privileged few of the older generation who knew him, the name recalls much more. Friendship came naturally to him. He had the rare and happy gift of making his visitors feel welcome; that their opinions mattered, and that his time was freely at their disposal. How comfortably he fitted into that distinguished and friendly group on the North American Continent which included Ralph Waters, Wesley Bourne, Emory ('Rovey') Rovenstine, Paul Wood and Harold Griffith. Their one objective seemed to be to further the progress of anaesthesia; and in the process they put their knowledge to the common good and liberally dispensed good fellowship."

Geoffrey Kaye, one of the great pioneers of anesthesia in Australia, has said of *Inhalation Anesthesia*: "I received my copy of this book from Dr. F. H. McMechan, on behalf of the I.A.R.S., at the New York Congress of 1938. The book impressed me greatly. Certainly, it had not a great deal to say about the technique of anaesthetic administration; rather did it deal with the pitfalls which await the novice-anaesthetist. Its precepts were full of what R. M. Waters describes as 'mule-sense,' the mule being a more sagacious animal than the horse. Impressive, and in many ways revolutionary, was Guedel's presentation of the 'signs of anaesthesia.'"

Kaye went on to list some of Guedel's other contributions to anesthesia: "The Cuffed Tube. The cuffed endotracheal tube arose, I think, from true collaboration between Waters and Guedel. It was Waters who sent me materials for the making-up of the first cuffs. Later, I saw a reenactment of the famous 'experiment of the dunked dog' at Wisconsin in 1938. News of the cuffed tube spread around the world with great rapidity. One was reminded of the spread of ether anaesthesia itself, first demonstrated publicly in Boston on October 16, 1846, and in use in Her Majesty's remote penal colony of Van Dieman's Land in June, 1847.

"The Pharyngeal Airway. Guedel's 'airway' was a definite advance upon those of Hewitt or Phillips. It was soft, atraumatic and of low respiratory resistance. It was so well-shaped anatomically that it was tolerated at a light plane of anaesthesia, without provoking 'gagging.' We used to demonstrate this fact to students at the University of Melbourne by passing the airway upon ourselves in presence of the class!

"'Controlled Respiration.' Essentially, the Guedel Technique was one of 'control of depth of anaesthesia,' rather than 'control by acapnia.' The former rather frightened me as coming too close to the histotoxic zone of the anaesthetics of that day. Unless I err, the acapnic technique was put forward by R. M. Waters, with Guedel a ready convert to it."

Guedel's fertile and energetic mind was into many other subjects pertaining to anesthesia, and his bibliography was absolutely gold-plated: there were no "pot-boilers" in it anywhere. His observations and opinions were checked and rechecked before he expressed them, so that he need not withdraw them later. He was also immensely pragmatic, and tended towards practical simplification rather than towards more complication of methods and concepts. This is well illustrated in a letter which he wrote to Ralph Waters in 1938:

"Self administration of nitrous oxide in labor is O.K. I told you that some twenty years ago. However, I do not like the idea of strapping a mask on the patient's face. There is too much danger of aspiration of vomitus. And even of asphyxia if the gas mixture goes wrong. Before I stopped doing obstetric anesthesia I had gone to the old McKesson machine because we had one at the hospital. I later developed a spring release mask for the Heidbrink but did not like it as well.

"For a number of years I spent a lot of time telling the patient just what to do and how to do it. Later I got tired of telling and there developed for me the best technique that I found. I would push the gas machine up to the patient, set the oxygen for twenty to thirty percent and tell the patient to take as much as she wanted whenever she wanted it. For the first twenty-minutes or half hour they would be taking it for most of the time whether they needed it or not. But they would do that anyway under the "Telling" system so it did not matter. After they had become sedated by the N_2O—after twenty minutes or half-an-hour—they would sleep between pains, awakening at the beginning of the pain. They would then put the mask to their face and breathe like the devil for a few breaths—six to twelve—and go to sleep until the next pain. I would let this go on for hours, in some cases up to the point of actual delivery, when I would take over. They would take care of their own anesthesia better and more safely than I could do it for them. After it was all over—the next day—they would invariably report that they were in labor but a short time. The hours were not noticed and they were happy. Keep the oxygen up. Don't strap the mask to their face. I used to strap it to their hand with adhesive tape so that they could find it easily when they wanted it. And don't pay too much attention to them."

Guedel's first published paper, in fact, was on the subject of the self administration of nitrous oxide in labor. It was entitled "Nitrous Oxide—Air Anesthesia. Self Administration in Obstetrics. A Preliminary Report." Guedel read this paper before the Indianapolis Medical Society, October 3, 1911, and it was printed in the *Indianapolis Medical Journal* for October, 1911. It is reproduced below.

NITROUS OXIDE-AIR ANESTHESIA. SELF-ADMINISTERED IN OBSTETRICS. A PRELIMINARY REPORT

ARTHUR E. GUEDEL

Indianapolis, Indiana

Read before the Indianapolis Medical Society, October 3, 1911

Printed in the Indianapolis Medical Journal, October, 1911

Revised by the Author, February, 1912

"The following report deals with the action of the gas (nitrous oxide) in obstetrical practice, and the encouraging results of its application.

*   *   *   *

"The extreme rapidity with which a state of analgesia closely followed by complete unconsciousness is produced, combined with its very transitory effect, —make it particularly applicable in this work. It has a not unpleasant odor, and is not at all irritating to the mucous membranes of the respiratory tract. . . . The only post-anesthetic effect is a pleasant restful drowsiness, nausea and vomiting being indeed rare. Also it is conceded, that, of all anesthetics now in use, nitrous oxide is by far the safest, both primarily and secondarily. —Another characteristic of the gas which makes it preferable to other anesthetics in obstetrics, is that it does not cause muscular relaxation.

The administration of nitrous oxide and air is very simple—the writer has secured in all but one case of normal labor, excellent results by allowing the patient herself to handle the inhaler. —The patient soon learns that her relief depends upon the result of a race between the action of the gas and the approaching pain, with the gas winning always if given an equal start."

1914

Published August and October, 1973

Faithful readers of "Classical File" will recall that an inquest was held at Winlaton, about 5 miles from Newcastle-upon-Tyne, on Tuesday, February 1st, 1848, to inquire into the death of Hannah Greener, a 15 year old girl who had died the previous Friday during a chloroform anesthesia.

Hannah's death, which occurred just 15 months after Morton's classic public demonstration of the efficacy of ether anesthesia at the Massachusetts General Hospital, and just 2 months after Simpson's introduction of chloroform as an anesthesic, excited great interest because it was the first mortality recognized as being due to anesthesia.

Although her general health was described as being good, Hannah had a good deal of trouble with her feet; and in the fall of 1847 she had become a patient in the infirmary at Newcastle-upon-Tyne, where one of her toenails was removed under ether anesthesia. She had made a reasonable recovery from the anesthesia and operation, but had complained for a number of days of a "heaviness in her head," "fretted" a good deal while in the infirmary, grew thinner while there, and continued to grow thinner after being discharged, and complained of pain in the chest, which she had never done prior to her hospitalization. Her stepmother attributed her ill health to the fact that she continued to suffer "much pain in her toes . . . . I think it was the pain being so great prevented her thriving."

By January of 1848, the pain in Hannah's toes was sufficient to again warrant medical attention, and Mr. Thomas Meggison, a surgeon at Wickham, was called into the case. He recommended that the toenail of the right big toe be removed, and the fateful operation was arranged for Friday, January 28th, 1848. Meggison has left us a description of the events:

"Hannah Greener died under my hands on Friday, while under the influence of chloroform, which I had given her for the purpose of producing insensibility during the operation of removing one of her toenails. She was suffering from onychia. She never complained of pain in the chest to me. The pain in her toes might cause her to become thinner. I seated her in a chair, and put about a teaspoonful of chloroform into a tablecloth, and held it to her nose. After she had drawn her breath twice she pulled my hand down. I told her to draw her breath naturally, which she did, and in about half a minute I observed the muscles of the arm become rigid, and her breathing a little quickened, but not stertorous. I had my hand on her pulse, which was natural, until the muscles became rigid. It then appeared somewhat weaker—not altered in frequency. I then told Mr. Lloyd, my assistant, to begin the operation, which he did, and took the nail off. When the semicircular incision was made, she gave a struggle or jerk, which I thought was from the chloroform not having taken sufficient effect. I did not apply any more. Her eyes were closed, and I opened them, and they remained open. Her mouth was open, and her lips and face blanched. When I opened her eyes they were congested. I called for water when I saw her face blanched, and I dashed some of it in her face. It had no

effect. I then gave her some brandy, a little of which she swallowed with difficulty. I then laid her down on the floor, and attempted to bleed her in the arm and jugular vein, but only obtained about a spoonful. She was dead, I believe, at the time I attempted to bleed her. The last time I felt her pulse was immediately previous to the blanched appearance coming on, and she gave a jerk. The time would not be more than 3 minutes from her first inhaling the chloroform till her death."

Mr. Lloyd confirmed Meggison's statements, and then Sir John Fife reported the autopsy which he had performed. His principal findings consisted of "a very high state of congestion" of the liver, kidneys, spleen, and brain, but particularly the lungs: "In my opinion the cause of death was the congestion of the lungs; and that congestion I ascribe to the inhalation of chloroform."

The jury agreed with Sir John: "We are unanimously of opinion that the deceased, Hannah Greener, died from congestion of the lungs, from the effect of chloroform, and that no blame can be attached to Mr. Meggison, surgeon, or to his assistant, Mr. Lloyd."

The ink was scarcely dry on this description of the inquest in the February 5th, 1848 issue of the *Lancet* before Dr. Simpson had sprung to the defence of the anesthesic drug which he had introduced. In an article titled, "Remarks on the alleged case of death from action of chloroform" in the February 12th, 1848 issue of the *Lancet*, Simpson wrote that he had "no desire to throw any—the very slightest—blame upon Mr. Meggison. Nothing could be possibly further from my wishes and intention"; and then he proceeded to belittle both Meggison and the coroner's jury. "The attempt at swallowing mentioned in the evidence was, I have no doubt, an attempt at breathing only, or at breathing combined with swallowing. But it was impossible for the patient, in her weak and torpid state, to inspire through a medium of water and brandy, any more than it would have been possible to inspire if the whole head and face had been inevitably submersed in the same fluid . . . the morbid appearances were not those resulting from chloroform; they were those resulting from asphyxia; and as I have already stated, the verdict should not have been, 'Died from the effects of chloroform,' but, 'Died from the effects of means used to restore her from the state of anaesthesia.'"

Within a fortnight, however, on February 23rd, a second death during chloroform anesthesia occurred, this one in America, when a Mrs. Simmons in Cincinnati, Ohio, died within a matter of minutes after commencing the inhalation of chloroform for dental anesthesia. Professor Simpson's glib explanation of the mechanism of Hannah's demise began to be doubted in a number of quarters. John Collins Warren, who had played such an important role in the Morton demonstration of ether anesthesia, wrote, "We were soon awakened from our dreams of the delightful influence of the new agent (chloroform), by the occurrence of unfortunate and painful consequences, which had not followed in this country on the practice of etherization."

Other deaths continued to occur, and by 1858, John Snow had collected and analyzed 50 cases of death from chloroform. The striking feature of some 40 of these deaths was the suddenness with which they occurred—early in the administration, and after only a "few drachms" of the drug. Reams were written in attempts to explain the mechanism of sudden death during chloroform anesthesia, almost always ending up with the same conclusion—overdosage. From their experience with ether, most anesthetists realized that, if that drug were given to excess, respiration would cease and death would occur from asphyxia; but the heart continued to beat after respiration ceased, so resuscitation was possible by stopping the administration. However, this sequence of events did not apply to the sudden chloroform deaths, so the overdosage explanation had to be altered to envision a sudden deep inspiration, which would develop a high concentration of vapor in the lungs, sufficient to cause overdosage and death.

Anesthetists went to great lengths in attempts to limit the concentration of chloroform and to administer as little of the vapor as possible at all times, but sudden chloroform deaths continued to occur. Silk, in 1892, presented statistics to show that between 20 and 36 deaths from chloroform had occurred annually in England alone from 1880 to 1890, and these figures did not include the deaths in Scotland or Ireland. Hayward wrote, "The truth is, that chloroform, when inhaled, acts on the system in a way that is not well understood, and may destroy life in spite of the utmost caution. Its effects are so sudden, that no foresight can prevent a fatal result."

In was, in fact, almost three-quarters of a century after Hannah Greener's death before the true explanation of sudden chloroform deaths was demonstrated. Dr. A. Goodman Levy performed a brilliant series of researches which he summarized in a presentation to the Section on Anaesthetics of the Royal Society of Medicine on May 1, 1914, titled, "Sudden death under light chloroform anaesthesia" (Levy, A. G., *Proc. Roy. Soc. Med.*, 7: 57–84, 1914). The first part of this paper is reprinted below, and the second part will be published in the October issue of *Survey*.

SUDDEN DEATH UNDER LIGHT CHLOROFORM ANAESTHESIA

A. GOODMAN LEVY, M.D.

Proc. Roy. Soc. Med., 7:57–84, 1914

* * * *

"Death from ventricular fibrillation under chloroform may be observed under any of the following and applied clinical conditons:—

(A) During the induction and early stages of the administration of chloroform, and exceptionally later in the administration: (i) during struggles and excitement; (ii) on removal of the chloroform; (iii) on abrupt re-administration of chloroform after removal, or its sudden increase during a period of very light anaesthesia; (iv) by any combination of these occurrences.

(B) During operation. By strong sensory stimuli under light anaesthesia.

(C) After operation. On removal of the chloroform, specially after a short operation."

* * * *

1915

Published February, 1965

Carbon dioxide holds unique positions in the life cycles of the flora and fauna of our planet, and indeed is essential to cellular and multicellular organisms in both aquatic and atmospheric environs. The geologic origin of carbon dioxide goes back well over a billion years, and the substance abounds in the earth's atmosphere, its rivers and lakes, its soil and its seas. The carbon dioxide of the atmosphere may have had its source from volcanoes or hot springs, or it may have been of biologic origin (if life, in fact, had *its* own origin in an anaerobic world). In either event, during the course of evolution, carbon dioxide became an essential part of the internal environment of all organisms; and some organisms which were unable to satisfy these internal needs by endogenous production of carbon dioxide became dependent upon the external carbon dioxide of the atmosphere. Thus, the substance plays a crucial role in the photosynthesis of plants, and an equally crucial role in the physiology of the more complex mammalian organisms.

In man, carbon dioxide excess provokes physiologic changes that can be of considerable moment. Respiratory stimulation is among the most prominent effects, and increasing the carbon dioxide content of the bloodstream increases both the rate and the depth of respiration, presumably due to excitation of the respiratory center(s). Carbon dioxide excess produces crisp and consistent tachycardia and hypertension, myocardial depression, increased cardiac output, and on occasion arrhythmias of serious import. These sometimes contradictory findings result from significant elevations of both epinephrine and norepinephrine levels, since carbon dioxide stimulates the sympathoadrenal system to release catecholamines. In similar fashion, the pituitary is stimulated by carbon dioxide (and the epinephrine which *it* releases) to increase the blood level of ACTH; and this, in turn, increases steroid production by the adrenal cortex and raises the concentration of arterial plasma 17-OH corticosteroids. Carbon dioxide increases cerebral blood flow and decreases cerebral vascular resistance, but high concentrations decrease the metabolic rate of brain tissue in response to the narcotic effect of carbon dioxide upon cerebral cells.

These physiologic effects can be of some considerable concern during the administration of anesthesia. Some provide defense against the chemical disturbances, while others are antagonistic reactions which tend to check or limit the primary action. It remains a moot point, however, whether moderate, short term degrees of hypercarbia are entirely harmful, for the homeostatic responses to carbon dioxide are certainly usually effective in the presence of hypercarbia of an extent ordinarily found in man during general anesthesia. Indeed, within the memory of a good many readers of *Survey* is the era when the anesthetized patient breathed spontaneously throughout operation and the application of a hand to a rebreathing bag was almost a sin! This, of course, was a sin in itself, and in time came to be recognized as such; but in any case, the advent of new and potent drugs made it mandatory to aid the body to rid itself of carbon dioxide, since this could not be accomplished by a drug depressed respiratory center and a paralyzed thorax. The anesthetist has accomplished this by assisting or controlling respirations to maintain sufficient alveolar ventilation to remove carbon dioxide excess from the blood stream, and by developing methods to then remove the carbon dioxide from the atmosphere within the anesthetic apparatus.

The anesthetist's interest in carbon dioxide goes back to the time of John Snow, who recognized that expired air contained carbon dioxide, and that breathing from a closed container made it necessary to remove the carbon dioxide. Snow self-experimented briefly with the concept of carbon dioxide absorption during respiration from a closed system; but throughout most of anesthesia's first seven decades, administration was from open or semi-open systems, and the problem of carbon dioxide accumulation was ignored—presumably because it was unrecognized. In 1915, however, Dennis E. Jackson, a pharmacologist concerned with the cost of research, developed a method of removing carbon dioxide from exhaled atmospheres of gaseous or volatilized anesthetic drugs which permitted continuous rebreathing from a closed container by the experimental animal, and which, incidentally, lowered the cost of nitrous oxide-oxygen anesthesia in Jackson's laboratory from about $2.50 per hour to 32 cents per hour. His studies were the immediate forerunners of the development of closed carbon dioxide absorption systems as they are known in clinical anesthesia today, and in 1963 the American Society of Anesthesiologists presented its Distinguished Service Award to Dr. Jackson in signal tribute to the significance of his contribution. His investigations were published under the title, "A New Method for the Production of General Analgesia and An-

aesthesia with a Description of the Apparatus Used" (Jackson, D. E.: *J. Lab. & Clin. Med.*, *1:* 1–12, 1915), and are reprinted below.

A NEW METHOD FOR THE PRODUCTION OF GENERAL ANALGESIA AND ANAESTHESIA WITH A DESCRIPTION OF THE APPARATUS USED

D. E. JACKSON, M.D., PH.D.

St. Louis, Missouri

J. Lab. & Clin. Med., 1: 1–12, 1915

"In the following paragraphs there will be described a method for the production and maintenance of prolonged general analgesia or anaesthesia by means of nitrous oxide, ethyl chloride, ether, chloroform, ethyl bromide, "somnoform," etc., with oxygen. The method involves a continuous process of rebreathing of the gaseous or volatized anaesthetics from which the exhaled carbon dioxide, etc., have been removed and to which oxygen is constantly added in proportions suitable to maintain the patient in a satisfactory condition. The method involves the use of special apparatus which is so arranged as to give the anaesthetist complete control of every phase of the anaesthesia at all times. In the apparatus here described great care has been taken to provide safety devices. So far I have had an opportunity to try this method only on animals, but there seems to be good reason to expect that in man results entirely comparable to those produced in animals may be readily obtainable. It is chiefly with this object in view that I have carried out a long series of experiments by this method."

*   *   *   *

1916

Published October and December, 1964

The adequacy of ventilation during anesthesia has become of widespread concern only during the last 20 years or so. Prior to that time, the mere presence of spontaneous respirations was often the major interest; and even the extremes of respiratory rate—profound bradypnea or profound tachypnea—were not always cause for urgent alarm. Thanks to Guedel, considerable attention *was* paid to the rhythm of respiration, the type of breathing, and the extent of intercostal as compared to diaphragmatic activity; but this was more to judge the depth of anesthesia than it was a concern over satisfactory respiratory exchange.

Today, the adequacy of ventilation during anesthesia is a matter of great concern, and it is a poorly equipped operating room suite that does not have facilities for the actual measurement of respiratory parameters. It is true that there are some anesthesiologists—particularly those of the older school—who regard anesthesia as an empirical art and who are content to make very few measurements of any type, relying, rather, on experience, intuition, and the feel of the bag; but the trend is away from "flying by the seat of the pants" in anesthesia as it is in aviation, and the present day anesthesiologist tends to seek a more scientific basis for his anesthetic practice and more objective means of following and controlling the progress of his patients. As a result, scientific tools that were the province of those engaged in research but a few years ago have become clinical tools that are now in daily use in the operating room.

The tools which measure the adequacy of ventilation, and more specifically the adequacy of *alveolar* ventilation, are a prime example. Only a few years ago, the determination of pH, carbon dioxide tension, and oxygen saturation in an anesthetized patient was a formidable procedure,

and one that was rarely performed except as a research exercise: it required an arterial sample of blood; a long and tedious analysis of the blood by a laboratory technician; and calculations, that were often beyond the ken of many of those who were administering the anesthesia, for the interpretation of the results. As more and more such studies were performed, however, it became evident that here was information of inestimable value in the conduct of clinical anesthesia. Anesthesiologists came to realize that knowledge of the acid-base status of the anesthetized patient's blood was a sensitive indication of the adequacy of alveolar ventilation, and that deviations from normal could provide an early and reliable warning of future trouble. Now, with the development of electrodes to measure pH, pCO_2 and pO_2, blood gas analysis has been tremendously simplified, and monitory of the acid-base status of the anesthetized patient has become a more commonplace procedure. This change represents a major advance in the application of objective measurement to clinical anesthetic practice and a giant step forward in the care of the surgical patient during operation.

Behind this development, and indeed fundamental to understanding the concept of acid-base equilibrium and its regulation, is the Henderson-Haselbalch Equation. Two of Henderson's papers, entitled, "Concerning the Relationship Between the Strength of Acids and Their Capacity to Preserve Neutrality" (Henderson, T. H.: *Am. J. Physiol.*, 21: 173–179, 1908), and "The Theory of Neutrality Regulation in the Animal Organism" (Henderson, L. J.: *Am. J. Physiol.*, 21: 427–448, 1908), are reprinted below. A translation of Hasselbalch's contribution, entitled, "Die Berechnung der Wasserstoffzahl des Blutes aus der freien und gebundenen Kohlensaure desselben, und die Sauerstoffbindung des

Blutes als Funktion der Wasserstoffzahl" (Hasselbalch, K. A.: *Biochem. Zeitschr.*, 78: 112–144, 1916) will be published in the December issue as the final "Classical File" in this year's volume of *Survey of Anesthesiology*.

CALCULATION OF THE HYDROGEN ION CONCENTRATION OF BLOOD FROM FREE AND BOUND CARBON DIOXIDE; OXYGEN BINDING AS A FUNCTION OF PH

K. A. HASSELBALCH

From the Laboratories of the Finsen Institute, Copenhagen

Received 7 October, 1916
With 12 Figures

Biochem., Zeitschr., 78:112–144, 1916

*   *   *   *

SUMMARY

"I. The hydrogen ion concentration of blood can be calculated more accurately by gas analysis, from the quantities of free and bound carbon dioxide, than by electrometry. Normally it is $10^{-7.33}$ at 40 mm. CO_2 tension.

"II. We now had to know the dissociation of carbonic acid at 38°. That carbonic acid at 38° is significantly more dissociated than at 18° we found to be in good agreement with Jul. Thomsen's thermochemical measurements.

"III. Bound CO_2 in blood is available solely as bicarbonate. With falling CO_2 tension, bound CO_2 decreases principally because oxyhemoglobin is to be considered a stronger acid in the presence of an alkaline reaction.

"IV. The amphoteric character of oxyhemoglobin in particular and, to a small degree, of the remaining blood proteins provides the uncommonly great stability of blood against shifts of pH. This stability applies as much to addition of acids as to influence of temperature and becomes even more important physiologically because the acid effect of oxyhemoglobin in the circulation due to increasing CO_2 tension is diminished by partial conversion to reduced hemoglobin.

"V. Using a larger human sample, we confirmed the correlation which Peters and Barcroft had demonstrated in one case between pH and constant K of Hill's formula for oxygen binding of blood. This principle apparently varied to some extent for beef, pig and pigeon blood.

"Reduced pH (pH at 40 mm, CO_2 tension) is decreased by about 0.03 in the blood of pregnant women."

Published October, 1972

Joseph Priestley was one of those who believed in the phlogiston theory.

Priestley was an erstwhile Unitarian minister who was driven from his pulpit—and his service to the church was abruptly terminated—by riots in which his house was pillaged and burned because of his known sympathies for the French Revolution. He eventually fled from England and settled in Northumberland, Pennsylvania, but not until after he had been elected 1 of the 8 associates of the French Academy of Sciences and a member of the Imperial Academy of Sciences at St. Petersburg. Which brings us back to the phlogiston theory.

The phlogiston theory, which was plausible, but erroneous, was first evolved by Joachim Becher in the latter half of the 17th century, and then was warmly championed and elaborated upon by his pupil, Georg Ernst Stahl. The theory postulated the existence of a mysterious element, "the material of fire," which was dubbed phlogiston by Stahl and which was supposed to be the essential constituent of all combustible bodies and play a part in respiration also. The fact that both life and combustion eventually became extinct in a confined space was held to be due to the air becoming completely saturated with phlogiston!

Priestley, like many of the physiologists, chemists, and philosophers of that day and age, subscribed wholeheartedly to the phlogiston theory; in the summer of 1774 he performed a series of experiments in which he produced an "air" by focusing a burning-lens onto a sample of mercuric oxide enclosed in a glass vessel inverted over mercury: "By means of this lens, air was expelled from it (the mercuric oxide) very readily. Having got about three or four times as much as the bulk of my materials, I admitted water to it, and found that it was not imbibed by it. But what surprised me more than I can well express, was, that a candle burned in the air with a remarkably vigorous flame."

He continued his experiments through the fall and winter, and by March of 1775 he was investigating the respirability of the "new" air. He discovered that, not only would a mouse live longer in the "new" air than in an equal volume of "common" air, but that there was "a diminution of 2/9 in a short time" of the residual air which the mouse had breathed. He concluded that this superiority of the "new" air lay in a greater capacity for absorbing phlogiston, and he reasoned that the gas originally contained less phlogiston than common air: accordingly, he named it dephlogisticated air, and a letter from Priestley about dephlogisticated air was read to the Royal Society on March 23, 1775.

It remained for Lavoisier to name the "new" air oxygen, and to show it was consumed during respiration; but it was almost a century before its importance in anesthesia was recognized, when, in 1868, Edmund Andrews, a Chicago surgeon, wrote the following. "Every surgeon has seen the prompt and pleasant anaesthetic action of the nitrous oxide gas, so much used by dentists, and has wished that in some way it might be made available in general surgery. The patient usually goes under the influence in 30 or 40 seconds, and wakes with equal promptness, without vomiting or other unpleasant symptoms, all of which is in striking contrast with the slowness, the nausea, and the discomforts of chloroform and ether. There have been, however, great obstacles to the use of the gas, owing to its evanescent action. The oxygen contained in it is in a state of chemical combination, so that it is not available for oxygenation of the blood; hence if any attempt is made to continue its action, the patient becomes purple in the face, showing all the signs of asphyxia; subsultus tendinum then supervenes, and shortly after he almost ceases to breathe, and, if allowed nothing but pure nitrous oxide, would doubtless die in a few minutes."

He went on to say, "I have for some time been experimenting, to see whether by the addition of free oxygen to the nitrous oxide, a mixture would not be obtained, by which a patient might be anaesthetized for an indefinite period without danger of asphyxia, and thus render gas available for the most prolonged operations of surgery. . . . It seems probable that the oxygen mixture will enable us to anaesthetize a patient for the longest as well as for the shortest surgical operations, and that it is safer and pleasanter than any anaesthetic known."

The absolute necessity for oxygen during general anesthesia, particularly general anesthesia produced by nitrous oxide, was documented in Courville's monograph-length classic in *Medicine*, "Asphyxia as a Consequence of Nitrous Oxide Anesthesia," which was published in 1936. Courville was a neuropathologist of great repute, and his descriptions of the pathologic lesions following anoxia are beyond compare. He was smart enough to recognize that there were a number of predisposing influences (idiosyncrasy, thymus lymphaticus, alcoholism, robust build, pulmonary conditions, heart disease, anemia, cerebral disease, and reflex effects) and also factors involved in the administration (impurities of the nitrous oxide, defects in the apparatus, poorly trained anesthetists, and obstruction of the upper airway), which could lead to anoxemia during nitrous oxide anesthesia. However, despite his brilliant account of the pathologic changes produced, Courville made the mistake of believing that the anoxemia state was an integral part of nitrous oxide anesthesia; for although it was some years before Faulconer proved it, anesthesiologists knew nitrous oxide was not inherently anoxic and that it was the amount of oxygen administered along with it which determined the anoxemic state.

There then followed the "if-a-little-oxygen-is-a-good-thing-why-then-a-lot-of-it-is-even-better" era of oxygenation. An oxygen tent was better than a nasal catheter because it promised higher tensions of inhaled oxygen, and an oxygen mask was best of all because it promised the most oxygen. In the same vein, cyclopropane was a much better anesthetic than nitrous oxide or ethylene because good anesthesia was obtainable at the same time that high concentrations of oxygen were being administered. One hundred per cent oxygen was the ultimate in oxygen therapy; when the internist ventured into the operating room (which he seldom did), he was absolutely delighted to see the anesthesiologist "giving all that oxygen."

The High Oxygen Era lasted until Terry's description of retrolental fibroplasia, and the role which oxygen played in its production, in 1942. At that point, some caution began to be practiced in regard to the long term treatment of the premature newborn infant with 100 per cent oxygen; however, it was not really until the resurgence of hyperbaric oxygenation in the 1950's that oxygen toxicity became more than an academic and/or military curiosity. It was then recalled that Paul Bert commented upon the toxic effects of oxygen in several different passages in his monumental book, *Barometric Pressure*, which was published in 1877; and that Lorraine Smith published a dissertation on the pathologic effects of increased oxygen tension in 1899. Perhaps the most comprehensive description of the pathology of oxygen toxicity, however, was Howard Karsner's paper, "The Pathological Effects of Atmospheres Rich in Oxygen" (Karsner, H. T.: *J. Exper. Med. 23:* 149, 1916), which is reprinted below.

THE PATHOLOGICAL EFFECTS OF ATMOSPHERES RICH IN OXYGEN

HOWARD T. KARSNER, M.D.

From the Nutrition Laboratory
of the Carnegie Institution
of Washington, Boston,
the Laboratories of Pathology
of the Harvard Medical School,
Boston, and the School of
Medicine of Western Reserve
University of Cleveland

J. Exper. Med., 23: 149, 1916

*   *   *   *

CONCLUSIONS

"In spite of numerous abnormalities or non-experimental lesions in the rabbit certain facts can be considered as established. It has been known for many years that pneumonia is produced by the more or less prolonged inhalation of high partial pressures of oxygen. The studies herein reported show that atmospheres containing 80 to 96 per cent oxygen under normal barometric pressure produce in 24 hours, or more commonly 48 hours, congestion, edema, epithelial degeneration and desquamation, fibrin formation, and finally a pneumonia, probably of irritative origin and to be described as a fibrinous bronchopneumonia. The important new points are the time relations of these changes and definition of the type of the pneumonia.

Other studies have noted slight passive congestion, but it is now established that this is to be accounted for in most cases by dilatation of the right side or of both sides of the heart. This congestion affects all the abdominal viscera and is accompanied by certain secondary changes such as cloudy swelling of the parenchymatous organs and phagocytosis of erythrocytes by endothelial cells of the mesenteric lymph nodes.

Although deficiency of oxygen may affect the hematopoietic system, the animals subjected to high oxygen percentages failed to show any demonstrable pathologic changes in blood, spleen, lymph nodes, or bone marrow, except for the presence of congestion."

1920

Published October, 1966

The syndrome of general anesthesia is characterized by a set of signs and symptoms which generally are rather constant. On occasions, however, as is true of other clinical entities, the signs and symptoms may vary widely from patient to patient. Furthermore, they may also vary in the same patient from time to time, owing to modification produced by premedication, the anesthetic drugs administered, the type of operation and the extent of the surgical stimulation, the effects upon respiration and circulation, and a large number of other factors. These inconsistencies in the signs and symptoms of the syndrome of general anesthesia, which are particularly apparent when modern drugs and techniques of anesthesia are employed, have led many to abandon attempts to analyze the depth of anesthesia (which is an ill-defined concept, at best) and simply to evaluate anesthesia as "too light, too deep, or just right."

This type of clinical intuition represents the art practiced by the experienced anesthesiologist, and is sufficient for his purposes. It lacks the precision necessary, however, if anesthesia is to advance beyond art to embrace science; and, more importantly, it does not provide aid or succor to the inexperienced anesthetist who has not developed such clinical intuition. The need, as Ralph Waters once stated it, is for "a simple and rapid means of teaching physical signs and danger signals which could be readily grasped by the uninitiated." This need to define the various "stages" of anesthesia and the signs by which they might be recognized has been understood from the very beginning. At the time of Morton's classic public demonstration of the efficacy of ether anesthesia, both Warren and Bigelow made note of the character of the pulse, the pupils, and the respiration, and of the behavior of the central nervous system and the musculature, although no attempt was made to classify these signs ac-

cording to depth of anesthesia. Within about 3 months of the introduction of anesthesia, Francis Plomley, in the January 30, 1847, issue of the *Lancet*, described one of the earliest classifications of depth of anesthesia, which was based in large measure on subjective mental sensations. He divided ether anesthesia into three "stages": "The first is merely a pleasurable feeling of half intoxication; the second is one of extreme pleasure, being similar to the sensations produced by breathing nitrous oxide, or laughing gas . . . . The third stage, the only one, I think, for performing operations in, is one of profound intoxication and insensibility." Within a matter of months after Plomley's communication, John Snow carefully divided the course of etherization into five "degrees," the first three of which occurred during induction and the other two during the period in which the patient was unconscious and quiet (*i.e.*, during "surgical anesthesia"). Snow's classification relied upon the anesthetist's objective observations of physical signs, and it is to Snow that we owe our recognition of the conjunctival reflex, deep and regular automatic breathing, the movement of the eyeballs, and the inhibition of the activity of the intercostal muscles.

Snow's classification has been improved upon but never really replaced, and from the time of Snow until World War I it was customary to divide anesthesia into four stages:

1. *Induction.* From the beginning of the administration until the loss of consciousness.

2. *The stage of struggling, or breathholding, or delirium, or dreams.* From the loss of consciousness to the onset of surgical anesthesia.

3. *Surgical anesthesia.* Characterized by deep, regular, automatic breathing and loss of the corneal reflex.

4. *Overdose, or stage of bulbar paralysis.*

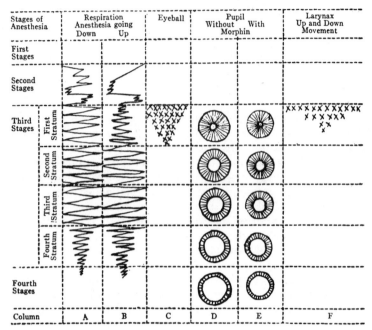

Stages of Anesthesia	Respiration Anesthesia going		Eyeball	Pupil Without With Morphin		Larynax Up and Down Movement
	Down	Up				
First Stages						
Second Stages						
Third Stages	First Stratum			◉	◉	
	Second Stratum			◉	◉	
	Third Stratum			◉	◉	
	Fourth Stratum			◯	◯	
Fourth Stages				◯	◯	
Column	A	B	C	D	E	F

Fig. 1. Schematic chart showing the significance of certain reflexes under various stages of ether anesthesia.

Shallow, irregular respirations, and dilated pupils which no longer react to light.

The exigencies of war brought great refinement to this broad and general classification. Arthur E. Guedel, "the father of modern anesthesia," found himself a member of the medical corps of the A.E.F., riding up and down the western front on a motorcycle from base hospital to base hospital, attempting to instruct and supervise untrained, inexperienced enlisted men in the art of anesthesia. To do this required abandonment of his own highly developed clinical intuition in favor of a charted set of physical signs and danger signals which could be utilized by his uninitiated personnel. These were published, in part, after the war under the title "Third Stage Ether: a Subclassification Regarding the Significance of the Position and Movements of the Eyeball," (*American Journal of Surgery*, *34:* 53–57, 1920), and are reprinted below with the kind permission of the publisher.

THIRD STAGE ETHER ANESTHESIA: A SUB-CLASSIFICATION

REGARDING THE SIGNIFICANCE OF THE POSITION AND MOVEMENTS OF THE EYEBALL*

ARTHUR E. GUEDEL, M.D.,

Indianapolis, Indiana

Am. J. Surg., 34:53–57, 1920

*   *   *   *

"VALUE OF EYEBALL AND PUPIL

In my experience, which includes over 10,000 cases conducted personally and by my assistants in France, the eyeball with its position and movements has afforded a sign which, in proper classification, is reliable and cannot be ignored. The oscillation marks the stage of ideal anesthesia after the first ten or fifteen minutes of administration has elapsed.

* Read before the Indianapolis Medical Society, April 1919; the Indiana State Medical Association, at Indianapolis, September, 1919, and the Sixth Annual Meeting of the Interstate Association of Anesthetists, at Cincinnati, September 15–17, 1919.

I have divided third stage ether anesthesia into four strata. The accompanying chart presents a correlation of the various signs found in the different strata of the third stage. Attention is called in this paper only to the third stage, inasmuch as there is nothing new to be said of the first, second and fourth stages. The chart consists of columns A, B, C, D, E and F, and takes into consideration various signs separately and in conjunction with each other."

* * * *

CONCLUSIONS

"1. This is a plea for lighter and better anesthesia.

2. It is a plea for better teaching of anesthesia in our medical schools and hospitals.

3. As long as we note any movement or eccentric position of the eyeball, aside from that which might be normal for the occasional patient, that patient has not had too much anesthetic; but after anesthesia has been well inaugurated, he has had quite enough.

4. The upper part of the third stage, namely, the first stratum, is anesthesia entirely as satisfactory to the surgeon as the second, third or fourth stratum of the third stage."

1921

Published August, 1968

It is intriguing how frequently the clinical usage of a drug may change with the passage of time.

Thiopental, for instance, is seldom employed by the competent anesthesiologist today except as a hypnotic to induce anesthesia. Through the years it has come to be recognized that thiopental is not only not a good analgesic, but is even antanalgesic—a most unfortunate term, but one which nevertheless manages to convey the message. Furthermore, it does not produce muscular relaxation, for although the pharmacologist has been able to demonstrate an action at the myoneural junction in the laboratory animal, this effect is of absolutely no clinical significance or usefulness. Finally, thiopental, rather than obtunding noxious reflex activity—as a good anesthetic should—actually enhances it, at least under certain clinical circumstances.

Yet when thiopental was introduced, it was advocated as, and employed for, total anesthesia. One of the early authoritative writings stated:

"From 2 to 5 cc. of a 2.5 per cent solution of pentothal sodium often is sufficient for induction of anesthesia; occasionally, as much as 0.25 gm. is required, rarely as much as 0.5 gm. . . . Once anesthesia has become established and the incision has been made, it is not difficult to maintain anesthesia by injection of 1 or 2 cc. of the solution whenever the patient phonates or moves. The largest doses that we have used have been in operations on the brain.

In one case a dose of 33 grains (2.2 gm.) was used and in two other cases, 45 grains (3 gm.). The operation in each case lasted about three and a half hours."

Succinylcholine is another drug whose usage has changed over the course of the years. When succinylcholine was introduced, it was hailed as the ideal muscle relaxant because its brief and fleeting action allowed it to be employed in a dilute infusion to provide controllable muscle relaxation. The latter persisted as long as the infusion was flowing, could be increased by speeding up the infusion, and terminated when the infusion was discontinued. One of the first clinical reports stated:

"The techniques by which succinylcholine has been employed have varied according to the degree and duration of muscular relaxation desired. Herein lies the great advantage of the drug—almost absolute controllability of both the degree and duration of relaxation. Muscular paralysis may be kept at a level just below that of normal muscular tone, may be carried to apnea and total flaccidity, or to any intermediate stage. Similarly, the desired degree of relaxation may be maintained for a minute or two, or may be sustained for many hours, and perhaps even longer."

The first change in the use of succinylcholine came when a number of cases of prolonged postoperative apnea began to be reported. These observations caused considerable concern; and when it was demonstrated that succinylmonocholine, one of the breakdown products of the hydrolysis of succinylcholine by plasma pseudocholinesterase, was in itself a muscle relaxant (much less potent, but much longer acting than succinylcholine), some anesthesiologists arbitrarily set a limit on the amount of succinylcholine which might be safely infused. The concept was that, as more and more succinylcholine was infused, more and more succinylmonocholine was produced and "piled up" in the bloodstream, all of which resulted in a prolonged neuromuscular block. At first the limit was set at 1 gram an hour; then it became 0.5 gram an hour; and finally it became 250 milligrams an hour.

At this point, a second change in the use of succinylcholine began to become evident. It was demonstrated that, with continued administration of the drug, the character of the block produced at the myoneural junction changed from a phase I to a phase II block, and it was considered that this change could account for the prolonged responses to succinylcholine which were sometimes encountered. The subsequent publication of data suggesting that phase II block (dual block, desensitization block) existed from the onset of the use of a drug such as succinylcholine led some anesthesiologists to abandon the use of the continuous infusion technique altogether and to use succinylcholine only for brief periods of relaxation (such as to facilitate endotracheal intubation), relying on a longer acting relaxant such as curare (for which there is a reliable antagonist) for the maintenance of relaxation.

It has been suggested that the recovery from dual block may be just as rapid as that from depolarization block, and that prolonged recovery is due not to the dual block but to frank overdosage. It has been further suggested that frank overdosage can be avoided by routine monitoring of the magnitude of the block with a peripheral nerve stimulator. This development could lead to yet a third change in the use of succinylcholine—a trend back to the continuous infusion technique!

Nitrous oxide is still another drug employed in anesthesia whose usage has changed drastically in the course of time. Nitrous oxide today is employed as a vehicle gas and for its analgesic properties, for it is recognized that it has limited potency and is not a total anesthetic. There was a time, however, when it was used as the sole anesthetic agent to produce total anesthesia—including all of the facets of anesthesia: hypnosis, analgesia, muscular relaxation, and obtundation of noxious reflex activity. The technique by which this end was accomplished was known as "secondary saturation": it was described by McKesson in a paper entitled, "Primary and Secondary Nitrous Oxide Saturation for Relaxation and as a Test of the Patient's Capacity for Operation" (McKesson, E. I.: *Can. Med. Ass. J.* 11: 130–136, 1921) and is reprinted below with the kind permission of the publishers.

PRIMARY AND SECONDARY NITROUS OXIDE SATURATION FOR RELAXATION AND AS A TEST OF THE PATIENT'S CAPACITY FOR OPERATIONS

McKESSON, E.J.

Can. Med. Assoc. J., 11: 130–136, 1921

A remarkable paper which begins with "In the primary, or induction stage of nitrous oxide oxygen anaesthesia, it is the usual practice to administer 100 per cent nitrous oxide to produce unconsciousness as soon as possible by a primary saturation of the blood with the anaesthetic gas. Very soon however, a small amount of oxygen must be mixed with the nitrous oxide to prevent the jactitations and other manifestations of acute anoxaemia. Now, if some fixed proportion of oxygen is decided upon it will be found too small for some and too great for others, since patients differ in their mixture requirements." . . . "In a primary saturation only the actively circulating blood is saturated before oxygen must be administered. There remains in the muscles, and in all other tissues, considerable volumes of nitrogen and oxygen, which in the early minutes of narcosis, enter the blood stream and dilute the nitrous oxide, thereby preventing deeper anaesthesia. In order to displace more of the nonanaesthetic gases in the body with nitrous oxide, the technic to be described as secondary saturation has been devised." These clinical observations on the uptake and distribution of N_2O antedate the chemical studies of Haggard on distribution of ether in the dog. The anesthetic technique described provided the case material for Courville's monograph on the pathologic brain lesions of hypoxia.

Published October, 1967

The existence of neurohumoral transmitter substances at the myoneural junctions of skeletal muscles, between autonomic nerves and their effector cells, and even within the central nervous system itself, is generally accepted by the majority of physiologists and pharmacologists; and the theory of neurohumoral transmission (that is, the concept that nerves transmit their impulses across most synapses and neuroeffector junctions by means of specific chemical agents, called neurohumoral transmitters) is the basis for the administration of a considerable number of drugs employed today in the clinical practice of anesthesiology.

In actual fact, however, the existence of these neurohumoral transmitters is knowledge of comparatively recent origin. Until the turn of the century, it was largely supposed that the transmission of excitation from the nerve terminals to effector cells was an electrical action current. One bit of evidence in opposition to this concept, however, was the "synaptic delay" which clearly occurs and is difficult to explain in terms of an electrical impulse. The first reference to the possibility that chemical substances might be concerned was contained in the suggestion by Dubois-Reymond in 1877 that transmission of the nerve impulse might be produced either electrically by action currents or chemically by exciting substances such as ammonia or lactic acid formed at the surface of the nerve endings. Then, in 1901, Langley pointed out that, when adrenal extracts were injected, the effects appeared to mimic the effects produced by the stimulation of sympathetic nerves. Three years later, in 1904, T. R. Elliott hypothesized that sympathetic nerve impulses release minute amounts of an epinephrine-like substance in immediate contact with effector cells, and that this substance was the chemical step in the process of transmission.

On the other side of the autonomic system, Langley, in 1904, on the basis of his studies with pilocarpine, and Dixon, in 1907, in more detailed studies with muscarine, recognized that the effects of these drugs mimicked the effects of stimulation of the parasympathetic nerves. Dixon postulated that "excitation of a nerve induces the local liberation of a hormone which causes specific activity by combination with some constituent of the end-organ, muscle or gland."

It was the brilliant researches of Otto Loewi, however, which established the first real proof of the chemical mediation of nerve impulses by the peripheral release of specific chemical agents; and he has described the circumstances surrounding the performance of the classical experiments which earned him a Nobel Prize in his autobiography which was published in 1960, the year before his death:

"As far back as 1903, I discussed with Walter M. Fletcher from Cambridge, England, then an associate in Marburg, the fact that certain drugs mimic the augmentory as well as the inhibitory effects of the stimulation of sympathetic and/or parasympathetic nerves on their effector organs. During this discussion, the idea occurred to me that the terminals of those nerves might contain chemicals, that stimulation might liberate them from the nerve terminals, and that these chemicals might in turn transmit the nervous impulse to their respective effector organs. At that time, I did not see a way to prove the correctness of this hunch, and it entirely slipped my conscious memory until it emerged again in 1920.

"The night before Easter Sunday of that year, I awoke, turned on the light, and jotted down a few notes on a tiny slip of thin paper. Then I fell asleep again. It occurred to me at six o'clock in the morning that during the night I had written down something most important, but I was unable to decipher the scrawl. The next night, at three o'clock, the idea returned. It was the design of an experiment to determine whether or not the hypothesis of chemical transmission that I had uttered seventeen years ago was correct. I got up immediately, went to the laboratory, and performed a simple experiment on a frog heart according to the nocturnal design."

This experiment, which became the foundation of the theory of neurohumoral or chemical transmission of nerve impulses, was described in Loewi's famous paper, "Uber humorale Ubertragbarkeit der Herznervenwirkung" (*Pfluger's Arch. ges. Physiol.*, 189: 239–242, 1921). "Classical File" and its readers are indebted to Dr. Carl S. Hellijas of the Department of Anesthesiology at Harford Hospital for his translation of this paper, which is printed below.

CONCERNING THE HUMORAL CONDUCTION

OF CARDIAC NERVE ACTIVITY

COMMUNICATION BY O. LOEWI

Performed with the Support of the Prince Liechtenstein Foundation

(With five illustrations; received March 20, 1921)

Pflüger's Arch. ges. Physiol., 189: 239–242, 1921

*   *   *   *

"*Discussion of Results.* The experiments show that, after stimulation of inhibitory and excitatory nerves, substances are demonstrated in the perfusion fluid of the heart which have the same type of effect as does nerve stimulation itself. Thus, under the influence of nerve stimulation, these substances are formed or given off, or they are formed beforehand and only then do the cells become responsive to them. There are two possible explanations for the meaning of these substances. They may arise as a direct result of nerve stimulation independent of the type of cardiac activity and may in their turn initiate specific cardiac reactivity to the nerve impulse, which would therefore be effective only indirectly. If their effect in this experimental design lags quantitatively behind that of nerve stimulation, it should be no surprise, for one must assume that only an infinitesimal amount of the substances formed in or on the cells, or given off by them, is transmitted to the perfusing fluid; in addition, this produces marked dilution. There is the second possibility that the substances are only products of the particular type of cardiac activity initiated by nerve stimulation; in this case, the identity of their effect with that of nerve stimulation would, to a certain extent, be fortuitous.

"Regarding the nature of these substances, the only thing we can exclude at the moment with respect to the products of vagal stimulation is potassium, because enhanced potassium activity is not inhibited by atropine, which was effective in our experiments."

Published June, 1961

Spinal analgesia, as an anesthetic technique, has enjoyed varying degrees of popularity that have alternated from overly enthusiastic acceptance to complete and total rejection. Curiously enough, there is nothing either strange or incongruous about this cyclical history of the popularity of spinal as a form of anesthesia, for it is the direct result of the fact that the technique possesses, at one and the same time, both superb advantages and devastating drawbacks.

Each wave of enthusiasm and acceptance has been generated by the very real benefits that spinal anesthesia can contribute to the operative care of the surgical patient. From the surgeon's point of view, perhaps no other form of anesthesia can provide such excellent muscular relaxation for pelvic and intraabdominal surgery, for not only is the reflex arc interrupted and the muscles of the abdominal wall paralyzed, but the gut is vigorously contracted by sympathetic blockade. From the patient's point of view, spinal anesthesia not only permits the retention of consciousness (which some patients dread to lose), but it also precludes the occurrence of secretions, excitement, postanesthetic nausea and vomiting, and somnolence during the immediate postoperative period that may be associated with general anesthesia. From the anesthetist's point of view, spinal anesthesia permits an approximate maintenance of the physiological *status quo* since it is accomplished by little disturbance of most metabolic processes; it also is nonflammable and so permits the use of cautery, x-ray, and other electrical appliances; and it is inexpensive in comparison with some other anesthetic agents and techniques of administration.

Nevertheless, and despite these very substantial advantages, spinal anesthesia has been accompanied on occasions by untoward results which, when they have occurred frequently, have ultimately led to a wave of rejection. Spinal anesthesia may be quite uncontrollable as to duration of block, so that on the one hand it cannot be terminated when deleterious effects do occur; nor, on the other hand, can it be extended (except by the use of continuous techniques or vasopressors) when the operation outlasts the anesthesia. Spinal anesthesia may also be uncontrollable as to the extent of block, and both respiratory depression (from high motor block) and distressing circulatory changes (from autonomic block) may result from its administration. The most malevolent disadvantage of spinal anesthesia, however, is the occurrence of postoperative neurologic changes, which may range all the way from simple postspinal headache to cranial nerve palsies, cauda equina syndrome, and ascending myelitis.

The frequency of untoward results, either immediate or late, following spinal anesthesia, is inversely proportional to the intelligence of application and the meticulousness of attention to detail employed by the anesthetist administering this form of anesthesia. The fact that spinal anesthesia has persisted in the anesthetist's armamentarium for over sixty years, despite occasional untoward results and subsequent waves of rejection, only serves to emphasize the inherent great advantages of the technique.

It is not surprising, then, that another regional technique, possessing many of the inherent advantages of spinal anesthesia, yet obviating a number of the more distressing and dire disadvantages, has become increasingly popular and in many instances has supplanted spinal anesthesia. The reference, of course, is to epidural anesthesia, which was employed with varying degrees of success by such men as Corning, Sicard, Cathelin, Tuffier and Heile in the period from 1885 to 1913, but was really developed by the Spaniard, Fidel Pagés, working at the General Hospital of Madrid in 1920 and 1921. *Survey of Anesthesiology* and its readers are indebted to Dr. Gordon P. Lowther and Dr. Juan Escudero for the translation into English of Pagés' article on spinal epidural anesthesia, entitled "Anestesia Metamerica", which was published in the June and July, 1921, issues of *Revista de Sanidad Militar* (Pagés, F.: *Rev. san. mil., Madrid, 11:* 351–365,

June; 385–396, July, 1921) and is reprinted below.

SEGMENTAL ANAESTHESIA

F. Pagés Miravé

General Hospital, Madrid

Rev. san. mil. Madrid, 11: 351–365 and 385–396, 1921

"Last November, whilst giving a spinal anaesthetic, it occurred to me to block the nerves between the intervertebral spaces and the meninges rather than pierce the dura. Instead of using the Stovaine which I had ready, I used a Type A Novocaine-adrenaline preparation containing 375 mg. of Novocaine and 25 ml. of normal saline in a galley pot, injecting it through the needle which was lying between the 2nd and 3rd lumbar vertebrae.

"On testing sensation five minutes later, pain appreciation was clearly reduced, commencing below the umbilicus and spreading to the antero-lateral surfaces of the lower limbs. At this time, however, there was no loss of sensation over the perineum and posterior surfaces of the lower limbs or the soles of the feet. Analgesia gradually increased until, twenty minutes after the injection, it was sufficient to permit the repair of a right inguinal hernia without the patient experiencing any discomfort.

"This result encouraged us to study the method further and we called it "Segmental Anaesthesia" since the loss of sensation could be confined to a limited number of spinal segments, leaving those above and below unaffected by the block."

* * * *

OPERATIONS CARRIED OUT UNDER SEGMENTAL ANAESTHESIA TO DATE

Repair of inguinal hernia	18
Repair of femoral hernia	3
Appendicectomy	4
Gastroenterostomy	2
Gastrectomy	1
Freeing of adhesions following appendicectomy	1
Cholecystectomy & exploration of common bile duct	2
Nephroplexy	1
Resection for drainage of effusions etc. (anaesthesia inadequate in one case)	2
Operation on calcaneum	2
Amputation of thigh	1
Arthrotomy of knee	1
Dislocated shoulder (anaesthetic failure)	1
Haemorrhoidectomy	1
Hydrocoele	2
Block dissection of glands of neck (analgesia complete but patient collapsed)	1
Total	43

"These results, considering that they represent the first cases in which segmental anaesthesia has been employed, are to my mind acceptable and justify further investigations."

1923

Published April, 1960

The florists of Chicago found carnations in curiously short supply in 1908. It was not that it was a "bad year" for carnations, for the growers had produced even more than in previous years, but the carnation growers had met with serious losses on their shipments to Chicago. The carnations which had been shipped to Chicago and placed in greenhouses seemed to "go to sleep." Buds of flowers which at the time of shipment showed petals and seemed destined to open into full bloom in the immediate future failed to do so. This strange behavior on the part of apparently normal carnations piqued the scientific interest of but few, although it was of considerable financial interest to the bewildered carnation growers. Two botanists of the Hull Botanical Laboratory, however, William Crocker and Lee Irving Knight, did go to work on the problem of these ailing flowers. Considerable research demonstrated that it was the illuminating gas which was used to heat the greenhouses into which the carnations were shipped from the growers that was the offender; and Crocker and Knight demonstrated further that ethylene, which comprises about 4 per cent of illuminating gas, was the major culprit.

The solution of this mystery received but passing attention, and then was buried deep in the pages of the *Botanical Gazette*. Buried, but not forgotten: for a decade later, Arno Benedict Luckhardt, University of Chicago physiologist, became intrigued with the fatal effects of ethylene on carnations, castor oil plants and sweet pea seedlings. Because of these toxic effects of ethylene on plants, Luckhardt began to study the effects of the drug on animals. These researches were interrupted temporarily by the Great War, but when resumed thereafter, in collaboration with J. B. Carter, confirmed the exciting discovery that ethylene did not kill, only anesthetized animals.

In retrospect, perhaps the discovery should not have caused that amount of excitement: Ludimar Hermann noted a mildly intoxicating action of ethylene as early as 1864; Eulenberg presented experimental evidence of the anesthetic qualities of ethylene in 1876; and Sir Benjamin Ward Richardson found ethylene to be an admirable agent for general anesthesia. Nevertheless, these reports were either hidden away in the German literature or had not been formally published; so Luckhardt *was* excited and sufficiently so to extend his studies to other animals, to Carter and himself, and to other volunteer workers. Luckhardt and Carter reported their preliminary experiences with ethylene as a gaseous anesthetic early in 1923, but the classic account of ethylene anesthesia was published by Luckhardt and Dean Lewis later that same year in the *Journal of the American Medical Association, 81:* 1851–1857, December 1, 1923, under the title of "Clinical Experiences with Ethylene-Oxygen-Anesthesia."

CLINICAL EXPERIENCES WITH ETHYLENE-OXYGEN ANESTHESIA

ARNO B. LUCKHARDT, PH.D., M.D.
AND DEAN LEWIS, M.D.

Chicago

J.A.M.A., 81: 1851–1857, 1923

"Several months ago, a preliminary report was published on the use of ethylene gas as an anesthetic in a series of 106 operative cases. A previous report presented a rather detailed study of the physiologic action of the gas on the usual laboratory animals, including a number of normal men. Since that time the number of operations performed at the Presbyterian Hospital, Chicago, has risen to some 800. In the preliminary communication on the clinical phases of the work, certain important facts received no mention at all, and others were ascertained only as the work progressed. Our attention was furthermore called to some earlier literature on ethylene which we had overlooked in spite of what we considered a thorough search. These reasons have prompted us to issue this report."

*   *   *   *

1924

Published October, 1957

The clinical utility of anesthetic agents usually has been appreciated months, years, or even decades, before the modus operandi of those agents has been understood. It has been for this reason that the Art of anesthesia has remained in the ascendancy over the Science of anesthetic administration, even today. One of the problems accounting for this unfortunate state of affairs in the past has been the lack of facilities, personnel, and adequate support, for the detailed laboratory investigations necessary to elucidate all the actions of a new drug before its introduction to clinical practice. A second, and equally important problem, has been the physician's reluctance to deny his patient the known benefits of a new drug, pending the total investigation of all of its attributes. Both of these problems, naturally, were more intense at the time of the introduction of clinical anesthesia in 1846; but even the most desultory scan of the current literature on such agents as Viadril, Fluothane, the Phenothiazine derivatives, and such muscle relaxant drugs as Mylaxen, suggests that both of these problems are still present today to plague the anesthesiologist in clinical practice.

In the case of ether, and despite the remarkably keen clinical observations of such men as Snow, it was almost a century before the fundamental physical and physiologic mechanisms of action were documented by sound scientific investigation. The 1924 volume of the Journal of Biological Chemistry contained Howard Haggard's brilliant series of articles on "The Absorption, Distribution, and Elimination of Ethyl Ether." They are papers which stand out as one of the landmarks of the introduction of scientific reasoning and understanding into the administration of clinical anesthesia.

THE ABSORPTION, DISTRIBUTION, AND ELIMINATION OF ETHYL ETHER

HAGGARD, H.W.

J. Biol. Chem., 59: 737–770 (April) 1924

J. Biol. Chem., 59: 771–802 (April) 1924

Haggard's series of 5 papers dealt with the absorption, distribution, and elimination of ethyl ether.

The sections were as follows:

I. "The Amount of Ether Absorbed in Relation to the Concentration Inhaled and its Fate in the Body" in which the laws governing the concentration of ether in air and its distribution between air and blood are discussed. Measurements were made of the concentration of ether in the arterial blood and in the urine.

II. "Analysis of the Mechanism of Absorption and Elimination of Such a Gas or Vapor as Ethyl Ether." A diagram illustrates the relations of respiration, circulation, and body tissue, the factors concerned in the absorption and elimination of ether. Mathematical analyses and the underlying principles were discussed. In addition, the increase in rate of induction and elimination of ether when used in conjunction with carbon dioxide was described.

III. "The Relation of the Concentration of Ether or any Similar Volatile Substance in the Central Nervous System to the Concentration in the Arterial Blood, and the Buffer Action of the Body." Measurement of the ether tension in the arterial blood and in the internal jugular vein is an index of basic concentration reached in the central nervous system which is the determining factor in the anesthesia action of ether.

IV. "The Anesthetic Tension of Ether and the Physiological Response to Various Concentrations." When the body is in complete equilibrium with any inhaled concentration, the ether content was shown to be similar in blood drawn from any site in the body.

V. "The Importance of the Volume of Breathing during the Induction and Termination of Ether Anesthesia" Prolonged induction of ether anesthesia is undesirable; by increasing the concentration, the induction can be greatly accelerated. More dilute concentrations of ether may be used to avoid pulmonary irritation, but the volume of alveolar air exchanged will be increased by the addition of dilute carbon dioxide."

1925

Published December, 1979

A good many anesthesia residents beginning their education today have the strange notion that anesthesia can only be induced with an i.v. drug. It is not strange that they have this strange notion, since almost all of the inductions which they have observed have been accomplished by the i.v. injection of a drug such as thiopental, or diazepam, or Innovar, or ketamine, or droperidol, or morphine, or the like; and they therefore quite naturally assume that this is the way that anesthesia is induced. As a result, having failed in the initial attempt at venipuncture, they will stab endlessly at the poor defenseless, insufficiently medicated, scared-to-death, and vasoconstricted patient in futile attempts to establish an i.v. line into which they can inject whichever of the above listed drugs they have chosen for the purpose of inducing anesthesia. While the resident struggles to achieve venipuncture, the patient becomes increasingly—and quite justifiably—upset; and the surgeon, fully gowned and gloved, paces the periphery of the operating room and also becomes understandably upset. Soon the rest of the surgical team, also fully gowned and gloved, naturally begin to share in the concern; and, in time, the feeling of tension in the room reaches the anesthesia resident, who becomes so frantic in his probings with the needle that every attempt is doomed to failure.

The idea of a mask induction to produce light inhalation anesthesia, with its abundant vasodilation—and an amazingly easy subsequent venipuncture—never crosses the resident's mind. The idea is completely foreign to the thinking of the resident, who has been imbued with the concept that, first and foremost, a venous line must be established. This is a dictum with which there can usually be little or no quarrel (there are, of course, exceptions to every rule); but the resident has not yet learned that the *when* of the initiation of a venous line is not carved in granite, nor cast in bronze, as having to be prior to the induction of anesthesia.

One of the reasons—probably *the* reason—that the resident does not consider an inhalation induction is that she or he has not become sufficiently confident of an ability to maintain an airway with just a mask and a pair of hands, aided and abetted perhaps with a pharyngeal airway. There is a prevalent belief abroad in the land of the novice resident that an endotracheal tube is essential to the maintenance of the anesthetic state, and that, if an endotracheal tube is not in place, it cannot be true general anesthesia. The use of massive doses of narcotics and muscle relaxants in today's anesthesia makes this concept true in a great many instances, of course; but until these drugs are used, and an endotracheal tube must be in place, the resident must be capable of maintaining an airway with the mask, a pharyngeal airway, and 2 hands.

However, if anesthesia is to be induced successfully with a mask and maintained without an endotracheal tube, the resident must have considerable *visual* knowledge of what constitutes normal respiratory movements, with the chest and abdomen rising in a smooth, synchronous fashion without either intercostal or xiphoid retraction. Only when this happy state of respiratory affairs is appreciated can the changes produced by inhalation anesthesia—and therefore the *respiratory signs* of inhalation anesthesia—be put to use in the management of the anesthetic state.

Knowledge and appreciation of the respiratory signs of inhalation anesthesia evolved rather slowly. The incomparable John Snow, in his classic 1858 volume, "On Chloroform and Other Anaesthetics: Their Action and Administration," pointed out that in deep chloroform anesthesia "the breathing is rendered difficult, feeble, or irregular, and is sometimes performed only by the diaphragm, whilst the intercostal muscles are paralyzed."

Guedel, in his classification of the signs of inhalation anesthesia which he presented in 1920, wrote: "There is no regularity or rhythm to the respiration of the second, or stage of excitement. From experience we recognize the transition from the second to the third stage, by the inauguration of respiration that is rhythmical and exaggerated. The exaggeration is marked and continues so, almost without change, provided there is a continuance of sufficient ether to carry the anesthesia progressively downward throughout the first, second and third strata of the third stage. However, as the fourth or deepest stratum of this stage is entered, the respiration shows beginning depression. This depression continues progressively downward through the fourth stratum until its complete cessation marks the transition into the fourth stage."

The man, however, who made the most precise and detailed analysis of the respiratory movements during inhalation anesthesia was Albert H. Miller of Providence, Rhode Island. Guedel wrote to Miller concerning the latter's contribution in relation to ascending respiratory paralysis:

"Dear A.H.:—

Thanks many times for sending me the R. I. Journal, and for your generous reference to my work. I do not feel that these stages of anesthesia are my work.

They are rather the work of my friends, and mine all run together.

It is too bad that our necessity for earning the dollar prevents us from getting together oftener. I have missed the contacts more and more because I have been able to attend meetings less and less. I promise myself that I will get around, and then when the time comes I find an excuse to stay at home. My loss.

I have often thought and I believe more as I study the question that your description of Ascending Respiratory Paralysis was one of the most helpful pieces of work we have had in this generation. I appreciate it very much.

Thanks again for your generosity, and with best wishes and highest esteem, I am

Sincerely
Art Guedel"

The observations by Miller to which Guedel was referring in his letter were presented in an article titled, "Ascending Respiratory Paralysis under General Anesthesia," which was published in the January 17th, 1925 issue of the *Journal of the American Medical Association* (84: 201) and is reprinted below.

ASCENDING RESPIRATORY PARALYSIS UNDER GENERAL ANESTHESIA

ALBERT H. MILLER

Providence, Rhode Island

J.A.M.A., 84: 201, 1925

"Under general anesthesia, the following types of respiration are to be noted: *Exaggerated Thoracic Type* (T.+). —Inspiration is produced by expansion of the chest without movement of the diaphragm or abdominal wall, or with retraction of the abdominal wall. This type of respiration —has been noted in some cases in which inflammatory lesions affecting the peritoneum of the diaphragmatic region were present.

"*Mixed, or Usual, Type* (M.). —During inspiration there is a synchronous expansion of the chest and protrusion of the abdominal wall.

"*Delayed Thoracic Type* (D.T.). —The chest expands during inspiration notably later in the respiratory cycle than occurs the contraction of the diaphragm.

"*Abdominal Type* (A.). —Inspiration is brought about entirely by the contraction of the diaphragm, with protrusion of the abdominal wall but without movement of the chest.

"*Exaggerated Abdominal Type* (A.+). —

During each inspiration, the abdominal wall rises while the chest retracts. Expiration is marked by retraction of the abdominal wall and expansion of the chest.

"These types of respiration, in the order given, result from a progressive ascending paralysis of the respiratory muscles."

1926

Published August, 1981

There was a time, not much more than a generation ago, when the use of more than 2 drugs during the administration of anesthesia was accused of being polypharmacy; and not only was polypharmacy considered to be bad, it was considered to be *very* bad. One could not tell what effects one was obtaining from which drug; and, much more importantly, one could not know when it was appropriate to add more of this drug, or less of that one. The Pharmacological Purists howled that polypharmacy was like the old-fashioned shotgun prescription, which threw in a pinch of most of the then-current pharmacopia in the hope that whatever the diagnosis might in truth be, one of the many ingredients of the prescription would halt the disease process.

The Technical Simplists had a different, but still accusatory, attack. They moaned that polypharmacy made the administration of anesthesia too complex, and that the complex in medicine is often more dangerous in the hands of the inexperienced and unknowing than is the simple. This is, of course, patently true; but it is less an argument against the use of several drugs during the administration of anesthesia than it is an argument—and a very good one, too—against the inexperienced and unknowing as the purveyors of anesthesia in any form.

The Pharmacological Purists and the

Technical Simplists had history on their side. First there was nitrous oxide, then sulphuric ether, then chloroform, and then chloric ether—each given singly as the sole and only anesthetic drug. Nitrous oxide was administered as the pure gas; whereas ether, chloroform and chloric ether were vaporized in air. This state of affairs persisted for almost a quarter of a century, until 1868, when Edmund Andrews, who was the Professor of the Principles and Practice of Surgery at the Chicago Medical College, advocated the addition of oxygen to nitrous oxide. "I have for some time been experimenting," he wrote, "to see whether by the addition of free oxygen to the nitrous oxide, a mixture would not be obtained, by which a patient might be anesthetized for an indefinite period without danger of asphyxia, and thus render gas available for the most prolonged operations of surgery. These experiments are not yet finished, but they have advanced far enough to show that the preparation, which I have named the Oxygen Mixture, is certainly available for a large part of our operations, and that for pleasantness, and probable safety, it is infinitely superior to chloroform, ether, or unmixed nitrous oxide."

Polypharmacy had begun!

It can be argued, quite justifiably, that the addition of oxygen to nitrous oxide administration is really not a mixture of anesthetic agents. Probably the first true combinations were the various preparations which incorporated both chloroform and ether, with or without the addition of ethyl alcohol. Such a mixture was suggested by John Gabb, of Bewdley, in the *Lancet* in May of 1848, just a few months after the introduction of chloroform. He proposed that it might be, "desirable to add a little of the stimulating effect of the ether to the directly sedative influence of the chloroform . . . Could this not be done by mixing the two agents in properly ascertained proportions? I should think . . . about one part ether to two parts chloroform would be the best proportion for the majority of cases." An almost immediate reply in a subsequent issue of the journal by Vaughan Jones, of Westminster, stated, "the administration . . . would not be found practicable, on account of the difference in specific gravity of the two agents."

The incomparable John Snow made the same point about a year later: "As the most desirable strength of a volatile narcotic liquid, not requiring great care in its use, is between that of chloroform and that of sulphuric ether, it might be supposed that by mixing the two medicines the desired end would be attained: but such is not the case: they have been so mixed by some practitioners, and I have tried them together, but the result is a combination of the undesirable qualities of both, without any compensating advantage. Ether is about six times as volatile as chloroform . . . When the two liquids are mixed, although they then evaporate together, the ether is converted into vapour much more rapidly; and in whatever proportions they are combined, before the whole is evaporated the last portion of the liquid is nearly all chloroform; the consequence is that at the commencement of the inhalation the vapour inspired is chiefly ether, and towards the end nearly all chloroform; the patient experiencing the stronger pungency of ether when it is most objectionable and inhaling the more powerful vapour at the conclusion, when there is the most need to proceed cautiously."

Snow's authoritative condemnation served to dampen any enthusiasm for such

mixtures until 1864, when the Committee of the Royal Medical and Chirurgical Society advocated a trial of George Harley's famous A.C.E. mixture: alcohol, 1 part; chloroform, 2 parts; and ether, 3 parts. By the 1880's, this combination had attained a considerable popularity. Indeed, the A.C.E. preparation was the first anesthesia known to the Mayo Brothers, as William Mayo has described: "My brother and I were brought up in medicine as farm boys are brought up on the farm. As fast as we were old enough, we were given tasks that had to do with medicine . . . Even at that time I helped Father with his surgical operations, acting as first assistant, and Charlie, at the ripe age of twelve, was forced into giving the anesthetic, the old ACE mixture . . . He was initiated at an operation for removal of a large ovarian tumor. Father was one of the first surgeons in America to undertake these operations. The operation in question was done in a private home, an old house with a stone barn about two miles southeast of Rochester on what is now Highway 52. In the midst of the operation, the doctor who was giving the anesthetic fainted. Charlie climbed up onto a cracker box and gave the anesthetic, and he did so well that from that time on he was the family anesthetist."

The A.C.E. mixture led in a rather roundabout way to the most important anesthetic combination developed during the first hundred years of anesthesia, the nitrous oxide—ether (or "gas-ether") sequence.

In the 1860's there was considerable concern in England over the mortality rates associated with the administration of chloroform anesthesia; and, in fact, this was precisely why the Committee of the Royal Medical and Chirurgical Society had been appointed. It was the Committee's charge, "to give their anxious attention to devise means for obviating such accidents;" and, as we have seen, they came up with the A.C.E. mixture as an alternative to chloroform. Their suggestion of the mixture, however, was inherently a suggestion for using ether as an auxiliary to chloroform, and this very much served to turn the attention of anesthetists back to ether, a drug which they had known since the halcyon days of the 1840's.

Also at this time, Europe was introduced to the revival of nitrous oxide as an anesthetic. After the tragic failure of the demonstration of nitrous oxide at the Harvard Medical School in 1845, the drug fell into disrepute and was not employed for many years. However, its use was revived by Gardner Quincy Colton with great success in 1862. Colton amassed a vast experience of 24,000 cases at the Colton Dental Association in New York City, which was established as an institution devoted exclusively to the extraction of teeth under nitrous oxide anesthesia. In 1867, Colton visited Paris to attend the International Exhibition and the First International Medical Congress. While in Paris, he met T. W. Evans, a fellow countryman who had practiced in the French capital as a dental surgeon for some years, and he instructed Evans in the preparation and administration of nitrous oxide. Evans was an apt and enthusiastic pupil, and he soon accumulated his own experience of upwards of 1,000 cases using the agent for dental extractions. The following year, in March of 1868, Evans went to London and gave several demonstrations at the National Dental Hospital. These demonstrations were attended by the leading metropolitan anesthetists and dentists of the day, including, of course, Joseph Clover, who had succeeded John Snow as the dominant figure in British anesthesia.

Clover was an original genius, like Snow; but whereas Snow's greatness lay in his power to grasp and formulate the physiologic processes of anesthesia, Clover's lay in his resourcefulness and his inventiveness in devising apparatus and methods of administration based on scientific principles. It was while watching Evan's demonstrations of nitrous oxide that Clover foresaw the possibility of modifying his own apparatus to permit the patient the pleasantness of induction with nitrous oxide and the potency of anesthesia with ether—and "gas-ether" was born!

It was not a long step—although it took a long time—from "gas-ether" to the classic gas-oxygen-ether sequence, or GOE. An-

drews, as we have already noted, had advocated the "oxygen mixture" of nitrous oxide and oxygen as early as 1868, and Clover had followed with the introduction of the nitrous oxide—ether sequence in 1876. What was missing was the mechanical apparatus by which the 3 drugs could be administered in combination. Sir Frederick W. Hewitt, in 1887, devised a machine for the administration of nitrous oxide and oxygen; but it was not until 1892 that he introduced the first practical gas and oxygen apparatus. The S. S. White Dental Manufacturing Company produced the first machine for anesthesia by the "non-asphyxial" method of Hewitt, and this became the prototype necessary for the development of apparatus for the administration of the gas-oxygen-ether sequence. GOE was the most important combination of inhalation agents employed during the first half of the present century and dominated the anesthetic scene for most of that time.

The most important non-inhalation drug used in anesthetic mixtures was morphine. The morphine story is told separately because it is different in both texture and substance. On the one hand, the drug was undoubtedly the first to be used intentionally for preanesthetic medication; and on the other hand, its use during general anesthesia can arguably be said to represent the first inkling of what we now call Balanced Anesthesia—although admittedly its use during anesthesia at that time was scarcely thought of in terms of the properties of hypnosis-analgesia-muscle relaxation-obtundation of reflex activity which we consider to be Balanced Anesthesia today.

Keys states that W. W. Greene, of the Maine Medical School, was the first to advocate, in 1868, the use of morphine during inhalation anesthesia as a procedure to prevent shock, delerium and nausea, and to shorten the anesthetic influence. However, Barbara Duncum records that, as early as 1864, Nussbaum of Munich accidentally discovered that an injection of morphine appeared to intensify and prolong chloroform anesthesia: " . . . he had already given chloroform for about an hour, during the extirpation of a malignant tumour, when, fearing to prolong the inhalation, he decided to substitute the use of morphine. The subcutaneous injection of 1 grain in solution not only provided satisfactory anaesthesia for the completion of the operation, as Nussbaum expected, but it also produced a long period of postoperative tranquillity. Nussbaum was much struck by this latter phenomenon and decided to turn it to account in future operations. The technique which he developed was first to establish chloroform anesthesia and then to inject, hypodermically, half a grain of acetate of morphine. This, he claimed, gave 'five or six hours of tranquil sleep' post-operatively, during which the patient was spared both pain and restlessness. A report on Nussbaum's work was made by a special committee appointed by the Versailles Medical Society. After experimenting on dogs the committee pronounced itself satisfied 'that the prolongation of chloroform anesthesia by means of hypodermic injections of the salts of morphia may be regarded as an established fact.'"

It was the great French physiologist, Claude Bernard, however, who did the definitive investigations on the use of morphine in conjunction with inhalation anesthesia. A chloroformed dog on which he was experimenting recovered consciousness, and Bernard injected what he knew to be an anesthetic dose of morphine. The animal not only became unconscious but, even more surprisingly, showed signs of renewed chloroform anesthesia. He repeated this experiment several times with the same results, and then he reversed the process: i.e., he injected the morphine first and then induced chloroform anesthesia. "When one begins with chloroform," he stated, "the unconsciousness produced is long drawn out as a result of the influence of the morphine, but by giving the morphine first . . . scarcely is the inhalation of chloroform interrupted before sensibility returns. Thus one had a rapid means alternatively to suspend and reestablish sensibility and this is important in certain cases . . . In giving an injection of morphine first and then administering chloroform a much

smaller quantity of the latter is needed. In this way one obtains anesthesia without so pronounced a stage of excitement and above all without running so great a risk of accident as one does with large and repeated doses of chloroform." These advantages, Bernard thought, should recommend the method, which he termed "mixed anesthesia," to surgeons.

The philosophy inherent in "mixed anesthesia" was carried one step further when the late George Crile, Sr., propounded his Theory of Anoci-Association in 1911. Crile, reasoning along physiologic lines, argued that, not only must the brain be protected against destructive psychic strain by the use of general anesthesia, but that local anesthesia must also be employed to exclude noxious impulses arising from the site of surgical interventions. He pointed out that, although such double protection could be achieved by deep general anesthesia produced with a single drug such as chloroform or ether, the cost to the patient in terms of deranged metabolism could be horrendous.

It remained for John Lundy, who adopted a similar line of reasoning, to coin the term, "Balanced Anesthesia," which he employed to designate the use of a combination of anesthetic drugs and methods so balanced that the burden for the relief of pain would be borne in part by the preliminary medication, in part by regional anesthesia, and in part by general anesthesia. Lundy first published the term, "Balanced Anesthesia", in a paper under that title in *Minnesota Medicine* in 1926 (Lundy, J.S.: Balanced anesthesia. *Minnesota Med, 9:* 399, 1926). It is reprinted below with the kind permission of the publisher.

BALANCED ANESTHESIA

JOHN S. LUNDY

Rochester, Minnesota

Minnesota Med., 9: 399, 1926.

"The average healthy man, other things being equal, thrives on a balanced diet. No one food will satisfy all his requirements and yet any one food taken in excess ultimately produces untoward results. The average healthy man is likewise usually able to take into his system a small dose of any of the anesthetic agents commonly used without untoward results, but a very large amount of any of these anesthetic agents ends unpleasantly. It seems logical that a combination of the various agents might be used, each one in small enough amount so that it would produce no unsatisfactory effect: whereas collectively these agents produce a balanced anesthesia after the fashion of a good diet.

"Balanced anesthesia for an average healthy man might be as follows: for an hour or an hour and a half before operation his nervous system is quieted by means of preliminary hypnotics without overdosage; at the time of operation sufficient local anesthetic may be employed either regionally or by infiltration without producing any marked reaction to the drug; nitrous oxide or ethylene anesthesia may next be superimposed on the foundation provided by the preliminary hypnotics and the local anesthesia and not be carried to the point where the patient's natural color changes; to these agents ether may then be added in sufficient quantity to produce the desired relaxation.

"It is proposed that anesthesia in this case be produced by the combined effects of a moderate amount of preliminary hypnotic, a moderate amount of local anesthetic, a moderate amount of nitrous oxide or ethylene, and an amount of ether sufficient to obtain the desired result. It is assumed that this person will have very little untoward effect from any one of the anesthetics here employed, but that when combined they will usually produce satisfactory anesthesia."

1927

Published April, 1972

The first issue of the *New England Journal of Medicine and Surgery and the Collateral Branches of Science* appeared in January of 1812. It contained "Remarks on Angina Pectoris," by Dr. John Warren: "Remarks on the Morbid Effects of Dentition," by Dr. James Jackson; "Case of Apoplexy with Dissections," by Dr. John C. Warren; "Treatment of Injuries Occasioned by Fire," by Dr. Jacob Bigelow; and "Remarks on Diseases Resembling Syphilis," by Dr. Walter Channing.

It was not the first journal of medicine in this country (the *Medical Repository* was published in New York in 1797 and continued for some 20 years; the *Medical Museum* was Philadelphia's contribution in 1804, discontinuing publication in 1813, only to be revived in 1820 and changed to the current *American Journal of Medical Sciences* in 1827; and Baltimore entered the journalistic lists with its short-lived *Medical and Physical Recorder* which appeared in 1809), but it was the first journal of medicine in the country, if not the world, which has continued, despite changes of form and name, in uninterrupted existence until the present day.

The Editorial Board of the *New England Journal of Medicine and Surgery and the Collateral Branches of Science* contained some unforgettable names of Boston Medicine: Dr. John Collins Warren, Dr. James Jackson, Dr. John Gorham, Dr. Jacob Bigelow, Dr. Walter Channing, Dr. George Hayward, Dr. John Ware, and Dr. John W. Webster. The 8 men formed a club which met each month to dine together and to read the papers submitted.

In 1824, the Editorship passed into the

hands of Drs. Walter Channing and John Ware—and capable hands they were, too. Dr. Channing had been born in 1786, had graduated from Harvard College in 1806, and in medicine from the University of Pennsylvania in 1809. In 1815 he was appointed the first professor of obstetrics and jurisprudence (what a combination of cognizances!) in the Harvard Medical School, a post which he held until 1847. Dr. Ware was born in 1795, received his degree in medicine from Harvard in 1816, and was the Hersey Professor of the Theory and Practice of Physic at Harvard Medical School from 1856 until 1858.

The *New England Journal* thrived under the Channing-Ware Editorship for only 3 years, when it combined with *The Boston Medical Intelligencer* in 1828 to become the *Boston Medical And Surgical Journal*. The *Boston Medical Intelligencer* was one of the first two medical weeklies in the world— the other was *The London Lancet*, under the Editorship of the incomparable Thomas Wakley—and was conducted by Jerome V. C. Smith from April 29, 1823 until February 12, 1826. The third volume was edited by James Wilson and the fourth and fifth by John G. Coffin, who continued as proprietor and editor until the last issue of the *Intelligencer*, which appeared on February 12, 1828.

The latter contained the following announcement: "On Tuesday next week, will appear the first number of the *Boston Medical and Surgical Journal*, as a continuation of this paper. When we consider the number, the talents and experience of the Editors of the forthcoming journal, and their abundant resources for matter, we cannot doubt that this paper will prove generally acceptable, because we feel an assurance that it must be interesting and useful."

Interesting and useful it was, publishing a number of milestones in medicine, not the least of which was Dr. Henry Jacob Bigelow's "Insensibility During Surgical Operations Produced by Inhalation" in the Wednesday, November 18, 1846, issue. But it also outgrew the confines of Boston, and in 1920 the Council of the Massachusetts Medical Society entered into negotiations for the purchase of the *Boston Medical and Surgical Journal*, and for its reorgani-

zation into the *New England Journal of Medicine*, since it was the official organ of not only the Massachusetts Medical Society, but also of the Boston Surgical Society, the New England Pediatric Society, the New Hampshire Surgical Club, and the New Hampshire and Vermont Medical Societies. As Dr. Robert M. Green wrote of it in 1923, "It represents the worthy survival of the fittest from the past of medical journalism in New England. It derives its form from the *Medical Intelligencer*, its substance from the *New England Journal of Medicine and Surgery*, its spirit from both." It has not betrayed this heritage, and today the *New England Journal of Medicine* is widely acknowledged as one of the leading publications in medicine in the world.

On December 29, 1927, in the very last volume of the *Boston Medical and Surgical Journal* before it become the *N. E. J. M.*, there appeared an article of uncommon semantic interest to the anesthesiologist. It was the President's Address, read at the Fourth Annual Meeting of the Eastern Society of Anesthetists, at Detroit, Michigan, October 3 to 7, 1927. It was entitled, "The Origin of the Word 'Anaesthesia,' (*Boston M. & S. Journal*, 197: 1218–1222, December 29, 1927) and is reprinted below with the kind permission of the publishers.

THE ORIGIN OF THE WORD "ANAESTHESIA"

ALBERT H. MILLER, M.D.

Boston Med. Surg. J., 197: 1218, 1927

"The word Anaesthesia is of Greek derivation and signifies lack of feeling or sensation. In 1718, it was used by J. B. Quistorpius in the title "De Anaesthesia". It first appeared in English in N. Bailey's Dictionary of 1721:—"Anaisthesia, a loss or Defect of Sense, as in such as have the Palsy, or are blasted".

* * * *

"Parr's Medical Dictionary, 1819, defined "Anaesthesia—Insensibility or loss of feeling, by touch. A resolution of the nerves occasioning a loss of feeling, generally a symptom of palsy, the same as Stupor."

There follows a detailed description of the events leading up to the successful etherization on October 16, 1846, at the Massachusetts General Hospital. In November, following a conversation with Dr. Morton, Dr. Oliver Wendell Holmes wrote Morton a letter, as follows:

"Boston, Nov. 21st. 1846.

"*My Dear Sir:*—Everybody wants to have a hand in a great discovery. All I will do is to give you a hint or two, as to names, or the name, to be applied to the state produced and the agent.

"The state should, I think, be called 'Anaesthesia.' This signifies insensibility, more particularly (as used by Linnaeus and Cullen) to objects of touch. (See Good—Nosology, p. 259.) The adjective will be "Anaesthetic." Thus we might say, the state of anaesthesia, or the anaesthetic state. The means employed would be properly called the anti-aesthetic agent. Perhaps it might be allowable to say anaesthetic agent, but this admits of question.

"The words, antineuric, aneuric, neuro-leptic, neuro-lepsia, neuro-etasis, etc., seem too anatomical; whereas the change is a physiological one.

"I would have a name pretty soon, and consult some accomplished scholar, such as President Everett or Dr. Bigelow, senior, before fixing upon a term, which will be repeated by the tongue of every civilized race of mankind. You will mention these words which I suggest for their consideration; but there may be others more appropriate and agreeable.

"Yours, respectfully,

"Dr. Morton."

"O. W. HOLMES."

*　　*　　*　　*

Published February, 1979

A rather undistinguished—and, in fact, an even less than mediocre—career as a football player came to an abrupt and inglorious end one bright Saturday afternoon in October of my senior year in high school when I was tackled from the side while returning a punt in the open field and my leg was broken. Athletic injuries in high school football are a dime a dozen, of course, but there were 2 rather distinctive features about this particular injury (quite apart from the fact that it was *my* leg being broken) which raised it a bit above the ordinary, plebeian high school athletic injury.

The first was the fact that the tackle was made, and the leg broken, by Endicott "Chub" Peabody, who 25 years later was to become the Governor of the Commonwealth of Massachusetts. Chub's subsequent Governorship was not the important point in making the injury distinctive, however. What made it so was the fact that, 4 years after he had broken my leg, Chub was to play guard on a very good Harvard football team and was to be named to the 1941 All-American Team by the Associated Press, the United Press, the International News Service, the All-American Board, the Collier's Magazine (for which Grantland Rice made the annual All-American selections); and that he was to receive the 1941 Knute Rockne Memorial Trophy from the Touchdown Club of Washington as "the nation's outstanding college lineman of the year." It has always been my contention that, if one is going to do anything as stupid and dull as having a leg broken in a high school football game, it might just as well be broken by the best, someone with class, style, and pinache.

The second distinctive feature about the injury was the nature of the injury itself, because Chub not only broke the leg but at the same time he also tore the medial meniscus in that knee. The leg healed quickly (it was just a fracture of the fibula), but that medial meniscus remained torn, and by the time the hockey season rolled around that winter the knee took to "locking" in the most frivolous of circumstances—while skating forward, while skating backward, while checking, while being checked, with an opponent being around, without an opponent being around, you name it. Whispered consultations between my family and a great friend of theirs, who was also an orthopedic surgeon and physician for Harvard's athletic teams, decreed that the offending piece of cartilage must be removed, and removed quickly "before arthritis set in." It was therefore decided that I would not spend Spring Vacation hitchhiking to Fort Lauderdale in Florida with my buddies, but in a hospital having the operation performed.

Why it was also decided that the operation should be performed under general anesthesia, rather than spinal anesthesia, in this healthy 17 year old undergoing a knee operation was never discussed in my presence, but that was the decision. In any event, when the appointed day came, I was given rectal Avertin and went off to sleep like a baby. As a subjective experience, the Avertin was several cuts above my previous exposure to anesthesia in that same hospital, which had occurred when my tonsils were removed at age 5 and the anesthetist had handed me a balloon, told me to "take a big, big breath and blow up the balloon," and arranged to have the big, big breath consist of straight ether vapor. By way of contrast, the Avertin was pure nectar, and I became an immediate and ardent devotee of rectal anesthesia, a devotion which lasted until I became an anesthesia resident. But that is quite another story.

The origins of rectal anesthesia go back a long way before the great events of the 1840's and the discovery of anesthesia, at least as far back as the Middle Ages, when the administration of narcotics by rectum was known to the School of Salerno. The formally documented history of rectal anesthesia, however, began a few months after Morton's epochal public demonstration of the efficacy of ether anesthesia on October 16, 1846. The following winter—just 5 months to the day—on March 16, 1847, Marc Dupuy (subsequently and frequently misspelled as "Duprey"), an intern of the Hospitals of Paris, presented a paper at the session of the Academie Nationale de Medecine titled, "On the Effects of the Injection of Ether Into the Rectum," which

was published the following month (April 1847) in *Comptes rendus hebdomadaires des seances de l'Academie des sciences*: "I wanted to investigate the possibility of bringing ether into the organism by another way than through the lungs, in order to avoid the inconveniences of the latter method. The experiments on three dogs and a rabbit showed that ether injected into the rectum was absorbed rapidly and caused a deep anesthesia.

"The change in color of the arterial blood which accompanies the inhalation of ether and which indicates the depth of the anesthetic plane did not take place when ether was administered via the rectum.

"*Research on a Dog.* I injected 15 gm. of ether mixed with 15 gm. of water (by shaking intensively) into the rectum of a small dog. The animal had been fasting for seven to eight hours. At the end of one minute there was a strong odor of ether on the animal's breath; a pronounced foamy salivation was observed. Four minutes later (from the beginning of the experiment) the animal appeared to be completely inebriated and was unable to stand on its feet, but could still drag its body on the floor. There was a complete loss of sensitivity of the skin, brought into evidence when the skin was pierced with a needle. The skin was incised with a knife, and incision did not produce any reaction of pain.

"After eleven minutes the dog was still inebriated; however, it tried to stand on its feet. At each attempt to walk the joints gave way. At the end of eighteen minutes sensitivity of the skin was still absent—the walk was steadier, but there was still some in-co-ordination—slowly, sensitivity of the skin returned, and there was a slight motor reaction when the skin was pierced with a needle. The animal remained indifferent to stimuli.

"Twenty-two minutes later sensitivity of the skin returned to normal and the dog could walk as usual, giving no further sign of muscular in-co-ordination. It vomited a small amount of a foamy liquid, examination of which disclosed nothing of significance.

"During the experimental period there

was no discharge from the anus. The secretion of saliva was increased, and the animal was swallowing continuously. At the end of the experiment the dog started to eat eagerly all the food given to him.

"It was concluded that the injection of ether and water caused only a slight irritation of the mucous membrane of the large bowel, since symptoms referable to the large bowel were at a minimum.

"*Research on a Rabbit.* I injected 10 gm. of ether mixed with 10 gm. of water in to the rectum of a rabbit. Three minutes later the animal was completely unconscious. I decided to examine the blood, and therefore I exposed and divided both femoral arteries. The blood was perfectly normal in appearance. Afterward, I opened the abdomen by an incision reaching from the thorax to the symphysis. Just as I was finishing the incision, the animal started to move a little, which suggested that anesthesia was waning. I repeated the injection of ether and water and obtained a most perfect anesthesia during the remaining experimental period. The bowel was removed from the abdominal cavity, and the aorta was exposed and cut through. The blood was flooding out of the vessel and was of a bright red color. I opened the thorax; the heart was still beating weakly, the lungs were pink and exhibited not the slightest amount of congestion. The spleen, liver and kidneys appeared normal. There was only a small amount of gas in the intestines, and the mucous membrane of the rectum did not show any vascular congestion.

"I think this proves quite conclusively that asphyxia is not a prerequisite of anesthesia, as some workers believe. The anesthesic effects of the inhalation of ether are not caused by suppression of oxygenation of the venous blood in the lungs. The finding of some investigators that arterial blood becomes dark under the inhalation of ether is simply an indication of incipient asphyxia due to insufficient aeration of the lungs. However, these investigators claim that anesthesia is preceded by the conversion of arterial blood to venous blood.

"If this were true, the color of arterial blood would have to be modified by an agent producing asphyxia before loss of consciousness would occur. Yet vaporized ether would be of no more value here than would any other asphyxiating gas.

"It seems to be the idea of these investigators that the primary cause of insensibility is asphyxia, and that ether facilitates asphyxia by displacement of oxygen in the respired air. I do not deny that asphyxia is in point of fact an excellent method of producing unconsciousness, but I doubt very much whether anyone will be tempted to try it out even once, for fear he might not have a second chance.

"Summary
1) Loss of consciousness is produced by injecting ether into the rectum.
2) The onset of the narcotic action of ether given by rectum is as rapid as when it is administered by inhalation.
3) There were no manifestations of asphyxia.
4) Rectal injection is a safer method of administration than that which consists in inhalation of vaporized ether.

"On this occasion M. Lallemand remarked that the opiates administered in the same manner have, as already noted by Dupuytren, a prompter and better action than when given by mouth, since they are absorbed more rapidly and are not submitted to any changes by the various digestive glands."

Almost simultaneously—and quite certainly without any knowledge of Dupuy's communication—Nikolai Ivanovitch Pirogoff published a paper in the same journal the next month (May, 1847) on rectal anesthesia entitled, "A New Method of Anesthetizing, with Ether Vapor, Patients Undergoing Surgical Operations":

"This method consists of the administration of ether by rectum. I was encouraged by the results obtained from experiments with animals to use this method for surgical operations, even in cases in which the inhalation of ether did not exert the least effect on patients.

"The lower part of the large bowel was cleaned by an enema and an elastic tube was introduced into the rectum. A locking syringe of the kind I use for the transfusion of blood is adapted to the distal part of the tube. This syringe is built in a sheet-metal container which is filled with water heated to 50°C. Due to this warm-water case, the liquid ether, which is aspirated into the syringe, changes instantly from the liquid to the vapor form, and it is this evaporated ether which enters the rectum by the elastic tube.

"The advantages of this method are obvious: the organs of respiration are unaffected. Ether anesthesia is completely independent of the patient's will power, and the action is much faster. I have the impression that this method will replace the inhalation of ether completely, which is very often inconvenient and disagreeable to the patient. Operations which are very difficult to do when anesthesia is produced by the inhalation method, such as operations on the face and mouth and in children, can be performed very easily with my method of anesthesia.

"The quantity of ether did not exceed 1½ to 2 ounces in all cases that I have observed to date. Full anesthesia was obtained after three to five minutes. No complications have been observed so far."

No useful purpose will be served by attempting to assign, from this distance in time, priority in the discovery and application of the method of rectal anesthesia as between Dupuy and Pirogoff. Dupuy was an intern who was never heard from before or after his historic paper. Pirogoff was an important Professor of Clinical Surgery in St. Petersburg, internationally known, and perhaps the most famous surgeon whom Russia ever produced. Indeed, it has been said, with a good deal of truth, that Russian surgery consists of 2 parts—pre-Pirogoff and post-Pirogoff. Pirogoff made numerous original contributions to surgery, particularly in the handling of amputations, gunshot wounds, and the surgery of bones. His name lives in the Pirogoff amputation, a method of osteoplastic amputation of the foot, which he devised in 1854; the Pirogoff amputation for hernia; and the Pirogoff (venous) angle. One of his great interests was topographic anatomy; and his famous research work, *Anatomia chirurgica*

truncorum arteriorum et fasciarum fibrosarum, not only brought him world-wide recognition, but did much to make anatomy the basis of surgery. It is little wonder, then, that the name of Pirogoff is immediately associated with such an innovation as rectal anesthesia, and that only serious medical historians have ever heard of Dupuy.

There was a second important difference between the 2 contributions quoted above, however, in addition to the comparative professional stature between intern and internationally renowned Professor: Dupuy used liquid ether, while Pirogoff employed ether vapor. Dupuy won this one hands down. The trail of the use of rectal ether vapor is strewn with bloody diarrhea, abdominal pain and distension, rupture of the intestine, colonic ulceration, and purulent peritonitis, not to mention respiratory depression, hypotension, and death. Little wonder that the history of rectal anesthesia consists of so many rejections of the technique, followed some years later by enthusiastic rediscovery and then further rejection. Indeed, it was not until Gwathmey's introduction of oil-ether rectal anesthesia in 1913 that the rectal route became widely accepted, and the installation of a liquid anesthetic agent—be it ether, tribromoethanol, trichloroethanol, paraldehyde, chloral hydrate, or the barbiturates—became firmly established as being far preferable to the rectal installation of a vapor.

Of all the drugs tried, Avertin (tribromoethanol in amylene hydrate) proved to be the most manageable and useful; and for a period of some 20 years, during the 1930's and 1940's, Avertin enjoyed great popularity. It was ultimately displaced by thiopental as an induction agent because the latter was less cumbersome and more manageable, while at the same time the barbiturate earned great patient (and therefore surgeon) acceptance.

Two papers published on consecutive pages in the April 22nd, 1927 issue of *Deutsche medizinische Wochenschrift*, one dealing with the pharmacology of Avertin (Eichholtz, F. "Rectal Anesthesia with Avertin (E 107) Pharmacologic Aspects," and one dealing with its clinical uses (Butzengeiger, O. "Clinical Experience with Avertin (E 107)," (*Deutsche med. Woch.*, *1:* 712, 1927) served to introduce the drug to the medical community. The latter paper is reprinted below.

CLINICAL EXPERIENCE WITH AVERTIN (E 107)

O. BUTZENGEIGER

Medical Director, Saint Mary's Hospital, Elberfeld, Germany

Deutsche med. Woch., 1:712, 1927

"The following remarks may be made about the use of E 107 anesthesia. The procedure offers the great advantage of an absolutely pleasant induction of anesthesia, which is not only not exciting but is also directly tranquilizing.—It is therefore of particular advantage in children and in patients who fear anesthesia more than the whole operation. The induction of anesthesia can be started in the form of an enema administered to the patient in his bed, without his knowledge that the procedure will result in anesthesia, since enemas are included in the routine preparation of patients for an operation. I believe that for this reason the procedure promises great advantages for Graves disease.

"Other advantages of the method are the absence of postanesthetic vomiting in most patients (this was true of 80 per cent of our patients, even after abdominal operations) and the relative well-being after the anesthesia and a remarkable amnesia for the preceding event."

*　　*　　*　　*

"Although I have great confidence in the method described, because I think its advantages represent an important step forward, I should like to emphasize the fact that each session of anesthesia actually is not a harmless incident, and that it must be managed with the greatest caution.—My own decision, for the present, is that I shall not attempt to achieve complete surgical anesthesia by means of E 107 until more and broader experience shall have accumulated."

1928

Published June, 1968

It is not entirely clear whether J. Leonard Corning or August Bier deserves the credit for the first spinal anesthetic. Corning was, of course, attempting to produce epidural anesthesia; but there are those who believe that he obtained spinal anesthesia instead, and they quote his first animal experiment in proof: "This was performed on a young dog. . . . I injected twenty minims of a two-per-cent solution of the hydrochlorate of cocaine into the space situated between the spinous processes of two of the dorsal vertebrae. Five minutes after the injection there were evidences of marked incoordination in the posterior extremities. . . . A few minutes later there was marked evidence of weakness in the hind legs, but there were no signs whatever of feebleness in the anterior extremities" (*Survey of Anesthesiology*, June, 1960). August Bier, on the other hand, was quite frankly in the business of gaining access to the cerebrospinal fluid: "I have attempted to render large areas of the body insensible to pain by introducing cocaine into the spinal cord. This was carried out in the following way: with the patient lying on his side, lumbar puncture is performed according to the familiar method of Quincke. The needle should be very fine. After the subarachnoid space is entered, the stilet of the needle is removed; the opening is immediately covered by the finger so that very little cerebrospinal fluid can escape. The desired amount of cocaine is then injected with the help of a 'Pravaz' syringe, which fits the needle tightly" (*Survey of Anesthesiology*, June, 1962).

Since the pioneer work of these two physicians, the popularity of spinal anesthesia has undergone a number of ups and downs, varying from wildly over-enthusiastic acceptance to total rejection. These waves of opinion have continued right up to the present day: the wave of rejection has almost always followed adverse experiences with the technique, and the wave of acceptance has almost always followed the "rediscovery" of the technique after a period of disuse. One of the causes of rejection, of course, has been neurologic sequelae. Another has been the consequences following inadvertent high spinal anesthesia.

The word "inadvertent" is most important, for intentional high spinal has found its advocates and its uses. Wesley Bourne and his colleagues in Montreal employed high spinal anesthesia quite intentionally for rib resections in the performance of extrapleural thoracoplasty and the induction of extrapleural pneumothorax. They performed the Etherington-Wilson technique: "In practice the chosen quantity of percaine solution, 1:1500, warmed to the patient's temperature, is injected slowly, continuously, and evenly, while the patient *sits as erect as possible*. The injection should take from 20 to 25 seconds. The *total time should be watched very accurately and must be from the beginning of the injection to the end of the sitting up*. At the end of the allotted number of seconds, the upright position is quickly changed to that of recumbency and the head of the table tilted slightly downwards." They considered premedication vital to the success of the technique: "Perhaps the most important part of the preparation of a patient for regional anesthesia is adequate sedation. We have made a habit of giving ¼ gr. of morphine with ¹⁄₁₀₀ gr. scopolamine 90 minutes before the time of operation and repeating these 60 minutes later if the patient is not

thoroughly bemuddled and langorous." In point of fact, any who gave anesthesia at the Grace Dart Home Hospital with Bourne in those days can vouch that the latter is an understatement: if the patient could reply to "good afternoon" when he was wheeled into the operating room suite, he immediately received another ⅙ gr. of morphine and ¹⁄₁₅₀ gr. of scopolamine *intravenously* on the spot! But perhaps the most important part of the technique was the fact that all of these patients had pharyngeal and laryngeal topical analgesia applied in the medical ward prior to coming to surgery, and artificial respiration with oxygen *via* an endotracheal tube was continued throughout the operation.

Another example of intentional high spinal anesthesia was as a technique of "controlled hypotension" employed by John Gillies and his colleagues in Edinburgh. The basic features of total spinal block as evolved by these workers consisted of a minimal injection of thiopental to induce hypnosis, the establishment of high spinal block by 150 to 300 mg. of procaine or 1.5 to 3.0 mg. of nupercaine administered intrathecally, and maintenance of light general anesthesia with nitrous oxide or cyclopropane. The patient was positioned meticulously to permit the operative site to remain superior, so that bleeding was minimal and the patient's blood volume remained constant. Since there was generalized arteriolar and postarteriolar dilation with considerable pooling of blood in the dependent portions of the body, emphasis was placed on the fact that the anti-gravitational resistance to venous return must not be allowed to be too great, lest the *vis a tergo* (already considerably reduced) be incapable of coping with the additional load. Venous return could be improved whenever clinical assessment of the state of the circulation dictated by altering the patient's position (particularly by raising the legs or tilting the table into Trendelenburg or reverse Trendelenburg, as the situation required), or by abolishing the vasodilation by the use of vasoconstrictor drugs which acted peripherally. As the vasoconstrictor paralysis wore off, normotension was reestablished: if this did not occur prior to closure, a vasoconstrictor drug was employed to reveal potential bleeding points. Gillies and his coworkers were the first to refer to their technique as "physiologic trespass"; but they could also point to hugely successful results when the technique was carried out in proper fashion.

But perhaps the most incredible experience with intentional high spinal anesthesia was that amassed by the Brooklyn surgeon, Koster. This work was published under the title, "Spinal Anesthesia. With Special Reference to its Use in Surgery of the Head, Neck and Thorax," in the December, 1928, issue of the *American Journal of Surgery* (Koster, H.: *Am. J. Surg.*, 5: 554–570, 1928) and is reprinted below with the kind permission of the publishers.

SPINAL ANESTHESIA WITH SPECIAL REFERENCE TO ITS USE IN SURGERY OF THE HEAD, NECK AND THORAX

Koster, H.

Am. J. Surg. 5:554–570, 1928

To prolong spinal anesthesia for abdominal operations, the author doubled the dose and volume of injection of neocaine and discovered his patients had "complete surgical anesthesia" without "respiratory nor cardiac embarrassment." He therefore used the technique for radical mastectomy, thyroidectomy, excision of tumors of the head, rhinoplasty and even mastoidectomy (performed by colleagues). Unfortunately he does not include the frequency with which these operations were performed. Of additional interest are his descriptions of operating room deaths he attributes to patients' disease and the neurologic sequelae he considers of little consequence. He concludes, "Besides the already emunerated advantages it should be remembered that this form of anesthesia can be administered and induced very rapidly, and by its use the surgeon is freed from the vageries of different anesthetists. This emancipation in itself is a definite advantage. All other factors remaining constant, the fewer the links in the operative team, the fewer the chances of trouble arising."

1929

Published October, 1970

The anesthesiologist learns during his first month of residency training that, following the administration of spinal anesthesia, the sympathetic blockade extends more cephalad than does the sensory loss, and that the sensory loss, in turn, extends more cephalad than does the motor paralysis. Block of the preganglionic sympathetic fibers results in a diffuse peripheral sympathetic vasodilation which generally extends some 2 to 4 segments above the sensory level; and it is usually the first block in onset and the last to disappear. The motor block, on the other hand, is generally 1 or more segments below the sensory loss.

If he was a good student during his medical school days, the anesthesiology resident will remember that the explanations for these phenomena are that nerve fibers can be divided into 3 major groups according to fiber size, and that fiber size can be correlated—to an extent, at least—with fiber function. He will also remember that local anesthetic drugs generally block transmission most easily in the smaller fibers, such as the thinly myelinated B fibers which carry sympathetic impulses, and the nonmyelinated C fibers which carry impulses arising in response to pinprick, whereas the A fibers, which subserve motor and proprioceptive functions, are the largest and the last to be blocked. Thus, sympathetic and slow pain sensation are usually blocked first in spinal anesthesia, followed by sensory block and motor paralysis, in that order.

If he was an exceedingly astute and interested medical student, he may even remember that the fact that nerve fibers are divided into 3 major groups on the basis of fiber size was demonstrated by Gasser and Erlanger, employing the cathode ray oscilloscope to record the spike potentials from a mixed nerve.

Joseph Erlanger was the son of Herman and Sarah Erlanger and was born in San Francisco on January 5, 1874. He received a B.S. degree in chemistry from the University of California, and the M.D. degree in 1899 from the Johns Hopkins University. After a year of internship at the Johns Hopkins Hospital, he was appointed to the department of physiology at the Johns Hopkins Medical School as an assistant. During the next 6 years he was promoted rapidly, first to instructor, then to associate, and finally to associate professor. In 1906, he left his alma mater to become the first Professor of Physiology in the newly established medical school at the University of Wisconsin. In 1910, Erlanger moved on to the Professorship in Physiology at the reorganized Washington University School of Medicine in St. Louis, where he remained until his retirement as Professor Emeritus in 1946.

Herbert Spencer Gasser was born the son of Herman Gasser and Jane Elizabeth Griswold Gasser in Platteville, Wisconsin, on July 5, 1888, just 14½ years, to the day, after Erlanger had been born. He attended the Wisconsin State Normal School and the University of Wisconsin, from which he received his A.B. degree in 1910 and his A.M. degree in 1911; it was at this time that he first met and studied physiology under Erlanger. In 1912 he began his medical school course at Johns Hopkins, receiving the M.D. degree in 1915. He returned to Wisconsin for a year in pharmacology,

and then went to the department of pharmacology at Washington University in St. Louis. He was appointed Professor of Pharmacology there in 1921. In 1931 he was appointed Professor of Physiology at Cornell University Medical College in New York City, and from 1935 to 1953 he was Director of the Rockefeller Institute for Medical Research.

It was while Gasser was in the department of pharmacology at the school of medicine at Washington University in St. Louis that he and Erlanger had such a fruitful collaboration on the problems of the electrophysiology of nerves—so fruitful, in fact, that in 1944 they shared the Nobel Prize. A major basis for that award, and one of the outstanding results of their collaboration, was a masterly piece of work published under the title, "The Rôle of Fiber Size in the Establishment of a Nerve Block by Pressure or Cocaine" (Gasser, H. S. and Erlanger, J.: *Am. J. Physiol.*, *88:* 581, 1929), which is reprinted below with the kind permission of the publisher.

THE ROLE OF FIBER SIZE IN THE ESTABLISHMENT OF A NERVE BLOCK BY PRESSURE OR COCAINE

GASSER, H.S. AND ERLANGER, J.

Am. J. Physiol., 88:581, 1929

This classic paper refutes the idea that a differing chemical composition of various nerve fibers accounts for the differential effect of cocaine and other local anesthetics on the modalities of sensation lost when applied to a mixed nerve. By relating fiber size, measured by conduction velocity, to rate of loss of nerve transmission, the authors clearly show that cocaine acts first on smaller fibers and that fiber size explains the order in which nerve functions are lost.

1930

Published February, 1981

During each of the past 2 years, there has been a Refresher Course Lecture presented at the ASA Annual Meeting on the subject of low flow anesthesia and closed systems; in addition, a book titled, "Low Flow and Closed System Anesthesia," has recently been published; and even an International Symposium on Low Flow and Closed System Anesthesia has been held.

To those of us who received our residency training in the late 1930's, the 1940's, or the early 1950's, the reaction to all of this is, "for goodness sakes—what's all the fuss about?" We grew up with low flow, closed, CO_2 absorption anesthesia, and it is as usual as putting the cat out at night and as comfortable as an old shoe. In fact, some of us still become a bit miffed to see a resident giving anesthesia day after day from an anesthesia machine with a canister in which the upper layers of soda lime are purple-blue and therefore partially exhausted. Why in heaven's name doesn't the resident change that soda lime? What happened to soda lime and the closed, CO_2 absorption inhalation anesthesia system anyway?

What happened was that halothane was introduced.

When halothane burst upon the anesthetic scene in 1956, the anesthesiologist was presented with a fully potent, nonexplosive, volatile anesthetic agent—and he took it and ran with it. Within a matter of a few short years, halothane was involved in about 80 per cent of all of the general anesthesias administered in this country, and it was administered in a semiclosed or a nonrebreathing system, with high flows of N_2O-O_2 as the carrier gases.

Two properties of the drug dictated these techniques. The first was halothane's immense potency, which made it possible to deliver precise amounts from a metered vaporizer into a large volume of carrier gases with great safety and consummate ease. In fact, high flow N_2O-O_2 halothane anesthesia was undoubtedly the simplest type of inhalation anesthesia to administer that the anesthetist had ever known. The second property was the minimal analgesia which halothane produced, at least in the low concentrations which were used to avoid the dose-related adverse cardiovascular and respiratory effects. The tremendous amount of analgesia added by the N_2O in this high flow technique was beautifully demonstrated in a classic study of the MAC of halothane, which was conducted by Saidman and Eger many years ago. Patients who received only halothane and O_2 had a MAC for halothane of 0.74 volumes per cent. If morphine was given as premedication prior to halothane-O_2 anesthesia, the MAC was reduced to 0.69 volumes per cent. However, if the morphine premedication was omitted, but N_2O was added to the O_2 as the carrier gas for halothane, the MAC fell to 0.29 volumes per cent. This change represented a 61 per cent decrease in the MAC of halothane when N_2O was used as compared to the use of halothane alone with O_2, and made the combination of N_2O's analgesia and halothane's potency the ideal anesthetic mixture in the minds of a good many people.

The use of high flow, semiclosed or nonrebreathing techniques, however, has certain inherent drawbacks. They are expensive, since both the carrier gases and the volatile agent are vented from the system and must be replaced with fresh carrier gases and vapor with each breath. They entail losses of heat, which not only is a considerable physiologic cost to the body, but requires the use of expensive accessory equipment such as blood warmers and hyperthermia mattresses. High flow techniques also entail large losses of body water, which must be replaced, and again with the use of added equipment in the form of humidifiers. The waste gases and vapors pose a health hazard (perhaps) to the operating room personnel, and this problem entails still further expense in the form of scavenging systems. There is a final cost to the patient—which will be hotly denied by every anesthesiologist, but by only some with complete justification—of loss of breath-by-breath attention to the patient's condition once the airway is secured, the ventilator properly set, and the vaporizer and flow meters dialed to safe and reasonable concentrations and amounts. All of these disadvantages are negated by the use of low flow anesthesia and the closed system, the keystone of which is CO_2 absorption.

It was just 3 years after the signing of the American Declaration of Independence in 1776 that the Abbé Felice Fontana announced that he had "discovered a new method of procuring to a sick person the benefit of breathing any quantity of dephlogisticated air (i.e., O_2) at a cheap rate." He went on to describe the use of a solution of lime for the purpose of absorbing what he called the "fixed air". This was probably the first reference—or at least one of the first references—to the clinical use of CO_2 absorption.

In 1849, Regnault and Rieset passed a current of O_2 into a small chamber, in which an animal was confined for the purpose of analyzing the changes produced in the air by the respiration of the animal. They used a strong alkaline hydroxide solution to absorb the CO_2 output of the animal, O_2 being added from a constant pressure reservoir. These principles were used by practically all workers studying respiratory metabolism thereafter.

Three-quarters of a century later, in 1916, Dennis Jackson, a pharmacologist at the Washington University Medical School in St. Louis, described a method by which he kept dogs anesthetized for long periods by filling a cabinet with N_2O, a pump being attached to circulate the N_2O through an alkali which absorbed the CO_2. A tank of O_2 was attached, which added O_2 slowly and thereby took care of the metabolic needs of the dogs as to O_2. The dogs could remain in the chamber in good condition for long periods of time. One of Jackson's chief interests in this work was in reducing the expense of running his laboratory, since continuous rebreathing from a closed container lowered the cost of N_2O-O_2 anesthesia in the laboratory animals from about $2.50 per hour to 32 cents per hour. However, his studies were the immediate forerunners of the development of closed, CO_2 absorption systems as they are known in clinical anesthesia today, and in 1963 the American Society of Anesthesiologists presented its Distinguished Service Award to Jackson in signal tribute to the significance of his contribution.

Ralph Waters, some 8 years later, designed a clinical apparatus based on the physiologic principles inherent in Jackson's laboratory mechanism, and successfully used a closed, CO_2 absorption technique to anesthetize human patients. Waters' appliance consisted of a mask with a well fitting rubber face cushion, a cylinder of granular soda lime $3\frac{1}{2}$ inches in diameter and 4 inches long, and a rebreathing bag with a tail, to which was attached tanks of N_2O and O_2. The patient inhaled from the reservoir bag through the canister into the lungs, and then exhaled through the canister back into the bag; and therefore, not unreasonably, his technique became known as the "to-and-fro" CO_2 absorption system. Waters pointed out the several practical advantages arising from this type of CO_2 filtration: the economy of anesthetic agents, the conservation of body heat and moisture, and the fact that there was no waste of drugs into the operating room—and therefore the disagreeable odors of drugs, such as ether and ethylene, could be kept away from the surgical team, and extremely volatile agents such as ethyl chloride were more easily controlled.

Waters noted that the limitations included the need for an extremely "tight connection with the air passages," and the fact that the design was therefore not suitable for nose and mouth work. Brian Sword, Waters' good friend, noted other pertinent limitations: the fact that having the canister and the rebreathing bag at the patient's face was unwieldy, too close to the field of operation, and inconvenient for repositioning the head during operation in the interests of maintaining the airway. Sword therefore designed, with the aid of Richard Foregger, the closed, "circle" CO_2 technique, which was reported in the September-October, 1930, issue of *Current Researches in Anesthesia and Analgesia* under the title, "The Closed Circle Method of Administration of Gas Anesthesia" (Sword, B.C.: *Anesth. Analg., 9:* 198–202, 1930), and is reprinted below.

THE CLOSED CIRCLE METHOD OF ADMINISTRATION OF GAS ANESTHESIA

Brian C. Sword

New Haven, Connecticut

Anesth. Analg., 9: 198, 1930

"By the closed circle method of anesthesia, an apparatus is so constructed that the inspiratory and expiratory phase run in the same direction. This requires a separation by means of valves and two tubes, one for inspiration and one for expiration connected by a "Y", so that it may be applied to a mask. The tubes (two feet in length and three quarters of an inch in diameter) are attached to a cannister by means of flutter valves. At the bottom of the cannister a rebreathing bag is placed. The soda-lime in the cannister should be dry and size for 8×10 mesh.

*   *   *   *

"After the patient has reached the stage of surgical narcosis,—the closed circle method of anesthesia is operated best between 300 and 400 cc. of oxygen per minute.

*   *   *   *

"I have used this method in about twelve hundred cases. Advantages:
1. Ease and rapidity of induction.
2. Flexibility.
3. The margin of surgical narcosis seems greater thereby insuring a smooth third stage of anesthesia.
4. Simplicity.
5. Economical.
6. The ease in changing from one anesthetic to another.
7. The removal of the bag and cannister from the field of operation."

1932

Published October, 1959

As might be expected, perhaps, the ether had scarcely dried from Long's towel and Morton's sponge before speculation arose as to the mechanisms involved in the production of the anesthetic state. A great deal of specious reasoning was done, and a favorite analogy was that between etherization and asphyxia. It is an analogy that still finds occasional supporters even today (sometimes with good reason!), but it was actually disposed of early in 1847 by the important series of experiments carried out by the French physiologist Flourens: "In ordinary asphyxia the nervous system becomes paralyzed through the action of . . . blood *deprived of oxygen;* during etherization the nervous system becomes paralyzed primarily through the direct action upon it of this singular agent."

There followed, through the years, a number of attempts to define the mode of action of anesthetic drugs on the basis of chemical or physical properties. One of the first of these was propounded independently in two separate laboratories by Meyer (1899) and Overton (1901). The Overton-Meyer Lipoid Solubility Theory was based upon the presumption that drugs having anesthetic action must be soluble in the fatty material or lipoids of the brain, and that their activity depended upon their high solubility in such lipoid material in relation to their solubility in water: *i.e.* on their oil-water solubility ratio. The objections to this theory have been numerous, including the complaint that water is not comparable to blood or lymph, and that olive oil is not comparable to the body fats; but the major failure of the Lipoid Solubility Theory has been that it holds true for aliphatic compounds only, and does not explain the action of numerous other chemicals which possess narcotic action, including heterocyclic substances, alkaloids and inorganic substances (such as bromide and magnesium).

A rather different explanation of anesthetic action was encompassed in Traube's Surface-Tension Theory (1904), based upon the parallelism which exists between the ability of drugs to lower the surface tension of a cell and their narcotic activity. He was able to demonstrate, in a series of alcohols, that there was a striking correlation between depressant activity and ability to lower surface tension. The objections to this theory have also been numerous, the most important one being the fact that there are substances which produce anesthesia which are surface-inactive, while at the same time there are many substances which lower surface tension (such as detergents) which have no anesthetic activity.

A third important theory of narcosis, the Cell-Permeability Theory, was first suggested by Hober in 1907, but really championed by Lillie during the following decade. This theory was based upon the fact that excitation could be shown to be accompanied by an increase in cell permeability, particularly to certain ions, and it was reasoned that depression would be accompanied by a decrease in permeability. In fact, Lillie, using Arenicola larvae, demonstrated that certain substances that caused muscular contraction also caused an increase in permeability to an intracellular pigment, while depressant substances, such as magnesium chloride and certain anesthetic drugs, decreased both activity and permeability. Again, however, the theory failed to stand up under careful inspection, for there is little evidence that anesthesia invariably is accompanied by a decreased permeability.

There were numerous other theories which also attempted to explain the nature of anesthesia on the basis of chemical or physical properties; but it became increasingly evident that no single property was shared by all drugs possessing narcotic activity which could serve as the basis for an explanation of such narcotic activity, and the necessity for a new approach to the problem began to focus attention upon the biological actions of anesthetic agents. Verworn, as early as 1909, had noted that narcosis was accompanied by diminished cellular oxidation, and at about the same time Warburg had also demonstrated that anesthetics inhibit oxidation; but the pioneer studies which really established the relationship between cellular metabolism and narcosis, and which led to much of the current work in this field, were those of J. H. Quastel and A. H. M. Wheatley, which were published in the *Proceedings of the Royal Society, Series B, 112:* 60–79, November, 1932, under the title of "Narcosis and Oxidations of the Brain."

NARCOSIS AND OXIDATIONS OF THE BRAIN

QUASTEL, J.H.,
AND WHEATLEY, A.H.M.

*Proc. Roy. Soc., London,
Series B, 112:60–79, November, 1932*

A series of experiments were described in which the uptake of oxygen by brain tissue was observed under various conditions and in the presence of a variety of narcotic agents. The conclusion was reached that narcotics have the general property of inhibiting the oxidation by brain of glucose, lactate and pyruvate, while leaving certain other oxidations unaffected. "It is suggested that a view of the mechanism of narcosis which fits most closely to the facts, is that the narcotic is absorbed from the blood at a specific area or centre of the nervous system. Here it brings about a diminution of the ability of the cells constituting the nervous centre to activate lactic or pyruvic acid, in this way inhibiting the oxidation by these cells of glucose, lactic and pyruvic acids. The access or activation of oxygen is quite unimpaired, but the diminished ability of the cells to oxidise glucose or lactic acid results in a lowering of the amount of energy available for the cells to accomplish their functional activities. Narcosis- or depression of the normal functional activity of the nervous centre in question- may then ensue."

1933

Published April, 1965

Diethyl ether, which is as old as the history of anesthesia itself, is a symmetrical, aliphatic organic oxide. It is a colorless, highly volatile liquid, which boils at 36.5°C. Its molecular weight is 74, and its specific gravity is 0.718 at 15°C., so that in liquid form it floats on water. It has an oil/water solubility coefficient of 3.2, an oil/blood solubility coefficient of 3.3, and an Ostwald, or blood/gas, coefficient of 15.08. It is highly flammable, with a flash point below 32°F.; and the range of flammability of ether is from 1.83 to 48.0 per cent when mixed with air, from 2.10 to 82.5 per cent when mixed with oxygen, and from 1.5 to 24.2 per cent when mixed with pure nitrous oxide. Ether oxidizes slowly in the presence of oxygen to form ethyl and other peroxides. It does not react with alkalis, and is not altered by soda lime or barium lime mixtures. The inspired concentration for surgical anesthesia varies from 3.5 to 4.5 per cent by volume, and the blood concentration necessary to produce (second plane) surgical anesthesia has been variously estimated as from 50 to 130 mg. per 100 ml. in man.

Ether inductions are slow and unpleasant, its vapor being irritating to the respiratory tract and producing breath-holding, coughing, laryngospasm, and secretions. Emergence is also slow, being the mirror image of induction, and postoperative nausea and vomiting are frequent, particularly if ether vapor is swallowed. It is a fully potent drug that can produce full muscular relaxation even in the presence of high concentrations of oxygen, but which also can produce severe physiologic disturbances.

Ethylene, on the other hand, a drug whose anesthetic properties were recognized only rather recently (in 1923), is an unsaturated (double bonded) aliphatic hydrocarbon, the simplest member of the olefine series. It is a colorless gas whose odor has been variously described as "sweetish," "musty," "nauseating," "ethereal," "pungent," and "foul." Its molecular weight is 28, and its specific gravity 0.97. It has an oil/water solubility coefficient of 14.4, an oil/blood solubility coefficient of 9.3, and an Ostwald coefficient of 0.140. It is highly flammable, with a flash point below 32°F.; and the range of flammability of ethylene is from 3.05 to 28.6 per cent when mixed with air, from 2.90 to 79.9 per cent when mixed with oxygen, and from 1.90 to 40.2 per cent when mixed with nitrous oxide. Ethylene may contain contaminants of manufacture such as carbon dioxide, nitrogen, oxygen, or, most dangerously, carbon monoxide. It is chemically stable under most circumstances, and is not altered by soda lime or barium lime mixtures. The inspired concentration for surgical anesthesia is 75 to 80 per cent, and the blood concentrations during (first plane) surgical anesthesia average from 120 to 180 mg. per 100 ml.

Ethylene inductions are rapid, since it is a comparatively nonirritating gas to inhale. Recovery is also rapid, with minimal nausea and vomiting. Muscle relaxation is insufficient for major surgery, however, and asphyxia is always a hazard since the concentration necessary to produce surgical anesthesia may cause suboxygenation. In the absence of the latter, though, it produces no deleterious effects on the circulatory, respiratory, or other systems or organs. The gas is somewhat more potent than nitrous oxide, and is therefore easier and safer to administer.

Chauncey Leake, after considering both the chemical structure and the anesthetic properties of each of these general anesthetic drugs, came to the conclusion that a compound incorporating the structural characteristics of diethyl ether (CH_3—CH_2—O—CH_2—CH_3) and ethylene (CH_2＝CH_2) would be a valuable anesthetic drug. Such a compound, divinyl ether, had been vaguely described by Semmler in 1855 as having been isolated from a species of allium, but it had never been synthesized and there was not even certainty that it had really been isolated. The problem was undertaken for Leake by two graduate students in the Department of Chemistry at Princeton University, Randolph Major and W. T. Ruigh, who were able to produce impure samples of the drug; and then, later, when they became associated with Merck & Company, they prepared pure divinyl oxide which they furnished to Leake for pharmacologic study and clinical trials. The reports of these investigations were published in the January, 1933, issue of *The Journal of Pharmacology and Experimental Therapeutics* (Gelfan, S. and Bell, I. R.: The anesthetic action of divinyl oxide on humans. *J. Pharmacol. & Exper. Therap., 47:* 1, 1933; Leake, C. D., Knoefel, P. K. and Guedel, A. E.: The anesthetic action

of divinyl oxide in animals. *J. Pharmacol. & Exper. Therap., 47:* 5, 1933), and are reprinted below.

THE ANESTHETIC ACTION OF DIVINYL OXIDE ON HUMANS

Samuel Gelfan
and Irving R. Bell

From the Department of
Physiology and Pharmacology,
University of Alberta,
Edmonton, Canada

Received for publication
April 5, 1932

J. Pharmacol. Exper. Therap., 47:1, 1933

*   *   *   *

"Divinyl oxide was first administered, very lightly and cautiously by the drop method, to one of us (S.G.) for a period of ten minutes. Nine minutes after the beginning of the introduction the subject was completely unconscious. A partial analgesia was present four minutes after the beginning of induction, and complete analgesia after seven minutes. There was practically complete muscular relaxation in the arms and legs after ten minutes, at which time the anesthetic was discontinued. Two minutes after the removal of the mask, the subject had fully recovered and was able to converse intelligibly. He immediately rose and walked about very briskly with perfect coordination. The pulse remained normal throughout. The breakfast, taken two hours before the anesthesia, was retained with no discomfort. Eight minutes after the removal of the mask, 150 cc. of water was ingested and retained. There was no nausea or vomiting at any time. About one hour later, lunch was taken with normal appetite and with no after effects. About 20 cc. of the anesthetic was used during the ten minutes."

*   *   *   *

THE ANESTHETIC ACTION OF DIVINYL OXIDE IN ANIMALS

C. D. Leake, P. K. Knoefel
and A. E. Guedel

From the Pharmacological
Laboratory of the
University of California
Medical School,
San Francisco, California

Received for publication
April 5, 1932

J. Pharmacol. Exper. Therap., 47:5, 1933

*   *   *   *

SUMMARY

"Pure divinyl oxide, although inflammable and explosive like ether, has definite advantages over ether which recommend it as a general inhalation anesthetic agent for clinical evaluation. It is more volatile than ether and more powerful and rapid in its anesthetic action. It is less irritating than ether and its general physiological actions are less severe. It has no significant pathological effect when administered without anoxemia. Recovery is more prompt than from ether and apparently less attended with nausea or other evidence of physiological distress. It may be administered by any technique used for ether. On the basis of the experimental evidence so far accumulated, divinyl oxide deserves clinical study to determine whether or not it has practical clinical advantages over the anesthetics now in common use. Divinyl oxide, on exposure to light and air, may polymerize or partially decompose with the appearance of formaldehyde and formic acid. Such material, of course, would be dangerous for anesthetic purposes."

Published October, 1981

Dr. Philip Bromage, whose almost 4 decades of experience with the technique and whose 2 books (the most recent weighing in at 746 pages) on the subject, have made him a world's authority on epidural analgesia, has this to say of the history of the method:

"Corning has been credited with being the first to use epidural analgesia in 1885. Corning had the idea that medications injected within the spinal canal might be taken up by the rich plexuses of blood vessels in the neighborhood and be carried into the substance of the spinal cord, thus allowing direct medication of the cord, either for treatment of neurological disease or for providing surgical analgesia. However, from his own description of the two experiments he carried out, it is evident that he neither intended nor achieved a genuine epidural injection. Nevertheless, it is ironic that Corning's hypothesis of spinal cord uptake was discredited and dismissed as unscientific. After the passage of nearly 100 years, the original idea now seems remarkably close to the truth, and all the available evidence points to the cord as an important site of action of epidural blockade.

"Epidural analgesia has been practiced, by one technique or another, since 1901 when Sicard and Cathelin of France independently popularized the caudal approach. After the favorable reports of Sicard and Cathelin, Tuffier attempted epidural analgesia by the lumbar approach later in the same year, but his lack of success, and the natural difficulties of locating a narrow space 2 to 4 mm. wide at a depth twenty times that amount, discouraged all further attempts for many years. In 1913, Heile tried to revive the idea of high epidural blocks by entering the spinal canal laterally through the intervertebral foramina instead of by midline puncture. Heile used this approach for surgical and therapeutic purposes, but his method does not seem to have had much following outside Germany. In the meantime, the caudal route became established as the only safe approach to the epidural space, and there was a tendency to limit the field of analgesia to the area supplied by the cauda equina (Läwen, 1911), since efforts to carry the block higher met with variable results, owing to the individual differences in the anatomy of the sacrum and its foramina.

"This state of affairs continued until 1921 when Fidel Pagés renewed interest in the midline lumbar approach, pointing out the increased ease of access and wider applicability of this route as compared with the caudal route. Pagés' method of identifying the epidural space was primarily tactile, demanding great dexterity from the operator in order to detect the "feel" of the needle passing from the ligamentum flavum into the epidural space. The degree of skill required for Pagés' method was clearly a limiting factor to the technique, and other workers set about establishing mechanical substitutes for manual dexterity. These refinements gradually developed, and it is now possible to obtain a very high success rate in lumbar epidural analgesia without possessing an unusual sensitivity of touch.

"Although the mode of action of epidural blockade remained conjectural, there was not lack of theories for its possible site of action, and for many years the technical aspects of epidural analgesia were dictated by clinical impressions and qualitative observations rather than by systematic measurements. There were notable exceptions to this, particularly in the works of Dogliotti (1939) and Gutierrez (1939), but the bulk of the literature on the subject was based on clinical results, without too much attention being paid to careful analysis of the many variables encountered between different drugs and different patients; therefore, it was not surprising that confusion and disagreement arose over details of technical management when the fundamental principles underlying these matters were so poorly understood.

"Thus, because the majority of practicing anesthesiologists came to regard the method as unreliable and even frankly dangerous in unskilled hands, it was relegated to the status of a museum piece, to be dusted and shown the light of day from time to time at examinations and scientific meetings, but for the most part not to be regarded too seriously except perhaps in the hands of a few enthusiasts who, some-

what inexplicably, made it their hobby" (Bromage, P. R.: *Epidural Analgesia*. Philadelphia: W. B. Saunders, 1978, pp. 1–2).

In the meantime, there was a growing concern over the dangers of general anesthesia in labor. The British reported a death rate from aspiration of vomitus as high as 1:3380 obstetric anesthetics; while a similar study in the United States showed a maternal death rate of 1:20,304 directly attributable to anesthesia, of which one-third were due to the inhalation of vomitus during general anesthesia, and about one-quarter the result of spinal anesthesia. In this country, Hingson led an almost-evangelical crusade to popularize caudal analgesia as an effective and safer alternative to general analgesia and anesthesia in obstetrics. The technique became hugely popular in certain sections of the country; but a 15 per cent failure rate, in the best of hands, because of both the variations in the anatomy of the caudal canal and the difficulty—indeed, often the impossibility—of identifying the caudal hiatus in the parturient at term made it something less than a panacea.

Furthermore, while successful caudal analgesia would produce perineal anesthesia and anesthesia of the lower birth canal, it did not provide relief from the pains of uterine contractions unless large doses were used, which added both to the possibility of toxic effects from the local anesthetic drug and to the likelihood that the higher level of anesthesia attained would greatly slow—or perhaps even stop—the progress of the first stage of labor. Spinal analgesia, which also could guarantee anesthesia of the perineum and of the lower birth canal, also would slow or even stop labor when the level of anesthesia was sufficient to control the pains of uterine contractions.

The fact of the matter was that the lack of definite knowledge concerning the paths of afferent nerves of the uterus to the cord prevented the scientific application of regional as an alternative to general anesthesia for the problem of obstetric analgesia and anesthesia. Today's highly successful answer to this problem, continuous lumbar epidural analgesia, rests firmly on the little-recognized but absolutely fundamental studies by Cleland, which specifically identified, for the first time, the pain pathways of labor.

Cleland began his 5 years of researches at McGill University in 1927, and then carried them to completion and conducted the clinical applications at the University of Oregon and the Oregon City Hospital. His investigations showed that the pain pathways for uterine contractions were T–11, 12 and those for cervical dilation were S–2,3,4. He reported his landmark work in the July, 1933, issue of Surgery, Gynecology and Obstetrics under the title of, "Paravertebral Anaesthesia in Obstetrics. Experimental and Clinical Basis" (Cleland, J. G. P.: *Surg. Gynecol. Obstet.*, 57: 51–56, 1933), which is reprinted below.

PARAVERTEBRAL ANAESTHESIA IN OBSTETRICS EXPERIMENTAL AND CLINICAL BASIS

J. G. P. CLELAND

Department of Physiology, University of Oregon, and Oregon City Hospital

Surg. Gynecol. Obstet., 57: 51, 1933

"The purpose of this paper is to survey the present status of our knowledge of uterine afferent nerves, to present experimental proof via visceromotor reflexes of the location of these paths in the dog, to correlate these findings in man, to explain the error of conclusions hitherto accepted, and to demonstrate that the pain of uterine contraction may be abolished without affecting the contractions by paravertebral block of only two adjacent nerves."

In a large number of complicated and meticulously-performed experiments in dogs and cats, it was shown that "afferent fibers from the uterus enter the spinal cord, in the dog, through the first and second lumbar roots."

*   *   *   *

"Although the analogy of the arrangement of afferent nerves in dog and man was well substantiated, the hypothesis that the lumbar nerve roots were numbered two higher in the dog than in man required experimental proof." This was ascertained in further experiments associated with afferent impulses from the fallopian tube of the dog. It could be deduced that the uterine afferent roots in the human are the eleventh and twelfth thoracic.

Clinical studies were carried out in five women in labor to corroborate the experimental findings. Local anesthesia was provided with procaine or nupercaine.

Typically, once labor pains were established, an area of hyperalgesia was found in the lower abdomen, the upper transverse boundary of which was one-third the distance from the umbilicus to the pubis, and the lower boundary of which was at Poupart's ligament, that is, the eleventh and twelfth thoracic.

When the eleventh and twelfth thoracic nerve roots on each side were injected paravertebrally with a local anesthetic, the pain of the uterine contractions ceased, and the area of hyperalgesia had disappeared, being replaced with analgesia.

The pain of dilation of the birth canal was abolished by a caudal block.

1934

Published April, 1959

Over the course of the years, cyclopropane has been many things to many men:

To the German chemist, August von Freund, who first prepared and identified the compound in 1882, cyclopropane was an isomer of propylene, made by reducing trimethylene dibromide with sodium in an alcoholic solution;

To the Canadian pharmacologists, Dr. Velyian E. Henderson and Dr. G. H. W. Lucas, cyclopropane was a contaminant of the propylene which they were employing as an experimental anesthetic, and suspect as the cause of the severe cardiac disturbances that they were encountering during those laboratory trials—when they had synthesized and purified the compound, they discovered its anesthetic properties, and then spent five years in carrying out a sufficiently diversified series of animal experiments to demonstrate the characteristics of the drug;

To patients, cyclopropane has been a relatively rapid and pleasant way to go to sleep, free from the terrifying, choking sensation that some had experienced with ether, and also, perhaps, free from the protracted sickness that some had suffered following ether anesthesia;

To surgeons, cyclopropane has been an anesthetic that provided moderately good working conditions, and has been particularly useful in the shocked or bad risk patient;

To the resident in the beginning phases of his training in anesthesiology, cyclopropane has been a tricky and terrifyingly potent agent, capable of taking the patient to the depths in a matter of a few breaths;

To the trained anesthesiologist, cyclopropane has been an anesthetic of precision—refined, advanced, civilized: "My conception of anesthesia with the older gases is that we administer the gas plus enough oxygen to keep the patient alive and in good condition. With cyclopropane, on the other hand, we administer oxygen with just enough gas to keep the patient asleep";

To insurance underwriters, cyclopropane has been a considerable hazard in the operating room, capable of lethal explosions from a small static spark;

To hospitals, cyclopropane has been a considerable expense, not alone because it is an expensive gas to manufacture, but even more importantly because of the tremendous costs of making all operating suites conform to the code for the prevention of fires and explosions;

To Dr. Ralph M. Waters and his associates at the Winconsin General Hospital in the early 1930's, cyclopropane was an anesthetic drug with enough promise to warrant careful clinical trials; these were reported by Drs. Stiles, Neff, Rovenstine, and Waters under the title, "Cyclopropane as an anesthetic agent: a preliminary clinical report" in *Current Researches in Anesthesia and Analgesia*, *13*:56 to 60 (Mar.–Apr.) 1934.

*   *   *   *

The present day anesthetist who is interested in reading a republication of the first clinical report on cyclopropane will likely be interested in some aspects of its background including significant, but little known, cooperative efforts between its Canadian discoverers and American workers.

Little did any of us realize the profound impact the introduction of cyclopropane anaesthesia would have in changing the attitude of American Medicine toward the anaesthetist as a medical specialist.

Ralph M. Waters, always endearingly referred to by his former residents as the "Chief," is in stature everything which the term implies. Even though, at his insistence, his name appears last on this important document, he did in fact engineer the entire project. As the junior resident in the department at the time, whose name more properly should have been last on this paper, I feel qualified to clarify certain matters of interest.

The anaesthetic properties of cyclopropane had been demonstrated to Dr. Waters on animals (cats) by Henderson, Lucas and Brown in the Pharmacology Laboratory of the University of Toronto and he was quick to appreciate its clinical potentialities. In fact, he was so impressed by the demonstrations that, immediately upon his return to the University of Wisconsin, he initiated measures for procuring cyclopropane. The first cyclopropane was very limited in amounts and, even by today's standards, very expensive.

Perhaps for the first time anywhere the departments of pharmacology, physiology, anaesthesia and surgery cooperated fully in a combined experimental and clinical undertaking. Dr. Walters and his residents worked in the departments of physiology, pharmacology or experimental surgery after completion of the clinical surgical schedules. Dr. M. Seevers, the well known pharmacologist, also had had clinical experience in anaesthesia under Dr. Waters.

The opportunity arose for me to make an "all expense paid" business trip back to Montreal. Because of this I was commissioned to stop over in Toronto and discuss cyclopropane developments with Brown, Henderson and Lucas. Dr. Waters had gone far enough with clinical studies to realize that cyclopropane would be a very important anesthetic. If conditions at the University of Toronto had changed, Dr. Waters was anxious that the first clinical reports should emanate from that institution. The Toronto group assured me that the same resistance by their surgical and anaesthesia departments to the clinical employment of ethylene precluded the introduction of cyclopropane into the surgical theatres in the forseeable future. Furthermore, they requested that the Wisconsin group under Dr. Waters proceed with their

studies as rapidly as possible and publish on what they believed to be the most promising inhalation anaesthetic of the time. Once again the discoverers of the anaesthetic properties of ethylene were obliged to look elsewhere for the clinical establishment of cyclopropane, whose anaesthetic qualities they discovered while purifying still another unsaturated hydrocarbon anaesthetic, namely, propylene.

It is very difficult to express in words the spirit of friendly cooperation which existed between the Canadian discoverers and the American workers. The important thing for the record is that it did exist.

WILLIAM B. NEFF, M.D.

CYCLOPROPANE AS AN ANESTHETIC AGENT; A PRELIMINARY CLINICAL TRIAL

STILES, J. A., NEFF, W. B., ROVENSTINE, E. A. AND WATERS, R. M.

Anesth. Analg., 13: 56–60 (Mar.–Apr.) 1934

This preliminary report described the administration of cyclopropane to 447 patients by the carbon dioxide absorption technique. It was found to produce adequate muscle relaxation. Although explosive, it was considered to be less so than ethylene, a commonly used anesthetic, and the incidence of postoperative complications compared favorably with other agents, particularly ether. The authors considered cyclopropane to be an experimental drug and believed it necessary to have a full year of carefully controlled observations before it could be introduced into general use.

Published June, 1973

"Daddy Warbucks lay close to death.

"Punjab stood guard at the doorway, utterly helpless to combat the chemical forces

at work inside his friend's body which were slowly disrupting the delicate balance within the nervous system which is essential

to life. The great Swedish neurophysiolog-
ical specialist was even then winging his
way across the ocean; but it was doubtful
that he could arrive in time, or that he
could stem the forced march of the Grim
Reaper even if he did arrive in time. Germaniotti's plot this time had been so devil-
ishly clever that all of the vast and far-flung
Warbuck's industrial complex was impo-
tent to combat it. The enemy's ruthless
scientists and henchmen had combined to
strike down the world's most powerful man
in one tantalizingly-brief second, and now
he was fighting for every breath.

"The doctors had explained the situation
to the Asp, and he in turn had tried to
make Annie understand the enormity of
the danger. The powerful ray gun, carefully concealed under the back seat of the
Warbucks limousine and activated by the
opening of the back door, released a stream
of Zirconium atoms which paralyzed the
transmission of acetylcholine within the autonomic nervous system ganglia, and the
pre-ganglionic cholinergic impulses could
no longer activate the synapses to produce
the propagated action potentials along the
post-ganglionic neurones.

"The cunning in Germaniotti's scheme
lay in its simplicity and finality. There was
no known (at that time) antidote to the
effects of the Zirconium atom, and only the
most transitory exposure was necessary to
produce almost total autonomic paralysis.
Furthermore, once the process was begun,
it was self-perpetuating, a vicious circle in
which initial paralysis begat further paralysis until, in time, paralysis was indeed total
and cellular respiration ceased."

The Germaniotti Incident, as it was to
become known to the followers of Harold
Gray's comic strip, "Little Orphan Annie,"
was neither the first nor yet the last science-
fiction episode in which the little redhead
and her faithful dog Sandy would be involved, but it was one based on firm pharmacologic principles—up to the point of
the stream of Zirconium atoms, at least.
Acetylcholine does indeed facilitate transmission within the autonomic ganglia; the
preganglionic cholinergic impulses do indeed activate the synapses; and this activation of the synapses does indeed produce

the propagated action potentials along the
postganglionic neurones.

The concept of ganglionic transmission
began with John Newport Langley, who
was born in 1852 and who died in 1926.

Langley "went up" to Cambridge University in 1871 with the intention of reading mathematics and history, but he soon
turned to natural sciences, probably influenced by the great physiologist, Foster:
"Langley first attended Foster's lectures
and practical classes in May of 1873 . . .
from that month until his last days, without
any break or important pause . . . he gave
all of his working life to the service of
physiology. In 1875 he took his B.A. degree and became demonstrator in physiology, and in 1903 he succeeded Foster to
the chair of physiology. Though Langley
was above all known as a prominent physiologist, he also dealt with pharmacological
problems. His two main fields of research
were the mechanism of secretion, and the
anatomy and function of the autonomic
nervous system."

And, of course, it was his concerns with
the autonomic nervous system which are of
interest to "Classical File."

In 1889, Langley and Dickinson pub-
lished a paper in the *Proceedings of the Royal
Society* entitled, "On the Local Paralysis of
Peripheral Ganglia, and on the Connexion
of Different Classes of Nerve Fibers with
Them," and which eventually led Langley
to the Nobel Prize which he shared with
Gaskell in 1918:

"Hirschmann has shown that after a
moderate dose of nicotin, stimulation of
the sympathetic nerve in the neck causes
no dilation of the pupil. He concludes that
nicotin paralyses the endings of the dilator
fibres in the pupil . . . it occurred to us that
the action of nicotin might be due to a
paralysis of the nerve cells of the superior
cervical ganglion, and not to a paralysis of
the nerve endings of the sympathetic nerve.
On testing this view, by stimulating the
sympathetic above and below the superior
cervical ganglion after injection of nicotin,
we found that, whilst stimulation below the
ganglion produced no effect, stimulation
above the ganglion produced a dilation of
the pupil and a constriction of the vessels

of the ear, as if no nicotin had been given. . . . If the alkaloid produces its effect by acting upon the nerve below the ganglion in consequence of any peculiarity of structure obtaining there, the local application of nicotin to the nerve should abolish its irritability. If, on the other hand, it produces its effect by acting upon the nerve cells in the superior cervical ganglion, the local application of nicotin to the nerve should have very little effect upon the nerve irritability, but the local application to the ganglion should abolish the effect of stimulating the nerve centrally of the ganglion. . . . In making the experiment on these lines, we isolate the sympathetic nerve in the neck . . . and . . . an inch and a half or so of the nerve is brushed over with a 1% solution of nicotin. . . . The central part of the nerve is stimulated several times at intervals of about two minutes; it produces the usual dilation of the pupil and constriction of vessels of the ear. The ganglion and the filaments proceeding from it are then brushed over with 1% nicotin; the sympathetic in the neck is again stimulated; it is found to be completely without effect; stimulation of the filaments running from the ganglion to the arteries produce the normal action. Hence, *nicotin paralyses the cells of the superior cervical ganglion.*"

The existence of ganglionic blocking drugs was a hugely useful experimental tool, but remained essentially of little therapeutic value until 1946, when Acheson and Moe published their definitive analyses of the effects of tetraethyl ammonium chloride (TEA) on the cardiovascular system and autonomic ganglia. In the meantime, however, a technique of conduction anesthesia was described which made it possible to block the transmission through autonomic ganglia by the injection of local anesthetic drugs. The regional anesthetic block of the stellate ganglion was described by LeRiche and his co-worker, Fontaine, in the May 23rd, 1934 issue of *La Presse Medicale* (LeRiche, R., and Fontaine, R.: L'Anesthesie Isolée Du Ganglion Etoile. Sa Technique, Ses Indications, Ses Resultats. *La Presse Medicale, 42:* 849–850, Mercredi, 23 Mai, 1934). *Survey* and its readers are deeply indebted to Miss Harmona Potter,

Assistant Librarian at the Hartford Medical Society, for the translation which is published below.

LOCAL ANESTHESIA OF THE STELLATE GANGLION

RÉNÉ LERICHE AND
RÉNÉ FONTAINE

Presse Médicale, 42: 849–850, 1934

"During the past nine years, we have carried out more than 200 procedures involving local anesthesia of the stellate ganglion, sometimes for diagnostic purposes and sometimes for therapeutic purposes.

"After numerous trials, we have adopted the following technique:

Anesthesia Technique for the Stellate Ganglion

"The patient is placed on a table, a pillow at the nape of the neck, and the head is turned in the opposite direction from the injection. The mid-clavicle is marked off and at this point, skimming the upper edge of the bone, a flexible platinum needle, 8–10 centimeters long and with a 6/10 diameter is inserted in the direction of the transverse process of the 7th cervical vertebra. When contact is made with the bone, the needle is moved in two directions. The hub is moved cephalad until the point of the needle has slipped in a downward direction the depth of one vertebra, and, at the same time, the hub is directed 30° laterally. At this moment, the needle is in contact with the stellate ganglion, and the injection of 10 cc. of 1% novocaine will produce anesthesia.

"In the cadaver, one can confirm this technique by injecting 10 cc. of methylene blue to color the stellate ganglion.

"In the living patient, a well-performed anesthesia of the stellate ganglion will, within a few minutes, produce the Claude Bernard-Horner Syndrome, which will last from one half hour up to several hours. At the same time, one will note vasodilatation and hyperthermia of the ipsilateral half of the face and of the hand.

"These physiologic manifestations are so constant that, if they are not present, the anesthetic procedure must be considered to have been unsuccessful. In other words,

infiltration of the stellate ganglion is correctly performed only when it is followed by the Claude Bernard-Horner Syndrome and by vasodilatation of the face."

Published August, 1974

When John Newport Langley won the Nobel Prize in 1918, it was largely as a result of his paper which was published in the 1889 issue of the *Proceedings of the Royal Society* titled, "On the Local Paralysis of Peripheral Ganglia, and on the Connexion of Different Classes of Nerve Fibers with Them." His interest in ganglion blockade was for its use as a physiologic and pharmacologic tool; but since that time, ganglion blockade has also become an important diagnostic and therapeutic measure, particularly in relation to the control of blood pressure.

Peripheral resistance resides mainly in the variably contractile arterioles and, to a lesser extent, in the capillaries and veins. The degree of contraction or tone of the arterioles, and probably also of the small veins, is maintained and controlled by several factors, of prime importance among which is the continuous stream of vasoconstrictor impulses which arise within the brain and pass down the spinal cord and out over the sympathetic fibers to the peripheral vessels. The peripheral resistance, therefore, can be reduced by an interruption of this pathway at any point in its course: by suppressing the formation of vasoconsrictor impulses, by blocking their pathway to the peripheral vessels, or by preventing the response of effector cells at the termination of the pathway.

Depression of the autonomic centers which are located in the midbrain will result in a decrease in the number and frequency of constrictor impulses arising in those centers; and it has been postulated that drugs such as hydralazine act in just this way—although present evidence suggests that a major action of hydralazine may also be direct relaxation of the smooth muscle of the vessel wall.

Depression of the vasomotor center in the medulla oblongata also will suppress

the stream of vasoconstrictor impulses. Central vasomotor depression of this type occurs to some degree with most narcotic and hypnotic drugs, and is known to occur quite consistently during deep levels of general anesthesia.

Reflex inhibition of the vasomotor centers (or stimulation of the vasodilator centers) will tend to detract from the effect that vasoconstrictor impulses have upon the peripheral vessels, and so will cause an increase in the cross-sectional area of the vascular bed and a fall of blood pressure. This is apparently the mode of action of the veratrum alkaloids.

Sympathetic blockade produced by blocking the preganglionic sympathetic fibers as they emerge from the spinal cord by one of the techniques of conduction anesthesia (spinal, epidural, or caudal anesthesia) has proven to be one of the most useful methods of reducing peripheral resistance.

Sympathetic blockade also may be effected by blocking the sympathetic ganglia themselves, either by paravertebral sympathetic ganglion blockade (which actually blocks the postganglionic, as well as the preganglionic, fibers) with a local anesthetic drug, or by the use of such systemically acting drugs as tetraethylammonium bromide or diiodide, hexamethonium salts (C6), pentamethonium salts (C5), mecamylamine hydrochloride (Inversine), Pempidine tartrate (Perolysen), Pendiomide, pentolinium tartrate (Ansolysen), phenactropinium chloride (Trophenium), trimethaphan camphorsulfonate (Arfonad), and similar drugs.

Sympathetic activity can also be interrupted at the sympathetic nerve endings as they terminate in the walls of the blood vessels by adrenergic blocking drugs. These compounds act by imposing a specific blockage between the effector cells and either the hormones of the adrenal medulla or the adrenergic mediator of the postganglionic nerves (*i.e.*, *l*-epinephrine or *l*-norepinephrine). Dibenamine and Dibenzyline are examples of this type of drug.

The response at the termination of the sympathetic pathway can be prevented by the direct action of drugs (such as the nitrites or nitrates, and certain ergot preparations) on the smooth muscle of the vessel walls themselves. These drugs are without adrenergic blocking properties, do not block sympathetic or parasympathetic ganglia, and have no effect on the hypothalamus or cortex. The site of action can be demonstrated by the intra-arterial injection of nitrites into a sympathectomized limb, and the recording of skin and muscle circulation.

Finally, there are 2 other classes of compounds which should be mentioned for the sake of completeness. They are the group acting by the inhibition of catecholamine synthesis (alpha-methyl-dopa), and those compounds acting by depletion of catecholamines from peripheral nerve endings in blood vessels, brain, heart, and from platelets (rauwolfia alkaloids).

While the anesthesiologist has utilized many of these methods of interrupting the continuous stream of vasoconstrictor impulses—and particularly, perhaps, the ganglion blocking drugs—he is historically associated with paravertebral lumbar sympathetic block. He has performed this block both for diagnostic purposes and in the treatment of a variety of peripheral vascular disorders. Rene Leriche described its use in the latter group of disease entities, and his technique, in an article which appeared in the November, 1934, issue of *La Presse Medicale* (Leriche, R. and Fontaine, R., Technic of Novocain infiltration of the lumbar sympathetic nerves. *La Presse Medicale 42:* 1843, 1934). *Survey* and its readers are deeply indebted to Miss Harmona Potter, Assistant Librarian of the Hartford Medical Society, for the translation which is published below.

TECHNIC OF NOVOCAIN INFILTRATION OF THE LUMBAR SYMPATHETIC NERVES

RENE LERICHE AND
RENE FONTAINE

Presse Medicale, 42: 1843, 1934

"Anesthetic infiltration of the lumbar chain produces in a few seconds both a subjective and an objective warming of the foot and leg, an increased oscillometric circulatory reading. To these indications of successful anesthesia there are almost always added special sensations that patients describe as a feeling of warmth going down into their legs. At the same time, pain if there is any, is considerably alleviated, or disappears, and vasomotor disturbances are modified. Movements of the toes and of the feet become easier and greater—if they had been either sluggish or limited—of course to the exclusion of any form of paralysis.

"The effect is unilateral. But there is reaction on the opposite side, and we were able to produce relief of pain phenomenon located on the right side by infiltrating the left sympathetic nerve, a fact common to all sympathetic nerve activity.

"The effect is temporary. However, it lasts longer than Novocain anesthesia. It frequently lasts for several hours; and by repeating the infiltrations, longer therapeutic action can be obtained. This fact has already been pointed out in speaking of anesthesia of the stellate ganglion.

"We have employed infiltration of the lumbar sympathetic nerve in varying situations:

a. In cases of arteritis, to alleviate pain and improve circulation.

b. In case of femoral embolism, where we have seen it cause disappearance of threatening and painful incidents—in a woman with cardiac embolism—to a point where it was no longer necessary to operate.

c. In cases of postoperative phlebitis, where it alleviated pain and caused the edema to recede.

d. In post-traumatic vasomotor syndromes with cyanosis, cold, functional disturbance, even osteoporosis, it has made it possible for us to avoid a periarterial sympathectomy.

e. In cases of painful arthritis, where it stops pain and contractures.

f. In cases of painful stumps, where its therapeutic effect is sometimes remarkable.

g. In cases of delayed resumption of function after operation on the lower extremity (operations on joints, ablation of the meniscus, etc.)."

Published August, 1970

The informed and experienced anesthesiologist is well aware that there are harmful effects associated with the use of controlled respiration, and that the technique involves considerable deviation from the normal physiologic mechanism of respiration.

The most obvious of these harmful effects is damage to the lungs because of the increased intrapulmonary pressure inherent in the method. In the absence of pulmonary bullae or blebs, and with properly performed manual controlled respiration, the danger is not great; in fact, the danger is probably less than during the simple act of coughing in which the intrapulmonary pressure developed may be as high as 80 to 90 cm. of water. The pressure produced in the lungs during manually controlled respiration, even with vigorous squeezing of the reservoir bag, seldom approaches these figures—it is more often in the range of 40 to 60 cm. of water. However, when mechanical ventilators are employed to produce controlled respiration, the possibilities of mechanical derangement make the danger of inadvertently high pressures and pulmonary damage very real.

More subtle are the harmful effects upon the cardiovascular system. Valsalva was the first to recognize the connection between increased intrathoracic pressure and decreased venous return: his seventeenth century experiment, still known to all second year medical students as "the Valsalva maneuver," clearly demonstrated that trying to expire against a closed glottis caused marked distension of the peripheral veins of the head and neck; and it is now well understood that, if continued, this exercise will cause a fall in blood pressure and even loss of consciousness as a result of cerebral ischemia. Furthermore, not only does the increased intrapulmonary pressure decrease venous return, but the loss of the usual negative pressure during inspiration abolishes the so-called "thoracic pump" mechanism which sucks the blood from outside the thorax into the great thoracic veins and the heart. The loss of this negative pressure, which at the height of inspiration amounts to -10 cm of water, further contributes to the decrease in venous return. Cardiac output suffers, not only because of these factors decreasing venous return, but also because of a tamponade effect upon the heart, since during the inspiratory phase of controlled respiration the heart itself is compressed to some extent between the inflating lungs. Finally, as the alveolar pressure rises above atmospheric, the pulmonary capillaries will also suffer compression, and the pulmonary capillary circulation will be decreased, putting an extra burden on the right ventricle.

The other unpleasant effects which may be produced by controlled respiration are related to overventilation, or its converse, underventilation. Overventilation will cause a fall in carbon dioxide tension and a rise in pH, or in other words, a respiratory alkalosis. Overventilation also leads to cerebral vasoconstriction and a potentiation of the anesthetic state, and although the mechanism whereby overventilation causes cerebral vasoconstriction is not entirely understood, it is undoubtedly to a large extent dependent upon the reduction of the level of carbon dioxide in the blood.

Despite this impressive list of harmful effects which may be associated with the use of controlled respiration, there is little question that the method represents one of the striking advances in anesthesia during the last quarter of a century. Prolonged respiratory assistance through endotracheal or tracheostomy tubes has saved lives which otherwise may have been lost. Controlled respiration, properly applied, can guarantee efficient ventilation, and the effects of respiratory depression can be offset, and life sustained, for days, weeks, months, and even years. It is no exaggeration to say that controlled respiration has taken the anesthesiologist out of the operating room and made him the primary physician in the practice of acute medicine, which is a role for which he is eminently suited.

All of these developments began simply enough as just a means of providing a quieter operating field in abdominal surgery—which specific work then was largely ignored for a number of years. In 1934, Guedel and Treweek published their article, "Ether Apnoeas," in the November–December issue of *Current Researches in Anesthesia and Analgesia* (*13*: 263–264, 1934), which is reprinted below with the kind permission of the publishers.

ETHER APNOEAS

GUEDEL, A. E.
AND TREWEEK, D. N.

Curr. Res. Anesth. Analg., 13: 263–264, 1934

This paper, based entirely on clinical observations, describes the relationship between blood levels of ether and carbon dioxide in maintaining spontaneous respiration during ether anesthesia. With higher ether levels higher carbon dioxide levels are required to stimulate respiration. Using a carbon dioxide absorption system, the authors describe two methods for obtaining high blood levels of ether and then reducing the carbon dioxide stimulus by "passive ventilation" which maintains apnea during ether anesthesia. They conclude "ether apneas are of no advantage except they present a quieter abdominal field . . . ."

1935

Published April, 1958

The combination of an animal waste product and an acid derived from apples to form barbituric acid was first effected almost a century ago in the historical city of Ghent by Adolf von Baeyer, the young assistant of the great chemist, August Kekulé. It was forty years thereafter, however, before the sedative actions of the barbituric acid derivatives were appreciated: in 1903, two of the titans of German organic chemistry—Emil Fischer and Joseph Von Mering—discovered the effectiveness of one of these compounds, diethylbarituric acid, in putting dogs to sleep.

That discovery opened the floodgates, and within months after the publication of their report, on "A New Class of Sleep-Inducers," the barbiturates began the ascent to a pinnacle of popularity that now finds American physicians prescribing an estimated three billion doses each year. More than twenty-five hundred different barbiturates have been synthesized during the past half century, and of these perhaps two dozen have achieved established positions in medicine. One of the most significant of these roles has been the intravenous use of the barbiturates for the production of anesthesia. Pernoston (or Pernocton), which was introduced in Gemany in 1927, was the first barbiturate to become widely employed as an intravenous anesthetic. Sodium Amytal, which was first synthesized in 1923, was used by Zerfas and McCallum of Indianapolis in 1929, and became the most successfully employed intravenous anesthetic on this side of the ocean. In 1931, Lundy reported the intravenous administration of Nembutal as an hypnotic agent; and the following year, Weese and Scharpff of Germany introduced Evipan (Evipal), a compound which represented a great improvement over the other barbiturates available for intravenous anesthesia.

The significant event from the anesthetic point-of-view came with the substitution of sulphur for the oxygen on the urea carbon in the barbituric acid molecule, giving rise to a homologous series of thiobarbiturates with distinctive pharmacological properties of unique use in anesthesia. It probably cannot be said that the thiobarbiturates revolutionized the practice of anesthesia to the extent that the muscle relaxants did, but it can be said they changed the practice of anesthesia in drastic fashion. The first detailed notice of the ability of the thiobarbiturates to effect such a change was contained in the paper by Lundy which was published in the August 21, 1935 issue of the *Proceedings of the Staff Meetings of the Mayo Clinic.*

INTRAVENOUS ANESTHESIA: PRELIMINARY REPORT OF THE USE OF TWO NEW THIOBARBITURATES

Lundy, J. S.

Proc. Staff. Meet., Mayo Clinic, 10: 536–543 (Aug. 21), 1935

The intravenous use of two new barbiturates was reported. While the intravenous administration of barbiturates had been found useful during general anesthesia for certain types of operations, the agents available were unsatisfactory because of their prolonged duration of action. One of these new agents (Barb. A.) is similar to pentobarbital with the exception that the oxygen molecule is replaced by sulfur. The advantages of the short-acting barbiturates was described and a table listed the types of operations in 700 cases in which "Barb. A" was used intravenously. It was concluded that the ideal agent for routine intravenous anesthesia has not been found yet but the available agents have been found to be satisfactory in certain types of cases.

Published June, 1957

The word "anesthesia" denotes, by its very definition, a *reversibility* of action; the connotation of the word has come to imply—to the clinical anesthesiologist, at any rate— a *controllability* of action as well. Much of the anesthetic progress of the past century has been in the achievement or improvement of this controllability, and the trend has been greatly accentuated during recent years. The development of short-acting anesthetic agents, such as cyclopropane, pentothal, and succinylcholine, represents increased controllability from the pharmacological point-of-view; and the utilization of induced hypotension, hypothermia, extracorporeal circulation, and mechanical ventilation during anesthesia, is an attempt to attain such controllability from the physiological standpoint.

The trend is scarcely new, however; control has been the concern of the anesthesiologist in regard to spinal analgesia for seventy years now. Of particular moment have been the duration of action of spinal anesthesia, and the extent of spread of the local anesthetic agent that is injected into the subarachnoid space. The duration of spinal analgesia depends chiefly upon the chemical nature of the local anesthetic drug and the dose in which it is employed, and to a much lesser extent upon the concentration of the solution in which it is employed—although the concentration of the drug is of great importance in relation to the *intensity* of anesthesia. Control of the level of spinal analgesia, on the other hand, depends upon a large number of factors, including the volume of the solution injected, the specific gravity of the solution, the position of the patient after injection, the site of injection, the dose of the drug,

the length of the spinal cord, the volume of the cerebrospinal fluid, and the curvatures of the vertebral column.

The paper published by Sise, in the December 1935 issue of the *Surgical Clinics of North America*, described the Lahey Clinic technique for spinal analgesia, a technique which utilized pontocaine to provide a duration of action sufficient for the contemplated surgical procedure and employed the effects of gravity on a weighted solution to provide control over the ascent of the level of anesthesia. It was by no means the first description of either the use of pontocaine for such a purpose or the employment of baricity to control the extent of spread of the local anesthetic solution; it was, however, a concise, clear, and rational description of a technique that has become, perhaps, the most important single method of producing spinal analgesia.

PONTOCAIN-GLUCOSE SOLUTION FOR SPINAL ANESTHESIA

SISE, L. F.

Surg. Clin. North America, 15: 1501–1511 (Dec.), 1935

Pontocaine solution is weighted with 10% glucose to make it easier to control the level of anesthesia produced by pontocaine. The technique involved the use in patients who are to be in a supine or head-down position, and the diffusion of the local anesthetic agent in the subarachoid space is described.

1936

Published October and December, 1958

For a variety of reasons, nitrous oxide comes very close to being the ideal anesthetic agent. It is nonirritating and free from disagreeable odor, and it provides a rapid and pleasant induction. It is not only hypnotic, but in addition is an excellent analgesic. It does not increase capillary bleeding. It diffuses rapidly through alveolar membranes, which permits a moment-to-moment control of the depth of anesthesia. It is excreted from the body rapidly and unaltered in structure, so that toxic degradation products do not form and accumulate in the body. It produces no significant changes in heart rate, blood pressure, cardiac output, or myocardial contractility. It does not depress the respiratory center, nor depress or exaggerate the respiratory movements. It has no significant effects upon liver function, renal activity or metabolism in general. Postanesthetic nausea and vomiting are unusual following its administration. It is nonexplosive and noninflammable with either oxygen or air. It is inexpensive and fairly simple to manufacture. It can be stored without undergoing chemical changes. It possesses, in fact, only one serious drawback: it is not a potent agent.

This lack of potency has been of tremendous importance throughout the history of nitrous oxide anesthesia. Among other things, it led Horace Wells to suicide. After a number of successful uses of nitrous oxide anesthesia in his own dental practice in Hartford, Wells was invited in 1845 to go to the Massachusetts General Hospital to demonstrate the method for the students of Dr. Warren's Harvard Medical School class. Because the drug is not fully potent, Wells failed to secure adequate anesthesia in the robust male patient being employed for the demonstration and the event turned out to be a total fiasco. He returned home a shamed and disgraced man, broken in health and spirit. Eventually he gave up

dentistry, traveled around the country with a troup of performing canaries, and reached the depths when he was jailed after bespattering a New York prostitute with sulphuric acid!

The lack of potency of nitrous oxide led the great French physiologist, Paul Bert, to his classical experiments in the effects of barometric pressure upon nitrous oxide anesthesia. He had, in 1878, completed a series of researches on the physiologic effects of variations in barometric pressure on the gases of the blood. He believed that the technique of administering 100 per cent nitrous oxide in order to achieve adequate anesthesia, which was the generally accepted technique of the time, made asphyxia inevitable; he suggested that if the gas, instead of being administered at normal atmospheric pressure, were administered under a positive pressure of two atmospheres, then 50 per cent air could be combined with 50 per cent nitrous oxide and adequate anesthesia without asphyxia would be possible. The result of this suggestion was the construction of a mobile, compressed air chamber serving as an operating theater in which a mixture of nitrous oxide and oxygen could be administered to the patient under positive pressure (the surgeon and his assistants were also subjected to the increased atmospheric pressure); this "anesthetic car" traveled around between the various hospitals in Paris for some time before it was abandoned as inexpedient.

Finally, and perhaps most importantly, the lack of potency of nitrous oxide led to the development of the technique of "secondary saturation," a method of controlled asphyxia that employed anoxia to compensate for the deficiency of lack of potency of the drug. The technique achieved tremendous popularity and widespread utilization, and represented an almost tacit admission by anesthetists that at least some of the anesthetic activity of nitrous oxide, when the drug was employed for total anesthesia, was dependent upon an anoxic action. The vast dangers of such anoxia were admitted, and then dismissed; but a gnawing awareness that anoxia was truly intolerable to the patient's safety grew and grew as anesthesiology began to blossom into a specialty. It remained for a neuropathologist to bring matters to a head by demonstrating that the lack of potency of nitrous oxide led to disasters which simply prohibited its continued use as a sole anesthetic agent; this Courville did in his superb monograph, "Asphyxia as a Consequence of Nitrous Oxide Anesthesia," which appeared in *Medicine, 15:* 129–245, May, 1936.

ASPHYXIA AS A CONSEQUENCE OF NITROUS OXIDE ANESTHESIA

CYRIL B. COURVILLE, M.D.

Department of Neurology,
College of Medical Evangelists
and Cajal Laboratory of Neuropathology,
Los Angeles County Hospital

Medicine, 15: 129–145, 1936

* * * *

SUMMARY

"This study is concerned with the problem of cerebral asphyxia or anoxia as a result of nitrous oxide anesthesia. It is based upon clinical and pathologic observations in a series of 13 cases, 9 of which terminated fatally. In all the fatal cases an autopsy was obtained and a more or less critical examination of the cerebral tissues was made.

"Cerebral manifestations following inhalation of nitrous oxide have been recognized for almost a hundred years. The immediate nervous manifestations usually consist of generalized convulsive seizures, muscular rigidity and persistent coma, at times terminating fatally with signs of "de-cerebrate rigidity." Delayed symptoms may occur in the form of a psychosis, a parkinsonian symptom-complex or disturbances of special sensation, particularly in the form of a partial or complete amaurosis. The patient may recover entirely after an anoxemic episode, may survive for a variable period with residual symptoms or may die within a few days. In fatal cases, death usually occurs within 2 to 7 days, but may occur only after an interval of weeks or months. Examples of each of these variations are to be found in the series of cases described herewith.

"Anoxemia following administration of nitrous oxide may be the result of an impure gas, a faulty apparatus, or a preexisting or suddenly developed pulmonary lesion. The possibility of faulty administration of the anesthetic and of individual idiosyncracy to this gas are also to be considered. Several factors may be present in a single case, all contributing to production of the cerebral lesion. Regardless of the exact source of the trouble, the clinical symptoms and the pathologic findings are the effect of *asphyxia* and are not due to any toxic effect of nitrous oxide itself.

"The mechanism in most instances seems to be one of two types,—(*a*) sudden circulatory and/or respiratory failure with consequent cerebral damage due to the immediate utilization of the remaining small amounts of available oxygen or (*b*) prolonged exposure of the brain to a dangerous degree of oxygen want.

"The resulting cortical lesion necessarily depends upon the degree of anoxemia and its duration. There may be (*a*) a sclerosis of scattered pyramidal cells, (*b*) an occurrence of discrete pale areas (*Herde*) in the cortex, (*c*) a patchy necrosis of superficial, intermediate or deep, or all cortical layers, (*d*) a subtotal destruction of the cortex, or if the patient survives for a sufficient interval, (*e*) a vascular scar may result due to the formation of new blood vessels. Changes in the nerve cells may be described as (*a*) sclerotic, (*b*) acute degenerative, (*c*) ischemic, and in chronic cases (*d*) "calcified" nerve cells. Lipoidal degeneration (*e*) is also a common form of cellular change.

* * * *

"A study of the brain in fatal cases discloses several interesting facts. Not all portions of the cortex are uniformly or symmetrically involved. This no doubt explains the variable clinical picture found in those cases surviving for several weeks or more. While it is possible to predicate the character of the lesion from the clinical history, one cannot always be sure of the severity of cortical damage. This is due to the great difficulty in evaluating all the possible causative factors. The earliest lesions are found about the pericellular and pericapillary spaces, which would suggest that the injury is a result of "tissue respiration"—a disturbed carbon dioxide-oxygen exchange between the tissue fluids and the cellular elements."

*   *   *   *

1937

Published August, 1967

For many years prior to the advent of pediatric surgery as a specialty, tonsillectomy, appendectomy, and a variety of orthopedic procedures were just about the only operations which were commonly performed on children; and these procedures were performed with the methods used on adults and by surgeons more accustomed to adult patients. The same situation held true regarding the anesthesia employed: reliance was placed upon the drugs, techniques, and methods used for adults, and it was administered by personnel who were more accustomed to adult patients. Indeed, in the first textbook of anesthesia, *On The Inhalation of The Vapour of Ether in Surgical Operations*, which was published in 1847, John Snow wrote, "I am not aware that any state of the patient with respect to age. . . .contraindicates the use of ether during a surgical operation. The patients whom I have given it have been of all ages, from early childhood to nearly eighty years. . . .the size of the patient is the only circumstance which I have observed constantly to influence the quantity of ether required to produce insensibility." In a much more recent text, published in 1943, Sir Robert MacIntosh and Freda Bannister wrote, "The drugs used to produce anesthesia and the methods of their administration are the same for children as for adults."

There was, however, a gradual awareness of the fact that children, and particularly infants, are not merely smaller editions of adult man. In 1903, Kopetzky, who then was anesthetist to the Harlem Hospital in New York, wrote in the *Medical Record*, "In selecting the anesthetic to be given to children, the anesthetist and the surgeon are confronted with a problem of grave import. . . .those who use chloroform continuously are most emphatic in warning against its dangers generally and especially in the hands of the inexperienced. The many operations to which children must frequently submit and which the general practitioner performs himself, with the aid of another no more qualified in its use than himself, cause the lives of these little patients to be endangered by the unhesitating acceptance of this too generally advocated procedure. . . . While it is true that the greater vascularity of the nervous system in children, combined with their inferior muscular development, as compared with the adult, would seem to render chloroform safe, yet the element of fear with its series of vasomotor phenomena is more than enough to counterbalance this. Children over two years of age are invariably frightened. . . . In the administration of ether, we are met at the outset with a series of objections. It is more disagreeable to administer. The irritation caused by it excites a flow of mucus which in the smaller bronchi of children is apt to cause obstruction and consequent danger."

The gradual awareness of the special problems of pediatric anesthesia found statistical documentation in the Beecher-Todd report: "The anesthesia death percentage is disproportionately high in the first decade of life. This indicates a great need for an attack on the anesthesia problems of infants and children. . . . Perhaps their immature organs are less able to withstand the stress of anesthesia than are those of healthy young adults. Doubtless, problems of ventilation are involved." The latter point had been brought up earlier by Gwathmey in his textbook on *Anesthesia* in 1914: "Nitrous oxid, unless given by some open method, is a very poor anesthetic for young children, as they do not seem to be equal to the task of breathing through valves." As pediatric anesthesia blossomed and flourished as a subspecialty, it became increasingly apparent that one of the major needs was for special equipment that could accommodate to the respiratory demands of the pediatric patient. Necessity being the mother of invention, a number of these gadgets were forthcoming. One of the most useful was Philip Ayre's T-piece, which he described in the July 1937 issue of *The British Journal of Surgery* (Ayre, P.: Anaesthesia for Hare-lip and Cleft Palate Operations on Babies; *Brit. J. Surg., 25:* 131–132, 1937), which is reprinted below with the kind permission of the author and the publishers.

ANAESTHESIA FOR HARE-LIP AND CLEFT PALATE OPERATIONS ON BABIES

PHILIP AYRE

Anaesthetist to Royal Victoria Infirmary and Newcastle General Hospital; Hon. Anaesthetist to Babies' Hospital, Newcastle upon Tyne

Br. J. Surg., 25: 131–132, 1937

"The anaesthesia employed for hare-lip and cleft palate operations at the Babies' Hospital, Newcastle upon Tyne, may be divided into two phases—the nitrous-oxide-oxygen phase and the oxygen-ether phase. In all cases the babies were intubated by the endotracheal technique of Dr. Magill, wide-bore rubber catheters being inserted through the mouth into the trachea just beyond the laryngeal opening. No especial difficulty was experienced in carrying out this procedure, except that on a few occasions the catheter entered a bronchus; this was manifested clinically by laboured respiration and jerky movements of the diaphragm. On slightly withdrawing the catheter, the breathing became normal.

"After prolonged trial, we found that, while nitrous-oxide-oxygen anaesthesia offered excellent results in adult patients, certain grave disadvantages presented themselves when the same anaesthetic was administered to infants. In the first place, the anoxaemia caused by nitrous oxide—and any proportion of oxygen below 20 per cent represents some degree of sub-oxygenation—appeared to be much more deleterious to babies than to adult patients. In the second place, it was extremely difficult to adjust the amount of re-breathing to the small proportions suitable for a baby. No matter how small the re-breathing bag, there was always too much "dead space," so that the respiratory exchange rapidly became hampered by the accumulation of excess products of respiration.

*   *   *   *

"In an endeavour to remedy the above distressing state of affairs (and spurred on by the caustic criticism of a candid surgeon!), the writer sought to devise a method by which the endotracheal technique could still be utilized without the drawbacks associated with nitrous oxide and excessive re-breathing. The following method is simple in the extreme, and has proved highly satisfactory during the last eighteen months at the Babies' Hospital.

"Briefly, the apparatus consists of a T-piece which is connected by a short piece of rubber tubing and a Magill angle-piece to a wide-bore Magill rubber catheter previously inserted into the trachea. Through one limb of the T-piece oxygen and ether vapour is delivered from a Boyle or other continuous-flow apparatus. The other limb remains open to the outside air; for convenience, a short piece of tubing may be attached and allowed to hang down beneath the operating towels. A strand of fine gauze, fixed with adhesive strapping close to the open end of the latter tubing, will wave to and fro with the patient's respirations, thus serving as a useful indicator to the anaesthetist.

"The advantages of this technique are as follows:—

1. The baby inhales fresh air and oxygen under as nearly normal physiological conditions as possible. The system is open to the outside air, without the intervention of a re-breathing bag, expiratory valve, or other obstruction to normal respiration. Sufficient ether vapour is added to the oxygen to maintain adequate anaesthesia, the baby being kept just short of "gagging." Deep anaesthesia is neither necessary nor desirable.

2. The 'dead space' is reduced to negligible proportions, while the continuous flow of oxygen at the rate of from 1½ to 3 litres a minute flushes out the lungs, and effectually prevents undue accumulation of respired products.

"The excellent colour and quiet, natural breathing of the babies have convinced us that oxygen and ether vapour, administered by the T-piece method, is the anaesthetic of choice for all hare-lip and cleft palate operations on babies and young children."

*   *   *   *

1940

Published June, 1969

The statement has been made that one of the greatest dangers of spinal anesthesia is the fact that it is so easy to perform. Anybody who can perform a lumbar puncture and then inject a solution of local anesthetic drug through the needle into the subarachnoid space can be a spinal anesthetist. Since almost any medical student—and certainly any doctor—can do these two things, there are a lot of potentially dangerous spinal anesthetists around, as anyone who has ever served on a Maternal Mortality and Morbidity Commission or an Anesthesia Study Committee can testify. But even in the most skilled of hands, the complications of spinal anesthesia are legion. Consider the following two case histories from the Anesthesia Study Committee of the New York State Society of Anesthesiologists:

"Case Report

A 29-year-old healthy female required elective cesarean section for cephalopelvic disproportion. Preanesthetic medication consisted of secobarbital 100 mg. and scopolamine 0.4 mg. hypodermically. On arrival in the operating room 90 minutes later, systolic blood pressure was 124 mm. Hg, diastolic 72, pulse rate 88. Spinal anesthesia was instituted with 1 per cent tetracaine (Pontocaine) 6 mg. and 10 per cent glucose 100 mg. With the patient supine the onset of sensory anesthesia was noted within 3 minutes; vital signs were unchanged. Two minutes later the level of sensory anesthesia was at the eighth and 5 minutes later at the sixth thoracic segment. Blood pressure determinations at 1-minute intervals during this period revealed progressive decline to 80 systolic, 50 diastolic; the pulse rate fell to 70 and then rose to 94. The patient was nauseated and perspiring. Oxygen by face mask and ephedrine 12.5 mg intravenously and 25 mg intramuscularly were administered. Testing with pin prick showed the level of sensory anesthesia remaining at the sixth thoracic segment. Within 3 minutes blood pressure had returned to preanesthetic levels and the patient was comfortable. The cesarean section was completed uneventfully."

"Case Report

A 35-year-old pregnant female, 4–0–2–2, was scheduled for elective cesarean section in her thirty-sixth week. She had had diabetes for 8 years, well controlled with diet and isophane (NPH) insulin. Following a protracted episode of vomiting in the twenty-sixth week of the present pregnancy, she had become hypoglycemic and required hospitalization for control of the diabetes. She was 5 feet tall and weighed 134 pounds, having gained 14 pounds in the 36 weeks of pregnancy. The diabetes was under control, with occasional glycosuria. Systolic blood pressure was 95 mm. Hg, diastolic 60; hemoglobin was 10 gm.

On arrival in the operating room with preanesthetic medication she was apprehensive, with a pulse rate of 120, blood pressure 90 mm. Hg systolic, 60 diastolic. The fetal heart rate was 140. Methoxamine (Vasoxyl) 20 mg. was injected intramuscularly. Fifteen minutes later tetracaine (Pontocaine) 7 mg. with glucose 70 mg. in a total volume of 1.5 ml. was administered intrathecally between the third and fourth lumbar vertebrae. She was then placed supine with a pillow under her head. Immediately afterwards blood pressure was 130 systolic, 70 diastolic. The patient whispered a complaint of dizziness and was seen to be breathing with difficulty; immediate testing revealed sensory anesthesia extending into the cervical region. Systolic pressure was now 70, diastolic 50, and breathing was reduced to ineffective, feeble, gasping efforts. The operating table was quickly placed in a moderate head-down position. Artificial respiration with oxygen by face mask was begun and phenylephrine (Neo-Synephrine) 0.04 mg. per ml. was added to the intravenous infusion. The fetal heart rate was 120. Within 3½ minutes systolic pressure had risen to 180, with diastolic 110, pulse rate 60. Phenylephrine administration was then terminated and blood pressure gradually declined to its preanesthetic level of 90 systolic, 60 diastolic.

Respiration was assisted by intermittent manual compression of the breathing bag until spontaneous ventilation was deemed adequate, 40 minutes after injection of the spinal anesthetic drug. Cesarean section was postponed and the patient taken to the recovery room where full motor and sensory function returned over the next 2 hours.

During the night she received pentobarbital 100 mg. She was somewhat apprehensive when returned to the operating room 5 hours later, although she seemed sleepy when undisturbed. Systolic pressure was now 140, diastolic 80, pulse rate 100, fetal heart rate 140. As before, methoxamine 20 mg. was administered intramuscularly about 15 minutes before lumbar puncture. This time, however, she was placed in a slightly head-up position, oxygen was administered by face mask, and a slow intravenous infusion of phenylephrine 0.02 mg. per ml. was started. Tetracaine-glucose was injected intrathecally through the same interspace, but the dose of tetracaine was reduced to 4 mg in a total volume of 1 ml. Blood pressure did not fall precipitously but declined gradually to 100 systolic, 70 diastolic, with pulse rate 80; the fetal heart remained at 140. Once again there was rapid development of sensory anesthesia to the cervical region, with intercostal paralysis and impaired but continued diaphragmatic activity. This time ventilatory assistance was required for only 15 minutes. Meanwhile cesarean section was performed and an infant weighing 2710 gm. delivered without difficulty. One-minute Apgar score was 10. Operation was completed within 35 minutes; subsequent recovery was uneventful."

In both of these patients, potentially disastrous complications from spinal anesthesia were expertly managed; but in the hands of the occasional anesthetist, who is unfamiliar with the problems which can arise and of the steps which must be taken in treatment of the problems, such situations can become tragedies. Which, of course, is the basis for the statement that one of the dangers of spinal anesthesia is that it is so easy to perform.

At least, it usually is easy to perform.

This statement is not true when there is extensive and well advanced hypertrophic osteoarthritis of the vertebral column or when the patient has had a fusion of the spine in the lumbar region. In these instances it may be utterly impossible to gain access to the subarachnoid space by the usual midline approach. The same thing is also true of patients who cannot, or will not, assume the standard postures for lumbar puncture, such as patients with ankylosed hips, inebriated patients, and medicated parturients. Either a different approach must be employed or spinal anesthesia abandoned. Romberger stated it well some 40 years ago: "To know only one of the many ways of inducing spinal anesthesia," he wrote, "*restricts* and *limits* the spinal anesthetist."

One of the most useful of the alternative approaches to the subarachnoid space is the lumbosacral. This technique was described by Taylor in 1940 in a paper titled "Lumbosacral Subarachnoid Tap" (Taylor, J. A.: *J. Urol., 43:* 561, 1940) and is republished below with the kind permissions of the author and the publishers.

LUMBOSACRAL SUBARACHNOID TAP

TAYLOR, J. A.

J. Urol., 43:561, 1940

A description of the lateral or Taylor approach to the subarachnoid space. His landmark for skin wheal was one cm. below and one cm. medial to the posterior superior spine and the needle was directed to enter the $L_5 – S_1$ interspace, avoiding the interspinous structures.

Published October, 1960

Pain has been defined as "a disagreeable sensation produced by the action of stimuli of a harmful nature." It is as old as human life itself—and almost as complex. Philosophers have often debated whether or not man would be happier in a world free of pain, and have argued that pain is a necessary contrast that permits pleasure to be appreciated.

From the physician's point of view, pain is the very cornerstone of the practice of medicine. It brings the patient to the doctor while there is still a chance for cure, and it frequently points to the location of the disease process. In an organism as highly developed as man, therefore, the sensation of pain acts as an important protective mechanism. In this respect, it is not the great enemy of mankind, but an ally— a protective aid in a world full of possible injurious influences.

Until fairly recently, pain was regarded as simply a feeling state, an emotional reaction like pleasure. It is now clear that pain is far more than an emotion: it is a specific sensation, provided with special and separate mechanisms for the detection of noxious stimuli and for the transmission of pain mechanisms. There are specific end-organs for pain, specific types of nerve fibers for the conduction of pain, specific neural pathways for its transmission, and even specific areas of the central nervous system for its perception. The neurophysiologist has labored valiantly against great obstacles in the study of the pain mechanism, and has done much to establish pain as a discrete physiologic entity.

Nevertheless, pain remains primarily a symptom, primarily subjective in nature. Consider only the myriad descriptive terms by which pain is characterized: dull, superficial, boring, pounding, deep, aching, twisting, cutting, griping, cramping, wavelike, compressing, constricting, vice-like, stinging, shearing, pricking, and many more. It is this subjective nature of pain that so often makes it difficult to evaluate medically, for while some types of pain can be distinguished physiologically, the *quality* of pain is usually a totally subjective concern, dependent upon the psychologic make-up (and the vocabulary!) of the patient.

A second, and overwhelming, problem in the study of pain is its *intensity*. Again, the subjective nature of pain has made objective, scientific evaluation a great difficulty. Depending upon an individual's psychologic make-up and pain threshold, pain of a given intensity may be interpreted all the way from "mild" to "severe." Yet fruitful research into pain mechanisms demands an objective measurement of the intensity, or degree, of pain. A significant contribution to the study of pain was made by James D. Hardy, Harold G. Wolff, and Helen Goodell, in the *Journal of Clinical Investigation, 19:* 649–657, 1940, under the title of "Studies on pain: A new method of measuring pain threshold; observations on spatial summation of pain," which is reprinted below.

STUDIES ON PAIN. A NEW METHOD FOR MEASURING PAIN THRESHOLD; OBSERVATIONS ON SPATIAL SUMMATION OF PAIN

J. D. HARDY, H. G. WOLFF, AND H. GOODELL

From the Russell Sage Institute of Pathology, in affiliation with the New York Hospital and Departments of Medicine and Psychiatry, Cornell University Medical College, New York

(Received for publication April 18, 1940)

J. Clin. Invest., 19: 649–657, 1940

* * * *

SUMMARY AND CONCLUSIONS

"1. A quantitative method for measuring pain thresholds in the skin by thermal radiation has been described. The method has the general advantage of measuring a physical quantity which is directly proportional to the changes occurring in the skin. The method has the further advantagaes of precision, simplicity of technique, rapidity of measurement, and the fact that the stimulus is innocuous upon repeated application except at high intensities. Further, any part of the skin surface may be studied and the size of the stimulated area varied at will.

"2. Pain thresholds measured in this way did not vary consistently with time of day, with the general effectiveness, or the emotional state of the 3 subjects.

"3. Individual threshold measurements for 3 subjects were 0.229, 0.231, and 0.233 gm. cal./sec./cm.^{2} and all measurements were found to be within ±12 per cent of their respective average values. The standard deviation for a single measurement was calculated to be ±2 per cent.

"4. Intense pain in any part of the body raised the pain threshold in the skin in other parts as much as 35 per cent.

"5. The senses of pain and heat, which were always stimulated together, were shown to be separate sensations through the action of acetylsalicylic acid. This drug lowered the heat threshold and raised the pain threshold.

"6. The peripheral structures responsible for pain sense were distinguished from those of temperature and touch by demonstrating that occluding the blood for 25 minutes did not directly affect the pain threshold in the ischemic hand, whereas other sensations could hardly be elicited.

"7. Pain sense was found to have no spatial summation in the sense that the pain threshold for many end organs was no lower than that for a few. This was observed to be the case for minimal stimuli and for supraminimal stimuli after morphine administration.

"8. The intensity of radiation which produced blistering in 3 seconds was observed to be twice that necessary for the bare perception of pain."

Published December, 1977

History has probably not recorded the details of the first malpractice suit against a physician; it certainly has recorded a vast accumulation of subsequent similar legal debacles.

A malpractice suit is an amazing bird,

with strange and wondrous anatomy, because it flies on so many wings.

There is the wing of true negligence, about which there can be no discussion.

There is the wing of alleged negligence, which is the basis of most of the nauseating malpractice suits today.

There is the wing of lack-of-rapport-with-the-patient, which is really the feathers of alleged negligence.

And so on until we come to the wing of the inadequate record—which, in the anesthesiologist's practice, is the anesthesia record.

Oh, there are other things in the hospital chart, of course, which are important to the anesthesiologist's defense against a malpractice suit. His preoperative evaluation and notes are important. His postoperative notes are important. The consultation notes are important. The laboratory data are important. The nurses' notes are important. History and physical examination are important. In fact, everything in the hospital record can be important. (So, too, can the lack of anything in the hospital record.) But there is probably no single item that is more important in most instances of a malpractice suit against the anesthesiologist than the anesthetic record.

Dr. Lucien E. Morris once wrote (in speaking of anesthetic charts) that, "many look on the making of records as an evil chore, whimsically required by remote Boards of Accreditation Examiners for accumulation in a dusty repository."

Dr. Morris was so correct. There are superbly competent anesthesiologists, who are also superbly trained physicians, and who take meticulous, considerate and concerned care of their patients—and what do you find in reviewing some of their anesthesia charts? No indication of what drugs were given, or when, or how, or with what result. The part of the chart which records vital signs says "o.k."

That will not go far with a jury in today's world.

The first anesthetic records were not records at all, really. They were narrative descriptions of what people thought that they remembered that they had done. The "anesthetic record" of the first chloroform death, for instance, consisted of Dr. Meggison's testimony at the inquest held following the death of the 15 year old girl, Hannah Greener, on the 28th of January in 1848. Hannah was to have had an ingrown nail removed from the great toe of her foot under chloroform anesthesia, and Dr. Meggison testified as follows:

"She appeared to dread the operation, and fretted a good deal: in fact, she commenced sobbing on our entering the house, and continued so until seated in the operating chair, and commencing the inhalation, which was done from a handkerchief on which a teaspoonful of chloroform had been poured. After drawing her breath twice, she pulled my hand from her mouth. I told her to put her hands on her knees and breathe quietly, which she did. In about half a minute, seeing no change in breathing, or alteration of pulse, I lifted her arm, which I found rigid. I looked at the pupil and pinched her cheek, and, finding her insensible, requested Mr. Lloyd to begin the operation. At the termination of the semilunar incision she gave a kick or twitch, which caused me to think the chloroform had not sufficient effect. I was preceeding to apply more to the handkerchief, when her lips, which had been previously of good color, became suddenly blanched, and she spluttered at the mouth, as if in epilepsy. I threw down the handkerchief, dashed cold water on her face, and gave her some internally, followed by brandy, without, however, the least effect, not the slightest attempt at a rally being made. We laid her on the floor, opened a vein in her arm, and the jugular vein, but no blood flowed. The whole process of inhalation, operation, venesection, and death, could not, I should say, have occupied more then two minutes."

These anecdotal accounts, however, were scarcely true anesthetic records.

The latter did not evolve until, beginning in 1895, two young house officers at the Massachusetts General Hospital began to keep detailed charts of their administrations of anesthesia. One of these young house officers was Harvey Cushing, who was to become the father of neurosurgery in this country; the other was Dr. E. A. Codman, a prestigious Boston doctor from a prestigious Boston family. The late Henry

K. Beecher, the first Henry Isiah Dorr Professor of Research in Anaesthesia at Harvard University, chronicled their achievements in an article entitled, "The First Anesthesia Records (Codman, Cushing)," which was published in the November, 1940 issue of *Surgery, Gynecology and Obstetrics* (*71:* 689–693, 1940) and is reprinted below.

TEXTS AND DOCUMENTS THE FIRST ANESTHESIA RECORDS (CODMAN, CUSHING)

HENRY K. BEECHER, M.D.

Boston, Massachusetts

Surg. Gynecol. Obstet., 71: 689–693, 1940

"With the rapid development of anesthesia in recent years, it is easy to lose sight of the fact that as the modern specialties go this one is old, with its origins in the first half of the nineteenth century. The introduction of anesthesia into the clinic altered the practice of medicine perhaps more than any other single advance; so it is of some interest to keep the historical account straight by recording the specific steps in the progression of the specialty when they can be identified, even though they be minor ones."

"It has been said that record keeping, the description and charting of the patients' course during anesthesia and operation, began in 1915. Since detailed anesthesia charts in the files of the Massachusetts General Hospital antedate 1915 by more than 20 years, it is of interest to record the fact that many of the Massachusetts General Hospital records bear the dates of 1894 or 1895. By that time two types of charts had been devised for the purpose and were in use.

"The later eminence of those who were concerned with this early record keeping adds to its interest. The details can be described by the letters of those who were responsible for the records. First, there is the letter from Dr. Codman to Dr. Harvey Cushing. This letter accompanied a collection of the early charts."

"Feb. 9th 20.
227 Beacon Street
Boston

Dear Harvey:

"Having nothing better to do lately I have been trying to put my effects into order again after the volcanic dislocation caused by the war and incidentally by the renting of our house.

"Katie, after my departure dumped all the accumulations of years into one pile. So during this snowy week I have had old diaries, letters and unpublished attempts at 'papers,' and mercilessly put them in the wastebasket. There are many things which remind me of you and show the stimulus you were to me. I am sorry that age now prevents me from reacting to your enthusiasm, and that I have ceased to cultivate my mind enough to follow your soarings in Pituitary realms.

"One of the things I cannot bear to dump in the wastebasket is a collection of ether charts which we made 30 years ago! In connection therewith I find a long *unpublished* paper on 'Etherization,' in which I described *vividly I think* but somewhat tediously the process as we then knew it. I must say I have never read anything better on the subject. I recall that the reason for not publishing it was that I took it to 'Coll' Warren, who regarded it as too frank for the good of the hospital, for it described in detail the case which I lost in the A. R. because I was paying attention to some tomfoolery which *you* (who had come in from the theatre), were entertaining us with, while the poor devil was inhaling vomitus! I also spoke of the case which stopped breathing under ether and interested you in Brain Surgery.

"So I send you these charts to destroy with some solemnity for you and I are the only persons that give a—for them. Do they give less ether per hour now?

Sincerely
E. A. Codman."

[Signed]

"Peter Bent Brigham Hospital, Boston, Mass.

February 10, 1920."

"My dear Dr. Washburn:

"I have just received the accompanying note [the preceding] from Dr. Codman with these old ether charts of the year 1895. So far as I am aware they represent the first attempt made anywhere to keep charts during anaesthesia, and the story is as follows:

"When Dr. Codman and I,[1] having entered the hospital together, were 'Junior House Pupils' I believe was the official term, or 'House Pups' the unofficial one, we gave the anaesthesia, as is the custom I believe now, twenty-five years later.

"I hesitate to recall what an awful business it was and how many fatalities there were.

"My first giving of an anaesthetic was when, a third-year student, I was called down from the seats and sent in a little side room with a patient and an orderly and told to put the patient to sleep, for Dr. — — — was to operate for the class. I knew nothing about the patient whatsoever, merely that a nurse came in and gave the patient a hypodermic injection. I proceeded as best I could under the orderly's directions, and in view of the repeated urgent calls for the patient from the amphitheatre it seemed to me an interminable time for the old man, who kept gagging, to go to sleep. We finally wheeled him it. I can vividly recall, even now, just how he looked and the feel of his bedraggled whiskers.[2] The operation was started and at this juncture there was a sudden great gush of fluid from the patient's mouth, most of which was inhaled, and he died.

"I stood aside, burning with chagrin and remorse. No one paid the slightest attention to me, though I supposed that I had killed the patient. The operation was completed in spite of the episode, as a demonstration to the class. I slunk out of the hospital, walked the streets of North Boston the rest of the afternoon, and in the evening went to the surgeon's house to ask

[1] Dr. Codman preceded Dr. Cushing by about 8 months.
[2] Curiously enough, it has been impossible to identify this patient in the hospital records.

if there was any possible way I could atone for the calamity to the man's family before I left the Medical School and went into some other business.

"To my perfect amazement I was told it was nothing at all, that I had nothing to do with the man's death, that he had a strangulated hernia and had been vomiting all night anyway, and that sort of thing happened frequently and I had better forget about it and go on with the Medical School. I went on with the Medical School but I have never forgotten about it.

"Now, to come back to these ether charts. Codman and I resolved that we would improve our technique of giving ether, which in those days in the large majority of cases meant crowding the patient to the second stage of anaesthesia as quickly as possible, and for the most part we used old sea sponges.

"In order to make a game of the task before us we made a wager of a dinner as to who could learn to give the best anaesthesia. We determined to let the test of satisfactory anaesthesia rest with the patient's behavior in the ward, and though I have forgotten just what was our scale of marking the cases, a perfect anaesthesia was supposed to be one in which the patient was sufficiently conscious to respond when left in the ward with the nurse and did not subsequently vomit. You will recall that in those days we had no ether recovery room in general use, except for the Saturday clinics.

"I think we both became very much more skillful in our jobs than we otherwise would have become, owing to this competition, but it was particularly due, I think, to the detailed attention which we had to put upon the patient by the careful recording of the pulse rate throughout the operation.

"Subsequently, on going abroad and getting interested in blood pressure, I discovered in use in Padua a simple recording instrument in Riva-Rocci's clinic. On returning home I came to utilize this always during the course of my neurological operations so that the procedure might be as comparable as possible to the records taken upon a kymograph during an experiment in the laboratory. A much more elaborate ether chart was thereupon prepared, on which not only pulse rate and respiration but the systolic blood pressure was recorded.

"On Dr. Councilman's instigation a paper was read here in Boston, January 18th, 1903 on the subject of The Routine Determination of Arterial Tension in Operating Room and Clinic. This was the beginning, I think, of the general use of a blood pressure apparatus in hospital wards, whether medical or surgical, for though the principle was not new the old Gärtner tonometer was most unsatisfactory because in cases of low blood pressure, the most important ones, it was utterly unreliable.

"I mention this because it is not uninteresting, in view of the universal adoption, subsequently, of instruments to measure blood pressure, to recall that the Division of Surgery appointed a committee to report on the subject. This report appeared March, 1904, *Bulletin No. 2 of the Division of Surgery*, and the final conclusion of this committee was as printed: 'The adoption of blood pressure operations in surgical patients does not at present appear to be necessary as a routine measure.' I find I have written on my reprint the verse from Dr. Holmes' Stethoscope Song:

'Now such as hate new fangled toys
Began to look extremely glum;
They said that rattles were made for boys
And vowed that his buzzing was all a hum.'

"I have always felt that this was one of the most interesting illustrations on record, of the reaction against the introduction of an instrument of precision into clinical use. It is precisely what happened in the case of the thermometer, the stethoscope, the X-ray, indeed of the watch itself, if one may regard Floyer's first use of the pendulum for this purpose as a watch.

"I have been moved to write all this because of the memories which have crowded in owing to a sight of these old charts, and,

simple as they are, you will see that Codman and I each got up our own type of chart. I am sorry that the final score is not given, nor do I remember who had to pay for the dinner. I am quite sure, however, that I did, for Codman usually managed to beat me in most things.

"I am sending this little bundle of things to you as it is a bit of ancient history, doubtless typical of many other bits of history that concern the succession of house officers who have rejoiced in their service at the Massachusetts General Hospital. It was undoubtedly a step toward improvement in what had been a very casual administration of a dangerous drug. We do much better with ether these days, but even so there remains much to learn.

"We are still, some of us, only too careless in its use, and stuch studies as Dr. Cutler, and Dr. Morton made during their term of residency at the M.G.H., pointing out the frequency of post-anesthesia pulmonary complications, are but a further step in the direction of improving our technique in its administration. I still feel that one of the most important elements in the giving of an anaesthetic is to have the anaesthetist keep during its administration a detailed chart of pulse, respiration, and blood pressure. At the time of his notable address some years ago on Ether Day, Dr. Keen, who took up this subject, intimated that too elaborate a record of this kind might take the administrator's mind from his primary job. I feel most emphatically that it keeps his mind on his job.

"Please put this in a corner of the Treadwell Library, where some day some young fellow may brush the dust from it and say: 'Who were these fellows anyhow, and what is this "ether" they are talking about? Do you mean that people used to be put to sleep by the inhalation of drugs in the 19th century?'"

"Very sincerely yours,
[Signed]HARVEY CUSHING"

1941

Published April, 1963

In 1864, a German chemist, Fischer, noticed that during the reaction of hexachlorethane with zinc and dilute hydrochloric acid to prepare tetrachlorethylene, another volatile substance was formed: he undertook to distill this substance and then identified it as trichlorethylene. Half a century later, in 1911, Professor K. B. Lehmann of Wurzburg University, while experimenting with the vapors of several different chlorinated hydrocarbons, discovered the anesthetic properties of trichlorethylene: he demonstrated that prolonged inhalation (3 hours) would produce light anesthesia in cats, and that even more prolonged exposure (5 hours) would produce deep anesthesia.

The drug, however, found little use except as an extracting agent in chemical laboratories until World War I, when it became widely used in heavy industry in Germany for the removal of grease from metal and machinery. This industrial usage led indirectly to the first clinical application of the drug: a syndrome of nausea, vomiting, vertigo, papilledema and analgesia of the area supplied by the trigeminal nerve occurred among factory workers who were handling the liquid, and 4 cases of this trichlorethylene poisoning were described by Plessner before a meeting of the Berlin Medical Society in 1915. One of his audience on this occasion, the neurologist Oppenheim, was struck by the fact that, although the patients had not been exposed to trichlorethylene for some 8 months, bilateral trigeminal nerve palsy affecting only the sensory root persisted, while all the other signs and symptoms had disappeared. He conceived that this effect might be utilized in the treatment of trigeminal neuralgia, for which surgical treatment at the time was both dangerous and unsatisfactory. Oppenheim proceeded to treat 12 patients with inhalations of trichlorethylene, and encouraged Plessner to do likewise in an-

other series of 14 patients. There followed a spate of papers on the treatment of tic doloureux with trichlorethylene, including one by Oljenick of Amsterdam who noted that the inhalations sometimes produced the effects of a narcotic, including giddiness and even unconsciousness.

The narcotic effects of trichlorethylene inhalations were also noted by Glaser in 1931, who suspected that the symptoms and signs described by Plessner had not been due to trichlorethylene at all. Glaser's paper attracted the attention of Dennis Jackson, Professor of Pharmacology at the University of Cincinnati, who was searching for a general analgesic that would be rapid, safe and retrievable. Jackson's experiments convinced him that the main, if not indeed the entire, action of trichlorethylene was upon the central nervous system, and that the cases of trigeminal palsy that had occurred in industrial workers were due to impurities. On the basis of Jackson's work, Striker and his colleagues at Cincinnati Medical School employed trichlorethylene, in the form of "trethylene," as an anesthetic-analgesic in a series of 304 patients with encouraging results; but the clinical use of the drug in anesthesia was terminated abruptly by a most condemnatory report of the Council of Pharmacy and Chemistry of the American Medical Association, which judged that the evidence, "does not justify the acceptance of trichlorethylene for use as a general anesthetic."

A major world war had led to the introduction of trichlorethylene as a therapeutic agent in clinical medicine, and a second world war led to its establishment as a useful anesthetic. The Blitz in England and other exigencies of military medicine pointed up the need for a nonflammable, inhalation anesthetic that could be used as a safe substitute for chloroform in warfare, and the Joint Anaesthetic Committee of the

Medical Research Council and the Royal Society of Medicine became interested in the unique properties of trichlorethylene in this regard. Langton Hewer, himself a member of this Committee, undertook the initial clinical investigation in 1940, and published the results under the title, "Trichlorethylene As An Inhalation Anaesthetic," in the June 21, 1941, issue of the *British Medical Journal* (Hewer, C. L., and Hadfield, C. F.: *Br. Med. J., 1:* 924, 1941), which is reprinted below.

TRICHLORETHYLENE AS AN INHALATION ANAESTHETIC

C. LANGTON HEWER, M.B., B.S., D.A.

Senior Anaesthetist to
St. Bartholomew's Hospital,
Hill End Hospital, St. Albans,
and St. Andrew's Hospital,
Dollis Hill; Anaesthetist to
the Brompton Chest Hospital

With a Prefatory Note
By
CHARLES F. HADFIELD, M.B.E., M.D., D.A.

Consulting Anaesthetist to
St. Bartholomew's Hospital;
Anaesthetist to the Emergency
Medical Service; Honorary Secretary
of the Joint Anaesthetics
Committee of the Medical Research
Council and the Royal Society
of Medicine

Br. Med. J., 1: 924–927, June 21, 1941

*   *   *   *

DETAILS OF PRESENT INVESTIGATION

"The number of administrations was 127 and, although this is admittedly a small series, an effort was made to choose representative cases. Most of the commoner major operations were performed under trichlorethylene anaesthesia, their duration varying from seven minutes to three hours ten minutes, the average being about forty-five minutes. The patients were either (a) air-raid casualties, (b) soldiers—most of whom were wounded evacuated from Dunkirk—and (c) ordinary hospital civilian patients. Their ages varied from 14 months to 81 years."

*   *   *   *

STAGES AND SIGNS OF ANAESTHESIA

"In most respects trichlorethylene resembles chloroform rather than ether, and the signs of the various stages of anaesthesia are similar to those encountered with nitrous-oxide-oxygen with chloroform as an adjuvant. Some degree of general analgesia appears to be present in the first stage, and this was proved to be due to trichlorethylene and not to the nitrous oxide by occurring when pure oxygen was used to vaporize the drug. The second stage was not usually marked, but in one or two patients violent excitement did occur. This can, of course, be avoided by starting with an intravenous barbiturate, but it was not done lest it should confuse the issue. The third stage was characterized by quiet automatic breathing and a variable degree of muscular relaxation. This was sufficient for the operative procedures except in three patients. The first was a muscular young man who was having a partial gastrectomy for ulcer; the second was a patient from whom a large malignant ovarian cyst was removed; and the third was a soldier who underwent manipulation of the spine. In each instance the addition of diethyl ether vapour for a short time secured the necessary relaxation."

*   *   *   *

1942

Published April, 1957

The introduction of curare by Dr. Harold R. Griffith represented a milestone of progress in anesthesia without equal since the classic public demonstration of ether more than a century before. The drug revolutionized the practice of anesthesia by permitting utter muscular flaccidity without the necessity of resort to deep and dangerous levels of general anesthesia. In the light of all that has followed, the story behind the introduction of curare is fascinating; it is best told by the man himself:

"Like everyone else, I knew that there was a need for better muscle relaxation during certain surgical procedures, so I pricked up my ears when, in 1940, Dr. Lewis Wright told me of his idea that curare might provide the relaxation. He told me of the work of Dr. A. E. Bennett in Nebraska, who had been using the new preparation, Intocostrin, to soften the convulsions of patients undergong shock therapy for psychiatric disease. Because curare had a fabulous reputation as a poison, I was only mildly interested; but I kept thinking about the possibilities.

I met Dr. Wright again in 1941, and asked him how he was getting along with his idea. He said he still thought that curare might be of value to the anesthetist, but he hadn't been able to get anyone to try it in the operating room. I argued to myself that if it did not kill Dr. Bennett's patients it could hardly do any serious harm to ours, because the major danger would be respiratory paralysis and even at that time we anesthetists were accustomed to maintaining controlled respiration over long periods: so I asked Dr. Wright to send me some Intocostrin.

On January 23, 1942, at the Homeopathic Hospital in Montreal (now the Queen Elizabeth Hospital), my resident, Dr. Enid Johnson, and I administered the first dose to a young man undergoing appendicectomy. The surgeon was Dr. George Novinger, now practicing in Knoxville, Tennessee. The following quotation is from the original anaesthetic record of that case:

"Intocostrin, Squibb (curare) 3.5 cc, given intravenously in 1½ minutes as operation started—no appreciable effect upon pulse or respiration. After 5 minutes, another 1.5 cc. of Intocostrin given. Apparently complete relaxation of abdominal muscles resulted and continued for 20 minutes, during which time cyclopropoane was lightened. At the end of this period, muscle tone returned, probably from wearing off of curare effect. Cyclopropane was then increased in concentration, and anesthesia continued in the usual way. There was no demonstrable change in pulse, blood pressure, or respiration."

The first case demonstrated that curare would actually relax abdominal muscles in patients under anaesthesia, and that this action was temporary and without cardiac depression. We then proceeded cautiously to test the drug in a variety of cases. Our first reported series was small, and would not be statistically significant if one were making a comparative study between similar drugs. But here the situation was quite different—this was a drug that did something entirely different than any drug then in use. It produced its muscle-relaxing effect in each case and we encountered no serious complication: so we decided that even after 25 cases we should make our work known and give other workers an opportunity to confirm or contest our findings."

The confirmations were not long in pouring in from all corners of the globe. Those who merely read the report, without themselves assessing Dr. Griffith's results clinically, were scathing in their condemnations and intimated that anyone who would administer such a poison to a patient was a very questionable character; those who read the report, and then went into the operating room for their own clinical trials, were unanimous in their support of the findings.

But the importance of Griffith's contribution lies not so much in the drug itself—good as it is—as in the fresh approach which it brought to anesthetic thought concerning the clinical pharmacology of anesthesia. No longer was it necessary to employ deep and toxic levels of general anesthesia in the hope that, like a shotgun blast, the pellets of the single agent would strike all the various physiologic systems of the body necessary in order to provide the essential facets of general anesthesia—hypnosis, analgesia, muscular relaxation, and the obtundation of noxious reflex impulses. Rather, it was possible to administer a specific drug to produce a specific effect, in just the quantity necessary to achieve that effect. This is the practice of clinical pharmacology, the introduction of science into anesthetic administration after a century of art. It is a concept that now has dominated the trend of the specialty for better than a decade; and more than the drug itself, it is the true measure of the magnitude of Griffith's contribution.

THE USE OF CURARE IN GENERAL ANESTHESIA

H. R. Griffith

AND

G. E. Johnson

Montreal, Canada

Anesthesiology, 3: 418–420, July 1942

"Every anesthetist has wished at times that he might be able to produce rapid and complete muscular relaxation in resistant patients under general anesthesia. This is a preliminary report on the clinical use of a drug which will give this kind of relaxation, temporarily and apparently quite harmlessly.

"The physiological action of curare as an interrupter of the neuromuscular mechanism has long been recognized, and its best known practical applications have been by South American Indians as an arrow poison and in the physiological laboratory. The crude curare of the South American forests contains numerous toxic substances, but it has been possible so to refine the drug that the elements of cardiac and respiratory depression are removed and only the "pure" curare effect remains.

"For several years this purified curare has been used experimentally in psychiatric hospitals to prevent traumatic complications in convulsive shock therapy. Bennett (1), Gray (2) and others have reported on the efficiency and harmlessness of curare when used for this purpose in quite a large number of patients.

"In January, 1942, at the suggestion of Dr. L. H. Wright, we began using Intocostrin (extract of unauthenticated curare, Squibb) in order to increase skeletal muscular relaxation in patients under general anesthesia. So far, we have given it to 25 patients, and in each case there has been rapid and complete muscular relaxation, which develops within one minute after intravenous injection of the drug and gradually disappears in from ten to fifteen minutes. In none of our patients has there been any serious depressing effect on respiration, pulse or blood pressure, and there was no demonstrable postoperative effect of any kind. Apparently the drug is very rapidly broken down and excreted almost as rapidly as it acts, although there is some evidence from the psychiatric experience that patients who are given a second injection on the same day require a smaller dose to produce the physiological effect.

"We administer the Intocostrin intravenously with a dosage of 10 to 20 mg. of the active curare per 20 lbs. of body weight. Intocostrin is prepared in solution containing 20 mg. of the active curare substance per cubic centimeter, so that an average adult dose is 4 to 5 cc. We have not given to any one patient more than 5 cc., and we make the injection rather rapidly, in less than a minute.

"It has not been necessary to administer artificial respiration or stimulants in any of our cases. As our patients are all under gas anesthesia, with means of resuscitation by oxygen immediately available, we do not fear this complication. Since Prostigmine is used as an antidote to curare, an ampule of this drug should always be available."

* * * *

SUMMARY

"A purified extract of curare (Intocostrin) has been administered intravenously to 25 patients under light general anesthesia. In each case temporary but complete muscular relaxation was rapidly produced with apparently no harmful effect."

Published August, 1958

Throughout the duration of human history—with the exception of the last hundred years or so—women have brought forth their children in pain, just as the Bible (somewhat retrospectively) said that they should. Not in ordinary pain, either; the Romans had a word for it: *poena magna*—the Great Pain of childbirth. Occasional forays into methods of relieving that pain have been made down through the ages. The early Chinese used opiates and soporific potions for the relief of pain during labor and delivery. The Greeks, of course, called on their gods, and there is that magnificent story of Actemia who, terrified by the suffering that her own birth had caused her mother, begged the favor of eternal virginity from the god Zeus; when she subsequently seduced Endymion, she was appropriately punished by a mythological superfecundation that made her the mother of fifty daughters at a single parturition! Even the Americans did their bit: Zerubbabel Endicott, physician in Salem, Massachusetts (and son of the famous Governor) prescibed, "For Sharpe and Difficult Travel in Women with Child Take a Lock of Vergins haire on any part of ye head, of half the Age of ye Woman in travill. Cut it very smale to fine Powder then taken 12 Ants Eggs dried in an oven after ye bread is drawne or otherwise make them dry and make them to powder with the haire, give this with a quarter of a pint of Red Cows milk or for want of it give it in strong ale wort."

The modern age of obstetrical anesthesia, of course, began with Morton's classical public demonstration of ether on October 16, 1846. The medical profession was quick to bestow the blessings of anesthesia upon women undergoing the pangs of childbirth. Sir James Y. Simpson, Morton's Scottish contemporary, first gave ether for this purpose in December of 1846, within weeks of Morton's Triumph. On April 7, 1847, the first woman in America to receive anesthesia during labor was given ether by Nathan Cooley Keep, a dentist. But it was Simpson, in November of 1847, who, after having first tried the new drug on his assistants, his wife, her niece, and a friend of the family, introduced the use of chloroform into obstetrics and thus ushered in the modern age of obstetrical analgesia.

Neither Simpson nor the cause of obstetrical analgesia had easy sledding after the initial introduction of the technique. Simpson himself was called a blasphemer, heretic, and agent of the devil by the strict Scottish Calvinists of his time, and the physicians of Edinburgh were circularized in the matter: "To all seeming, Satan wishes to help suffering women but the upshot will be the collapse of society, for the Fear of the Lord, which depends upon the petitions of the afflicted, will be destroyed. For tens of thousands of years births have taken place without any means of allaying pain. Has not Nature disclosed the wisdom of God in her conduct of the process of birth?" The clergy then quoted *Genesis 3:* 16 from the pulpit: ". . . in sorrow thou shalt bring forth children"; to which Simpson, himself a student of the Bible, replied (from *Genesis 2:* 21): "And the Lord God caused a deep sleep to fall upon Adam, and he slept: and he took one of his ribs, and closed up the flesh instead thereof." Queen Victoria settled the issue for both Simpson and obstetrical analgesia at the time of the birth of her eighth child, Prince Leopold: ". . . . the Queen had chloroform exhibited to her during her late confinement . . . It acted admirably. It was not at any time given so strongly as to render the Queen insensible, and an ounce of chloroform was scarcely consumed during the whole time. Her Majesty was greatly pleased with the effect and she certainly never has had a better recovery."

Methods of inhalational analgesia remained in ascendance in obstetrics for many years; until, in fact, the onset of "Twilight Sleep", that "state of clouded consciousness" induced by the combination of morphine and scopolamine, in 1906. Considerable furor followed, as it had in the instance of chloroform analgesia. The opponents cited that "the expulsion period averaged 6 hours and 15 minutes against the normal 1 hour and 45 minutes", and concluded that "Scopolamine causes protraction of birth and causes asphyxia". Carl Gauss, the initiator of Dämmerschlaf (or "Twilight Sleep") defended the technique by pointing out that its failures were due to misuse: "If you could trust to having an average woman, you could use an average dose; but the dose is easier to standardize than the woman"—an aphorism that remains true of obstetrical analgesia to the present day.

It became evident that, whatever salutory effects "Twilight Sleep" might have on the mother's pain threshold, they were at least offset by the disastrous effects upon her infant's respiratory mechanism, and other drugs and combinations of drugs were tried for analgesia during labor. The barbiturates gained rapidly in favor; and there then followed the usual controversy over the effects upon labor and the newborn in the form of the "Battle of the Barbiturates", which was largely lost when Irving reported that apnea neonatorum occurred in from 35 to 65 per cent of the babies (depending upon the drugs used) as compared to 2 per cent for a series with no analgesic drugs. The urgent need was obviously for a method of obstetrical analgesia and anesthesia that spared the mother pain but also spared the infant's respirations.

As early as 1901, Kreis of Germany had used spinal anesthesia for operative delivery; and the use of caudal and epidural anesthesias for obstetrical deliveries followed, albeit some years later. There was little doubt that conduction anesthesia did decrease the incidence of asphyxia neonatorum, but there remained the problem of prolonging the action of conduction anesthesia sufficiently to obtund not only the pain of delivery, but also the excruciating pangs of labor itself. There were a number of workers who contributed to the solution of this problem, and there were a number of innovations of importance; but perhaps none was acclaimed by such widespread adoption as the technique of continuous caudal anesthesia, described by Edwards and Hingson in the *American Journal of Surgery. 57:* 459–464, September, 1942.

Published August, 1980

Simpson, chloroform, and obstetric anesthesia form a triad in the history of anesthesia which seem just naturally to go together, but there is more to that statement than appears on the surface.

There appears to be no doubt whatsoever that James Young Simpson, who held the Chair of Midwifery at Edinburgh, was the first to apply the "Yankee Dodge" of ether anesthesia to the practice of obstetrics. He was a great opportunist, with a mind that was both receptive and perceptive, and he welcomed the new idea at once as soon as he heard about it. Furthermore, he acted on it; and on January 19, 1847, 3 months after Morton's introduction of ether anesthesia, and just 2 months after its first use in the British Isles, Simpson employed ether for internal podalic version and the delivery of a dead fetus from a patient with severe pelvic contracture. This operation, of course, required full ether anesthesia with unconsciousness; and this became Simpson's way of conducting obstetric anesthesia, not only for patients requiring forceps or operative deliveries, but also for normal deliveries.

On March 19, 1847, just 2 months to the day after his first use of ether anesthesia in obstetrics, Simpson published his first paper, "On the Employment of Ether in the Practice of Midwifery", in the *London Medical Gazette.* But even as he was publishing his first paper on ether in midwifery, Simpson was casting about for an inhalation agent that would not have all of ether's drawbacks: "The disagreeable and very persistent smell, its occasional tendency to irritation of the bronchi during its first inspirations, and the large quantity occasionally required to be used"—but particularly the giddiness, nausea and vomiting.

His search was straightforward and primitive, and consisted of self-experimentation: he and his assistants, Doctors Matthews Duncan and George Keith, would gather around the dinner table in the evening after supper and test, by the rough and ready but practical method of inhalation, a variety of volatile substances including Dutch liquid, acetone, nitric ether, benzin, and iodoform vapor, as well as chloride of hydrocarbon, aldehyde, and bisulphuret of carbon. The suggestion to try chloroform came from David Waldie, a Scotsman who, like Simpson himself, had been born in the Royal Burgh of Linlithgow, and who at the time was chemist at Apothecaries Hall in Liverpool. In fact, Waldie was one of the few men then living who knew anything about chloroform, and without his suggestion Simpson would never have heard of the substance at all, because at that time it was only a chemical curiosity. It had been discovered and described, simultaneously and independently, in the fall of 1831 by 3 chemists, Samuel Guthrie in the United States, Eugene Soubeiran in France, and Justus Liebig in Germany. In 1834, the famous French chemist, Jean Baptiste Andre Dumas, determined the chemical nature, physical properties, and true formula, and named the chemical chloroform.

The ultimate experiment, which was conducted by Simpson and his young assistants, and which proved the anesthetic properties of chloroform in man, was described by Professor James Miller, a surgeon who was a colleague and neighbor, who used to look in each morning at nine o'clock to see how the enthusiasts had fared in the experiments of the night before:

"Late one evening, it was the 4th of November, 1847, on returning home after a weary day's labour, Dr. Simpson with his two friends and assistants, Drs. Keith and Duncan, sat down to their somewhat hazardous work in Dr. Simpson's dining-room. Having inhaled several substances, but without much effect, it occurred to Dr. Simpson to try a ponderous material which he had formerly set aside on a lumber-table, and which on account of its great weight he had hitherto regarded as of no likelihood whatever; that happened to be a small bottle of chloroform. It was searched for and recovered from beneath a heap of waste paper. And with each tumbler newly charged, the inhalers resumed their vocation. Immediately, an unwonted hilarity seized the party—they became brighteyed, very happy, and very loquacious—expatiating on the delicious aroma of the new fluid. The conversation was of unusual intelligence, and quite charmed the listeners—some ladies of the family and a naval officer, brother-in-law of Dr. Simpson. But suddenly there was talk of sounds being heard like those of a cotton mill louder and louder; a moment more and then all was quiet—and then crash! On awakening, Dr. Simpson's first perception was mental—"this is far stronger and better than ether," said he to himself. His second was to note that he was prostrate on the floor, and that among the friends about him there was both confusion and alarm. Hearing a noise he turned round and saw Dr. Duncan beneath a chair—his jaw dropped, his eyes staring, his head bent half under him, quite unconscious, and snoring in a most determined and alarming manner. More noise still and much motion. And then his eyes overtook Dr. Keith's feet and legs making valorous attempts to overturn the supper table, or more probably to annihilate everything that was on it. By and by Dr. Simpson having regained his seat, Dr. Duncan having finished his uncomfortable and unrefreshing slumber, and Dr. Keith having come to an arrangement with the table and its contents, the *sederunt* was resumed. Each expressed himself delighted with this new agent, and its inhalation was repeated many times that night—one of the ladies gallantly taking her place and turn at the table—until the supply of chloroform was fairly exhausted."

The gallant lady who took her place at the table was Miss Petrie, a niece of Mrs. Simpson's. Usually a retiring young woman, she began shouting with ecstacy and excitement, "I'm beginning to fly! I'm an angel, oh, I'm an angel!"

Simpson's proclivity as an opportunist was never demonstrated better than during the next 8 days. On November 5, the day after the evening of sniffing, Simpson employed chloroform for childbirth with spectacular success. On November 10th, Simpson reported the use of chloroform as an anesthetic in a paper read before the Medico-Chirurgical Society of Edinburgh. On November 12th, this paper was published under the title of, "An Account of a New Anaesthetic Agent as a Substitute for Sulphuric Ether in Surgery and Midwifery." By November 15th, Simpson had accumulated a total of 50 cases of chloroform administrations, and he published this fact in an addendum to his November 12th paper. Thus, in the course of 11 days, Simpson had experimented on, introduced, reported, and published on chloroform anesthesia—clearly, he didn't suffer from the reticence of a Crawford Long.

Nor was there any reticence in Simpson's own report of the first use of chloroform in childbirth on that November 5th:

"The lady to whom it was first exhibited during parturition, had been previously delivered in this country by perforation of the head of the infant, after a labour of three days' duration. In this, her second confinement, pains supervened a fortnight before the full time. Three hours and a half after they commenced, and ere the first stage of the labour was completed, I placed her under the influence of the chloroform. The child was expelled in about twenty-five minutes after the inhalation was begun. The squalling of the child did not, as is usual, rouse her; and some minutes elapsed after the child was removed by the nurse to another room, before the patient awoke. She then turned round and observed to me that she had enjoyed a very comfortable sleep, and would now be more able for the work before her. In a little while she remarked that she was afraid her sleep had stopped the pains. Shortly afterwards her infant was brought in by the nurse from the adjoining room, and it was a matter of no small difficulty to convince the astonished mother that the labour was entirely over, and that the child presented to her was really her own living baby."

Simpson's great triumph of obstetric anesthesia with chloroform was not regarded as such in all quarters. Many influential members of the medical profession—including Charles D. Meigs of Philadelphia, Francis H. Rainsbotham in the British Isles, and Frederick W. Scanzoni of Germany—objected to the use of anesthesia in obstetrics; but, particularly, the Scottish Calvinist clergy were outraged, for the gospel itself, in *Genesis, iii,* 16 contained God's malediction to mothers: "In sorrow thou shalt bring forth children." Simpson, himself a pious Christian, was in his turn outraged that the ministers of religion could think that God was a vindictive God, and he quoted *Genesis, ii,* 21 right back at his accusers: "And the Lord God, caused a deep sleep to fall upon Adam, and he slept: and he took one of his ribs, and closed up the flesh instead thereof"—what God himself did could not be sinful. The preachers had a ready answer in that the creation of Eve out of the sleeping Adam took place before the Fall, and the curse pronounced upon Eve and her daughters was not uttered until our parents had been driven forth from Paradise. Simpson countered this

with *James, iv,* 17: "Therefore to him that knoweth to do good and doeth it not, to him it is sin."

The quarrel raged on for 6 years, ending abruptly when suddenly loyalty to the throne was invoked on the side of chloroform, and Simpson unexpectedly found an ally whom none of the clergy dared answer, the Head of the Church of England, Queen Victoria. During her seventh confinement at the time of the birth of Prince Leopold on April 7th, 1853, Her majesty was suffering the usual pangs at the end of the First Stage of Labor when the Royal Accoucheur, James Clark, recommended the use of Simpson's discovery. The Queen readily agree, and for all intents and purposes the conflict as to whether painless childbearing could be acceptable to God Almighty, or was necessarily sinful, was ended. Victoria wrote later: "Dr. Snow administered the blessed chloroform and the effect was soothing, quieting and delightful beyound measure." On April 18th, 1857, upon the occasion of the birth of Princess Beatrice, Her Majesty again inhaled chloroform during the confinement; and the *Lancet*, which had loudly pontificated just 4 years earlier that, "in no case could it be justifiable to administer chloroform in normal labour," routinely reported that "Her Majesty was delivered safely of a Princess . . . on Tuesday last . . . the anaesthetic agent perfectly succeeded in the object desired." Simpson's last sweet measure of triumph in the struggle with his foes came when Queen Victoria placed a Sir in front of his name and a Bart. after it. He chose as his coat-of-arms the rod of Aesculapius over the motto *Victo dolore* (Victory over Pain).

Even as Simpson was founding the subspeciality of obstetric anesthesia—indeed, within 3 months of his first use of ether for obstetric anesthesia—another chapter was being written, the chapter on obstetric analgesia. The credit for the introduction of obstetric analgesia must go to a dentist, Nathan Colley Keep, who was the first Dean of Harvard's School of Dentistry, where he had been one of Morton's teachers and, before that, had probably been the man to whom Horace Wells had been apprenticed for the study of dentistry. On April 10, 1847, Keep wrote the following letter to the Editor of the *Boston Medical and Surgical Journal:*

"Dear Sir,

On the 7th inst. I administered the vapor of ether in a case of natural labor. The patient was in good health and in labor of her third child. Five and a half hours having elapsed from the commencement of the labor, her pains, which had been light, but regular, becoming severe, the vapor of ether was inhaled by the nose and exhaled by the mouth. The patient had no difficulty in taking the vapor in this manner from the reservoir, without any valvular apparatus.

In the course of twenty minutes four pains had occurred without suffering, the vapor of ether being administered between each pain. Consciousness was unimpaired and labor not retarded. Inhalation was then suspended, that a comparison might be made between the effective force of the throes with and without the vapor of ether. No material difference was detected, but the distress of the patient was great. Inhalation was resumed, but the progress of labor was so rapid that time could not be found for sufficient inhalation to bring the system perfectly under its influence; still the sufferings of the last moments were greatly mitigated. From the commencement of the inhalation to the close of labor, thirty minutes. Number of inhalations, five. No unpleasant symptoms occurred, and the result was highly satisfactory.

Yours, etc.
N. C. Keep"

This was the original description of an attempt to provide a technique of anesthesia particularly adapted to obstetrics, synchronizing the intermittent administration of the anesthetic with the regularly recurring contractions, and it became the principle upon which obstetric analgesia with both ether and chloroform was founded. It was the manner in which John Snow had administered chloroform for 53 minutes to Queen Victoria at the time of the birth of Prince Leopold, in 15 minim doses (0.9 ml.) intermittently on a handkerchief, a technique which ever thereafter was known as *chloroform a la rèine.*

Snow, as early as 1849, wrote that, "when the practice of inhalation in midwifery was first introduced by Dr. Simpson, he very naturally adopted the plan which is usually followed in surgical operations, making the patient unconscious at once, and keeping her so to the end of her labour. It was soon found however, by other practitioners that this is not necessary: and indeed it would not be safe in protracted cases. Drs. Murphy and Rigby were, I believe, amongst the first to state, that relief from pain may often be afforded in obstetric cases, without removing the consciousness of the patient. And I soon observed the same circumstance. Some persons indeed, have alleged that the pain of labour can always be prevented, without making the patient unconscious of surrounding objects; whilst others have asserted that no relief can be afforded unless unconsciousness is induced. But both these opinions are directly opposed to experience. There are comparatively few cases in which the suffering can be prevented throughout the labour without interfering with consciousness. although there are very many cases in which it can be in this way prevented in the early part of labour. This difference depends, in some measure, on the constitution of the patient, but chiefly on the severity of the pain to be prevented."

For much of the first hundred years of anesthesia, ether and chloroform were the mainstays of both obstetric anesthesia as well as obstetric analgesia. In 1880, N_2O was used for the first time for pain relief in labor by Klikovich and, administered by inhalation at the commencement of contraction, proved a very effective analgesic technique. The first parenteral technique for obstetric analgesia was that of "twilight sleep," produced by Gauss and von Steinbuckel of Frieburg in 1902, and consisted of the combined injection of morphine and scopolamine. Since it combined sedation and analgesia with almost complete amnesia for the entire period of labor, it was hugely popular with the clientele (the parturients) and came to control many an obstetric practice. There was no significant increase in maternal mortality with "twilight sleep," but the effect on infant mortality was very apparent: the all-too-frequent birth of "blue babies," some of whom died, induced thoughtful obstetricians to search for a substitute for morphine. They tried, successively, Pantopon, heroin, and then the synthetic narcotics, like meperidine and alphaprodine; but a narcotic is a narcotic, and the price of fetal respiratory depression always had to be paid. "Twilight sleep" was then changed to a barbiturate-scopolamine regime, with the thought that the barbiturates would be less depressant on the fetal respiratory center than the narcotics; but this was only partially true, while the maternal restlessness, which had been a major problem even with the narcotics, increased to such an extent that in at least one well-known lying-in unit, football helmets were standard protective equipment for the obstetric patient in the Labor Room.

Rectal anesthesia with ether for surgery had never achieved any great popularity for such good and sufficient reasons as bloody diarrhea, abdominal pain and distension, rupture of the intestine, colonic ulceration, and purulent peritonitis, not to mention respiratory depression, hypotension, and death. Gwathmey's oil-ether colonic anesthesia, however, overcame the irritation of the mucosa by the addition of olive oil to the ether, and developed into a successful method for the relief of pain in childbirth in the hands of the careful physician—when left to the untutelaged, it maintained the same capacity for disaster as any other technique placed in the hands of the unknowing.

The great breakthrough in both obstetric anesthesia and obstetric analgesia came when these 2 objectives could be combined in a technique which *ordinarily* would provide pain relief during both labor and delivery with minimal systemic effects upon mother or fetus, with few or no complications to either, with high maternal acceptability, and with a happy anesthesiologist and an equally happy obstetrician. Edwards

and Hingson provided the groundwork for all of this with their adaption of Lemmon's technique for continuous spinal anesthesia to the caudal route in the paper titled, "Continuous Caudal Anesthesia In Obstetrics," which was published in the September, 1942, issue of the *American Journal of Surgery* (Edwards, W.B. and Hingson, R.A.: *Am. J. Surg., 57:* 459, 1942), and is reprinted below with the kind permissions of the authors and the publishers.

CONTINUOUS CAUDAL ANESTHESIA IN OBSTETRICS

EDWARDS, W. B.
AND
HINGSON, R. A.

*Am. J. Surg., 57: 459–464
(Sept.) 1942*

"Continuous caudal anesthesia, or the extradural introduction of fractional doses of anesthetic substances through the sacral hiatus into the sacral canal, has been practiced by us at the U.S. Marine Hospital, Stapleton, Staten Island, New York since early January, 1942. We consider this form of anesthesia to be an improvement over the conventional type of peridural anesthetic administered by a single injection. In this latter procedure the time limit of satisfactory anesthesia is from forty-five minutes to two and a half hours, while with continuous caudal administration, the anesthesia can be safely prolonged indefinitely. The maximum time of effective anesthesia during labor, in our experience, has been thirteen hours."

*   *   *   *

"We realize that our series is too small to make all inclusive assertations as to its merit, but we do suggest—the method is worthy of further study in the larger clinics in which an accurate evaluation can be obtained."

1943

Published June, 1972

Man has always been exposed to the extremes of environmental temperature, the nature of the extreme during a number of milleniums now depending for the most part upon how close to, or how far from, the Equator he was, or how far above or below sea level that he happened to be. By and large, he has regarded these extremes as merely the normal facts of his existence, and his life styles through the eons have developed in such a way as to facilitate his existence in his own particular climate. Occasionally, if he moved about and into a new clime, with a different extreme of temperature than that with which he was familiar, he regarded the experience as not only unpleasant and a drag, but a threat against which he must take preventive measures if he was to survive. And even more occasionally, he noted the effects of these extremes of temperature upon his physiologic status quo or that of other organisms in the same environment. His concern with these effects has been greatly increased during the past few years due to the development of the Space Race, for in outer space he is subjected to the ultimate in extreme cold with which he has had to contend; and during reentry into the earth's atmosphere, perhaps the ultimate in heat—although there were those present in Hiroshima and Nagasaki during August 1945, who, for a fleeting moment, could probably have argued the latter point.

There is no imaginable way at the present time that man can put the extremes of temperature to use for his physiologic advantage; but exposures to moderate increases or decreases in temperature are a different story. The use of cold as a therapeutic tool, for instance, while often regarded as a fairly recent development, is by no means new, for the numbing effects of cold have been recognized throughout the ages, and occasional use has been made of this knowledge in medicine for centuries. Hippocrates advocated the use of snow and ice to check hemorrhage; and he was also aware of the analgetic action of cold, for he wrote in his *Aphorisms*, "swellings and pains in the joints, without ulceration, those of a gouty nature, and sprains are generally improved by a copious affusion of cold water, which reduces the swelling, and removes the pain; for a moderate degree of numbness removes pain."

The Saxon Leechbook, now known as the *Lacnunga*, was transmitted to writing by an unknown Anglo-Saxon monk about 15 years before the Norman Conquest (*i.e., circa* 1050) and contains a host of incantations and charms for the treatment of disease. The vast majority of these recipes and invocations are largely superstitious in nature; but the *Lacnunga* also contains perhaps the first recorded suggestion of the use of cold for refrigeration anesthesia—chilling a part of the body by the application of cold water to deaden the pain of incising and draining an abcess: "Again, for eruptive rash. Let him sit in cold water until it be deadened; then draw him up. Then cut four scarifications around the pocks and let drip as long as he will."

There then began the continued cycle of rediscovery and the neglect of the use of cold as an anesthetic which has been the history of the technique. There was another surge forward in 1595 when Johannes Costaeus (de Costa) of Venice published his *De Igneis Medicinae Praesidiis*, in which there is the briefest reference to the use of cold—in the form of water, snow, or ice—to relieve the pain of surgical incision. Half a century later, Severino of Naples, the father of comparative anatomy, demonstrated refrigeration anesthesia to Thomas Bartholin (the discoverer of Bartholin's glands), when the latter visited Naples in 1646. Fifteen years later, Bartholin devoted almost an entire chapter in his book, *De Nivis Usu Medico*, to Severino's use of snow as an anesthetic: "Before treating ulcers of the limbs by cauterization, the rubbing-in of snow produces insensitivity. Marco Aurelio Severino, my old teacher and friend, who is the foremost surgeon of our time, taught me this at the University of Naples. As a general rule, he put the snow in a capacious vessel . . . and applied it to the skin. He told us that, if we were not afraid of gangrene, we could apply it under narrow, parallel bandages; in a quarter of an hour, the nerves will be numbed, and it will be possible to make an incision at that point without causing pain. The surgeon can employ this method successfully even when opening up the area between the thighs, close to the perineal arch, for lithotomy;" and then he added, in proof that the mystique of the bedside manner was an early acquisition of medicine, "when he wishes to conceal the nature of the treatment, in order to make the results seem more astonishing, the aforesaid Severino dyes the snow with ground ultramarine or some other colouring matter."

Refrigeration anesthesia was rediscovered once again in 1807 when, after the battle of Preuss-Eylau, Baron Dominique-Jean Larrey, Napoleon's Surgeon General, noted that there was no pain during amputations performed on soldiers who had lain in the snow on the battlefield at below freezing temperatures. The use of refrigeration anesthesia was increased considerably in 1866 when once again it enjoyed a revival, this time due to Benjamin Ward Richardson's (Richardson was John Snow's biographer) introduction of his ether spray for the purpose of producing local anesthesia by freezing tissues. This technique was later modified by the use of ethyl chloride which, because it evaporates more quickly, is more effective than ether for this form of anesthesia.

The really definitive work on the use of local refrigeration anesthesia for surgery, however, was that performed by Dr. Frederick M. Allen, beginning in about 1937. He published a number of papers on the subject, but he first attracted widespread interest in the technique with a paper entitled, "Refrigeration Anesthesia for Limb Operations," which was presented before the American Society of Anesthetists in New York City in April of 1942 (Allen, F. M., *Anesthesiology, 4:* 12, 1943) and is reprinted below with the kind permission of the publisher.

REFRIGERATION ANESTHESIA FOR LIMB OPERATIONS

FREDERICK M. ALLEN, M.D.

Anesthesiology, 4: 12, 1943

*   *   *   *

CONCLUSION

"Refrigeration differs fundamentally from all other known forms of anesthesia in that it abolishes reactivity not only in the nerves but also in the entire protoplasm. It thus has a unique value in the prevention of shock. Its usefulness in respect to pain, edema, thrombosis, infection, tissue vitality and other conditions is also discussed."

1944

Published April, 1979

All wars are stupid, of course.

But high on the list of the absolutely most stupid wars of all times was the Crimean War, fought in 1854 by the Turks, the British and the French against Russia.

Russia, ambitious for a gateway to the warm Mediterranean, had built a vast naval base at Sevastopol. The British and French had watched carefully, and had waited until the last nail had been hammered, and the last capstan had been set in place on the docks—then they attacked with the object of destroying the whole shebang.

Outside of its unquestioned standing in the Top Ten listing of the absolutely most stupid wars of all times, the Crimean War would have long since been forgotten except for 2 little things.

The first was a lunatic battle ordered by an imbecile British junior officer, for no conceivable purpose: a nonsensical charge into a massively fortified cul-de-sac which was immortalized by the English poet, Alfred Lord Tennyson, in the epic poem which recounted the tragic carnage, "The Charge of the Light Brigade":

> Half a league, half a league,
> Half a league onward,
> All in the valley of Death
>   Rode the six hundred.
> "Forward, the Light Brigade!
> Charge for the guns!" he said
> Into the valley of Death
>   Rode the six hundred.
>
> "Forward, the Light Brigade!"
> Was there a man dismayed?
> Not though the soldier knew
>   Some one had blundered.
> Theirs not to make reply,
> Theirs not to reason why,
> Theirs but to do and die.
> Into the valley of Death
>   Rode the six hundred.
>
> Cannon to right of them,
> Cannon to left of them,
> Cannon in front of them
>   Volleyed and thundered;
> Stormed at with shot and shell,
> Boldly they rode and well,
> Into the jaws of Death.
> Into the mouth of hell
>   Rode the six hundred.
>
> Flashed all their sabres bare,
> Flashed as they turned in air
> Sabring the gunners there,
> Charging an army, while
>   All the world wondered.
>
> Plunged in the battery-smoke
> Right through the line they broke;
> Cossack and Russian

> Reeled from the sabre-stroke
>   Shattered and sundered
> Then they rode back, but not,
>   Not the six hundred.
>
> Cannon to right of them,
> Cannon to left of them,
> Cannon behind them
>   Volleyed and thundered;
> Stormed at with shot and shell,
> While horse and hero fell,
> They that had fought so well
> Came through the jaws of Death,
> Back from the mouth of hell,
> All that was left of them,
>   Left of six hundred.
>
> When can their glory fade?
> Oh, the wild charge they made!
>   All the world wondered.
> Honor the charge they made!
> Honor the Light Brigade,
>   Noble six hundred!

The second thing for which the Crimean war will always be remembered is the role which it played in revolutionizing nursing—and, indeed, sparking the foundation of modern nursing—by the greening of Florence Nightingale.

Florence Nightingale was born in the city of Florence, Italy (the city from which she derived her name) in 1820.

She was the daughter of a wealthy and aristocratic British family, who had connections at the highest levels of government and society.

Her early life was a round of suitors and parties and foreign travel. But the suitors did not suit her, the parties seemed frivolous, and from the age of 17 her all-consuming ambition was to be a nurse.

Her family was appalled. Their distress was quite natural, for the vocation of nursing, in England at that time, was almost always the calling of women of the lowest standards and class, and the conception of nurses that the public harbored was that of "tipsy, promiscuous harridans." Under the circumstances, the Nightingales simple forbade their daughter to pursue her dream, and the subsequent struggle was long and bitter. Denied entry into direct nursing, the daughter compensated by visiting every hospital which she could to observe nursing in action, visited the religious orders on the continent to observe the nursing techniques of the Sisters of Charity and other such groups, and studied sanitation in its largest sense. She was indefatigable in her reading and observations, and made copious notes of all that she encountered in these fields. She was 33 years of age before the family admitted that she was not going to "marry and settle down," and she was permitted to pursue her chosen vocation.

But it was the Crimean War which really launched her on her chosen career.

The reports from the Crimea were of unbelievable lack of care for the wounded British soldiers, and this raised a public outrage in Great Britain. The Secretary At War, Sir Stanley Herbert, who was an old family friend, asked Miss Nightingale to head a contingent of 38 nurses to Scutari, a suburb of Constantinople, where 2 abandoned Turkish barracks served as the hospital for the British armies.

Her group arrived at Scutari in November, 1854, and found the most appalling conditions: 1800 patients, many on the floor, all cold and without adequate covering, inedible food, non-existent sanitation, poor ventilation, rats and mice running free, dysentery and fever rampant, and "not a basin, not a towel, not a bit of soap nor a broom could be found." Her determination and administrative ability, not to mention her personal financial resources, cut through Army red tape to reach the highest centers of British government, and soon she had clothing, fresh water, an adequate sewage system, food, beds, remodeled wards and—most importantly—the grudging admiration of Army doctors who had been implacable against the participation of women nurses in war.

She lowered the death rate at Scutari from 40 to 2 per cent, she and her small contingent were blessed by thousands of soldiers, and she returned to England a national heroine. Queen Victoria requested an audience with her, and a "Nightingale Fund" was raised by a large group of influential citizens to allow her to set up the model school of nursing of which

she dreamed. This school was started at St. Thomas' Hospital in London, which fulfilled all of her requirements since it came complete with a medical school connection, was large and influential, and was both a charitable and a long-established institution. She planned a 4-year course of instruction and clinical training for young women, not less than 25 nor more than 35 years of age, who were to be selected for "fitness and character." The first 15 probationers began their studies on June 24, 1860: the first modern nursing school was off and running, and 4 years later the Nightingale Nurse began to appear on the medical scene.

Miss Nightingale continued to work to consolidate the gains made in Army Nursing which the Crimean War had produced, and she wrote extensively. One book, called "Notes on Nursing," was published in 1859 and became a classic (it is still available in reprinted forms in many languages); and that same year a second book, "Notes on Hospitals," was also published. "Notes on Hospitals" contained the following statement: "Small wards for casualty cases should be built separately and be separately administered . . . if the cases be as bad as possible, all the more necessity is there for care in placing them where they may have a moderate chance to recover." Her knowledge of hospital administration and hospital design was derived from her on-the-job training at Scutari; and it was from the overcrowded, reeking, disease-ridden old Turkish barracks-turned-hospital that she had developed her sure instinct that the worst cases needed to be congregated in a small area where they could be given specialized nursing and attention.

This was not, however, the first reference to a recovery area. The most complete history of the evolution of the modern Recovery Room is in an unpublished account entitled, "The Historical Development of Postanesthetic Recovery Rooms," which was written by Ms. Nancy Thiel, R.N., the Recovery Room Supervisor at the University of Minnesota Hospitals (who became Mrs. Frederick Van Bergen in 1964 when she married the Professor and Head of the

Department of Anesthesiology, University of Minnesota Medical School).

Ms. Thiel, with help from Dr. Albert Faulconer, Jr., who was then Head of the Section of Anesthesiology at the Mayo Clinic, unearthed probably the first documented reference to a Recovery Room, which preceded the publication of Miss Nightingale's book by almost 60 years. It is to be found in the account of the plans for the expansion and renovation of the Newcastle Infirmary (which had been founded in 1751), which was published in 1801 and which contained the following statement: "The fourth story of the building was to contain the operating room and five 2-bedded rooms, . . . reserved for patients who were dangerously ill or had recently undergone a major operation. Each room was to contain only one patient in a serious condition, the other bed being occupied at night by a nurse or a convalescent patient acting as a nurse." Ms. Thiel cogently observed that this is a remarkable idea coming from a hospital planning committee some 45 years before the discovery of anesthesia, and demonstrated the great perspicacity of the Committee in recognizing that the postoperative patient needed special and close observation, even if it was through the untrained eyes of a fellow patient.

Very little more was heard about the recovery room (or wards, or areas) until around the end of the nineteenth century and the beginning of the twentieth century, when hospital architects began referring to them in the literature. It was noted by Ms. Thiel in her monograph that a book on hospital construction, published in 1907, contained plans of the operating suite of the Augustana Hospital in Chicago, Illinois, which included designs for a recovery room. The authors stated that its purpose was to segregate patients who were recovering from surgery so that they would not ". . . disturb or be disturbed by other patients." The New York Hospital, one of the earliest in the United States, Ms. Thiel observed, included recovery rooms in ". . . 1907 when the newly reconstructed operating theater of the hospital was finished and opened for service. The interesting part of the reconstruction was the provision

of two recovery room suites . . . (which) were obviously planned to isolate the patient emerging from the depths of anesthesia from the other patients in the public wards."

There are also available a number of word-of-mouth descriptions pertaining to recovery rooms, recovery wards, or recovery areas in this era (1910–1940), which usually begin, "When I was a student at the University, I remember there was a recovery area . . .", or "When I first came to Elsewhere Hospital, they were just building a recovery section in the new renovation . . .", but details as to specific purposes and the uses are seldom offered in these ruminative remembrances. The integrity of the commentators and the continuing lucidity of their minds leave no doubt, however, that a number of large medical complexes did have recovery "somethings" at this time, and unquestionably some were employed for the recovery of postoperative patients.

It was World War II, though, that really put recovery rooms—as it did anesthesiology itself—firmly into place on the medical scene. . . . The "Shock Tent" in the combat zone provided maximally efficient pooling of personnel, equipment, and organization in one centralized area, and was the obvious solution when qualified personnel and essential equipment were at a premium. In these battlefield "shock tents," not only could the equipment, the drugs, and the personnel be gathered to treat massive numbers of patients in shock, but triage could be performed even as the shock was being treated. The success of this approach was so evident that the concept spread rapidly back from the front lines to military base hospitals, and then almost as rapidly to military hospitals back in the States. From there it was only a matter of time before the "Shock Ward" would attract the interest of civilian hospitals; and, indeed, in 1941, Dr. John Lundy, while visiting a large army hospital, saw such a ward in which all patients who had undergone operation received postoperative care. "The purpose of the ward was to concentrate in one place all patients who, after the operation, required measures such as catheterization, change of dressing, removal of drains, administration of parenteral therapy, and special nursing care."

Lundy seized upon the concept, but as an anesthesiologist he adapted it to the specific needs for care in the transition from the anesthetized state to a conscious state in the postoperative surgical patient, and for this reason he called it a Post-Anesthesia Room. The initial founding of such a "P.A.R." was described in an article entitled, "'P.A.R.' Spells Better Care for Postanesthesia Patients," which was published in the November, 1944 issue of *Modern Hospital* (Lundy, J.S. and Gage, R. P.: *Modern Hospital, 63:* 1944) and is reprinted below.

"P.A.R." SPELLS BETTER CARE FOR POSTANESTHESIA PATIENTS

John S. Lundy
AND
Robert P. Gage

Section on Anesthesiology and Section on Biometry and Medical Statistics, Mayo Clinic, Rochester, Minnesota

Modern Hospital, 63: 1944

"The possibility of having a special room, or ward, for patients who have been anesthetized and who for a brief period need special attention has been largely side-stepped. However, with manpower becoming progressively reduced as the result of the war, it becomes increasingly clear that some provision must be made for care, immediately after anesthesia, of patients who have undergone operation under a general anesthetic.

"On March 17, 1942, a room was established at St. Mary's Hospital that was designated as the "postanesthetic observation room." —The name of this room gradually became abbreviated until it was called the "P.A.R.".

*   *   *   *

"If the patient is completely unconscious, he is sent to the P.A.R. and there he will stay for anywhere from one to three hours. Often his stay in this room is comparable to the length of his anesthesia.

*   *   *   *

"It was found that in the P.A.R. a minimum of one bed per operating room was undesirable and that a few more beds could be used advantageously. —A staff of three, consisting of two nurses and one orderly, was able to take care of some 4,000 patients in the course of the year.

*   *   *   *

"The P.A.R. is equipped with suction apparatus, oxygen, carbon dioxide, stimulants, intravenous sets, fluids, blood plasma, lighted laryngoscopes, intratracheal tubes and any other necessary special equipment."

*   *   *   *

Published August, 1957

There are only three anesthetic requirements for good direct laryngoscopy and endotracheal intubation. The first of these is cooperation on the part of the patient; in a surprising number of conscious patients such cooperation will be willingly supplied and will permit intubation under topical anesthesia, but cooperation is most easily obtained by the simple expedient of anesthetizing the patient. The second requirement is sufficient relaxation of the jaw to permit exposure of the glottis and larynx: again, in the exceptionally cooperative patient, this can be achieved in the conscious state, but is most reasonably produced by anesthesia, either by the production of deep levels of general anesthesia or by the use of muscle relaxant drugs. The final requirement is said to be control over reflex activity from the pharynx and larynx, either by the application of topical anesthesia in the conscious patient or the lightly-anesthetized patient, or by resort to deep general anesthesia.

These requirements are generally fulfilled in a satisfactory, or nearly satisfactory, fashion. Yet endotracheal intubation remains, on occasion, difficult, time-consuming and even traumatic. A lack of an appreciation of the dynamic anatomic relationships involved is the usual problem. Chevalier Jackson, the foremost contributor to the field, described the classical position for the exposure of the larynx in 1913: "the patient's head must be in full extension, with the vertex firmly pushed down toward the feet of the patient, so as to throw the neck upward and bring the occiput down as close as possible beneath the cervical vertebrae." Thirty years later, Jackson revised his earlier views and described what is now referred to as the "amended" position, in which the head is raised at least 10 cm. above the level of the table and is then slightly extended at the atlanto-occipital joint. The absolute necessity of the correct anatomical alignments provided by the "amended" position for the

performance of endotracheal intubation were emphasized neatly and dramatically in the invaluable paper by Bannister and MacBeth entitled, "Direct Laryngoscopy and Tracheal Intubation", which appeared in the November 18, 1944 issue of the Lancet.

DIRECT LARYNGOSCOPY AND TRACHEAL INTUBATION

BANNISTER, F. B.
AND
MACBETH, R. G.

Lancet, 2: 651–654
(Nov. 18) 1944

The anatomical principles which render laryngoscopy and intubation easy are explained by means of diagrams and x-ray photographs. These illustrate the correct and incorrect methods of exposure.

1945

Published June, 1971

Dr. William T. Lemmon, in reviewing the results of some 2000 spinal anesthesias in 1939, noted that his 2 most common difficulties were "its failure to take" or failure to produce anesthesia, and "its wearing off too soon" or the return of pain and muscular contraction before the operation had been completed, necessitating supplementation with ether, nitrous oxide, cyclopropane, hexobarbital, or local anesthesia. He rationalized that, if the spinal needle were left *in situ* in the subarachnoid space, he could continue to administer doses of local anesthetic drug until he achieved a "take," or he could administer further

doses of the drug as his initial dose began to "wear off."

He presented these ideas, and a technique based on them which he developed, in a paper entitled, "A Method for Continuous Spinal Anesthesia," which he read before the Philadelphia Academy of Surgery on December 4, 1939, and which he subsequently published in the January 1940, issue of Annals of Surgery. Lemmon's results attracted immediate attention, since they provided a method for adapting spinal anesthesia to lengthy abdominal surgery. The duration of spinal block could theoretically be extended indefinitely, and the advantages of spinal anesthesia could be obtained wherever they were desired without being restricted to the duration of action of a single injected dose of local anesthetic drug. Surgeons who had experienced the difficulties of attempting to close upper abdominal incisions when it was impossible to get patients relaxed under general anesthesia, when, in fact, the closure was more difficult than the operation itself, almost drooled at the thought of closures performed under perfect muscular relaxation and with collapsed intestines. Lemmon had a most receptive audience that December night in Philadelphia when he made his pitch to the Academy of Surgery.

His technique was thoroughly ingenious and was based on 2 special pieces of equipment, a malleable German silver needle (18 gauge) and a specially designed mattress. The mattress was 5 inches thick, 18 inches broad, and 6 feet long, with a gap 7 inches long which was beneath the lumbar spine when the patient was supine and was continuous with another gap which came to the side of the mattress. The spinal puncture was made with the patient lying on the side and after the use of an introducer to establish a puncture hole in the skin and a track on into the subarachnoid space, so that the malleable spinal needle would not bend before it could be forced through the skin or the ligaments farther along in its course. As soon as the spinal puncture had been completed and cerebrospinal fluid was seen to be escaping from the end of the malleable spinal needle, the air in about 3 feet of rubber tubing was displaced by injecting the local anesthetic solution through it; the distal end of the tubing was attached to the end of the spinal needle; and the proximal end was attached to a syringe loaded with the local anesthetic solution.

An initial dose of local anesthetic solution was then introduced into the subarachnoid space from this syringe, and the patient turned on his back with the needle still left in the spine, the needle being so placed that it was in the center of the gap in the mattress. It was not allowed to touch the table

or the mattress at any time; and in this regard Lemmon emphasized the importance of the use of the malleable silver spinal needles, since in 2 instances ordinary non-malleable needles were broken off in the spine when patients suddenly bent or moved out of position. These broken needles constituted a serious accident, and their retrieval could be extremely difficult.

The results of this technique, when everything went right, were impressive. If analgesia was not present within 10 minutes of the initial injection, an additional dose could be given, or even a third dose, if that was required to produce a "take." The level of analgesia could be controlled by the position of the patient, the dilution of the local anesthetic drug, the total dose used, the total volume injected, and the force of injection. Lemmon made the point that some patients require more intrathecal local anesthetic drug than others and that the drug should be given as needed. He compared the situation to the fact that there is no set dose of ether for a given patient, but rather that ether is given under control as needed, and the dose varies greatly, not only from patient to patient, but in the same patient at different times. The same is true in operations under spinal anesthesia.

However, despite the obvious advantages of the continuous, or fractional, technique, it also had its disadvantages, the most important being that it was cumbersome. The movement of the patient from his side to his back was crucial: an inch or two mistake in placing the lumbar spine, with several inches of the malleable silver needle sticking out of the patient's back, precisely over that essential gap in the mattress was a critical maneuver. It was not surprising, therefore, that modifications would be devised to obviate the difficulties of the malleable needle and the split mattress. Dr. Edward S. Tuohy's was the most important, and one of the papers introducing his innovation was entitled, "Continuous Spinal Anesthesia: A New Method Utilizing A Ureteral Catheter." This was published in the August 1945 issue of the *Surgical Clinics of North America (25: 834–840, 1945)* and is reprinted below with the kind permission of the publishers.

CONTINUOUS SPINAL ANESTHESIA; A NEW METHOD UTILIZING A URETERAL CATHETER

Tuohy, E. B.

Surg. Clin. North America, 25:834–840, 1945

The author describes in great detail the technique for catheter spinal anesthesia much as it is practiced today. He does not report its success in any specific group of patients, but states that complications are no greater than with conventional spinal anesthesia.

1946

Published December, 1966

In his book, "On Chloroform and Other Anaesthetics; Their Action and Administration," published posthumously in 1858, John Snow wrote:

"The direction which it is usually requisite to give beforehand, to the patient who is to inhale chloroform, is to avoid taking a meal previous to the inhalation; for chloroform is very apt to cause vomiting, if inhaled whilst there is a quantity of food in the stomach. . . . The best time of all for an operation under chloroform is before breakfast. . . . Moving the patient as the effects of the chloroform are subsiding is very apt to excite vomiting when it might not otherwise occur; it is therefore desirable, when convenient, to allow the patient to lie for half an hour or so, without moving his head from the pillow. By this means, even when a feeling of nausea is present, it often subsides without the occurrence of vomiting. It is advisable also not to give the patient anything to eat or drink till about an hour after the inhalation, and, as a general rule, not even then, unless there is some inclination for it; for if anything is taken into the stomach before the effects of the chloroform have entirely subsided, it is apt to excite vomiting. . . . The most usual time for the vomiting to commence is when the inhalation has been discontinued, and the effects of the chloroform are passing off. In many cases, it occurs before the patient has become quite conscious, and he does not know it has occurred unless he is told. In a few cases, especially where there is a good deal of food in the stomach, the vomiting comes on before the operation is finished, or even before it is commenced."

Snow did not attribute any great danger to the occurrence of vomiting during anesthesia, except to note that it could interfere with the inhalation and that the patient might wake up before the inhalation could be recommenced. Four years later, however, in the Edinburgh Medical Journal, Dr. G. W. Balfour published an article entitled, "New Cause of Death Under Chloroform."

"The case occurred during the Burmese war in 1853; and was related in a letter from John Balfour, Esq., D.I.G., then field-surgeon to the army in Burmah. A soldier received a gunshot wound through the upper part of the thigh, and secondary haemorrhage repeatedly recurred. It was supposed that the profunda or one of its branches was injured, and it was determined to tie the femoral artery above and below the origin of the profunda;—this was done while the man was under chloroform. In the course of the operation the man, who had had his dinner previously, became sick and vomited. He subsequently sank and shortly died from exhaustion, as was supposed. On examination of the body, the profunda was found cut across by the ball, and a false aneurism formed at the seat of injury, and *the trachea was found filled with vomited matters*. Dr. Balfour remarked that, though an extreme case, this was but a sample of one very common source of danger in the use of chloroform, arising from its anaesthetic properties interfering with the natural actions of the nervous system. . . . Remarks were made by various members as to the inconvenience and occasional danger of administering chloroform to patients who had been taking food shortly before; and cases in point were adduced. . . . Dr. Thomas G. Balfour stated, in reply to Dr. Sidey's last remark, that he had once been called to see a healthy, plump little child, who had gone to bed quite well and had been found dead in the morning. The child had taken a hearty meal of porridge in the evening, and had shown no symptoms that could afford any clue to the cause of its sudden death. On opening the trachea, however, a quantity of its food was found lodged there, the starchy nature of which was proved by the usual iodine test."

Today, regurgitation and vomiting, followed by aspiration, is recognized as one of the leading causes of mortality associated with the administration of anesthesia. In a study of one thousand mortalities reported by the Association of Anaesthetists of Great Britain and Ireland, no less than 110 (11 per cent) were due to regurgitation or vomiting. Furthermore, and of great significance, in 92 of these 110 patients, the nature of the vomited or regurgitated material was fluid. The importance of this fact had been recognized previously and very clearly by Mendelson, who distinguished between the obstructive symptoms resulting from the aspiration of solids and the commoner asthmatic-like reaction of those who inhaled liquids from the stomach. Indeed, the syndrome of pulmonary edema, bronchospasm, cyanosis, tachycardia and hypotension which follows the aspiration of liquid gastric contents is now associated with Mendelson's name. His experimental approach to this anesthetic problem was published under the title of "Aspiration of Stomach Contents Into The Lungs During Obstetric Anesthesia" (Mendelson, C. L.: *Am. J. Obst. & Gynec., 52:* 191–205, 1946) and is reprinted below with the kind permission of the author and the publisher.

THE ASPIRATION OF STOMACH CONTENTS INTO THE LUNGS DURING OBSTETRIC ANESTHESIA

Curtis L. Mendelson, M.D.

(From the Department of Obstetrics and Gynecology, Cornell University Medical College and New York Hospital)

American Journal of Obstetrics & Gynecology 52: 191, 1946

"In most texts on pulmonary complications, aspiration of stomach contents into the lungs during general anesthesia is considered under the heading of postanesthetic pneumonia. Aspiration of infected material is said to produce atelectasis, pneumonia, and lung abscess.

*   *   *   *

"There have been sixty-six instances of aspiration of stomach contents into the lungs in 44,016 pregnancies at the Lying-In Hospital from 1932 to 1945. The incidence of this complication is 0.15 per cent.

An analysis of the cases is presented and followed by experimental work to clarify the pathology of aspiration, and thereby gain insight into its diagnosis, prevention, and treatment.

*   *   *   *

"Aspiration was recorded as having definitely occurred in the delivery room in 68 per cent. In 32 per cent this complication went unrecognized until later. The character of the aspirated material in the 45 recorded cases was liquid in 40 and solid in five.

*   *   *   *

CONCLUSIONS

"1. Gastric retention of solid and liquid material is prolonged during labor.

2. Aspiration of vomitus into the lungs may occur while the laryngeal reflexes are abolished during general anesthesia.

3. Bronchial configuration favors right-sided aspiration. Massive aspiration, however, readily involves both lungs.

4. Liquid material is more frequently aspirated than solid.

5. Aspiration of solid material usually produces the classical picture of laryngeal or bronchial obstruction.

6. Aspiration of liquid produces an apparently hitherto unrecognized asthmatic-like syndrome with distinct clinical, roentgenologic, and pathologic features. This syndrome is due to the irritative action of gastric hydrochloric acid, which produces bronchiolar spasm and a peribronchiolar exudative and congestive reaction.

7. Aspiration of stomach contents into the lungs is preventable. The dangers of this complication as an obstetric hazard may be avoided by: (a) withholding oral feeding during the labor and substituting parenteral administration where necessary; (b) wider use of local anesthesia where indicated and feasible; (c) alkalinization of, and emptying the stomach contents prior to the administration of a general anesthetic; (d) competent administration of general anesthesia with full appreciation of the dangers of aspiration during induction and recovery; (e) adequate delivery-room equipment, including transparent anesthetic masks, tiltable delivery table, suction, laryngoscope, and bronchoscope; and (f) differential diagnosis between the two syndromes described, and prompt institution of suitable therapy."

Published October, 1974

A colleague made the remark to me in 1952, "I've tried your succinylcholine. I don't like it as well as curare. You have to breathe for them."

It seems like an incredible remark today; but it was really quite a natural remark to make in 1952, because it reflected the attitude in this country concerning the respiratory effects of curare. Anesthesiologists, by and large, believed that curare could produce adequate abdominal relaxation without impinging upon ventilatory exchange to any marked degree. There were several reasons for this misconception.

The first, probably, was contained in Griffith's classic article, "The Use of Curare in General Anesthesia," which reported the first use of a muscle relaxant during anesthesia (*Anesthesiology, 3:* 418, 1942). Griffith and Johnson wrote, "In none of our patients has there been any serious depressing effect on respiration, pulse or blood pressure, and there was no demonstrable postoperative effect of any kind." In truth, with the relatively crude methods of measurement available at the

time, there probably were not. They used 3 to 7 ml. of the Squibb preparation, Intocostrin, and they used it to "top off" the relaxation produced by a fully potent anesthetic agent such as cyclopropane. It was scarcely a paralyzing dose: the curare was used mainly to produce more muscle relaxation than would otherwise have been present at the depth of the relatively low concentration of inhalation anesthetic which was being employed.

In time, it occurred to those who had not forgotten all of their anatomy that the motor branches of the intercostal nerves supply not only the intercostal muscles (the respiratory muscles), but also the muscles of the abdomen; and that relaxation of the abdominal muscles should therefore also be accompanied by relaxation of the intercostal muscles, with a commensurate decrease in respiratory effort.

Absolutely logical—but there was also an explanation for this. A very precise sequence of the relaxing effects of curare had been documented. First, the small, rapidly moving muscles such as those of the fingers, toes, eyes, and ears were involved; then the muscles of the limbs, neck, and trunk; next the intercostal muscles, and only ultimately and finally the diaphragm was paralyzed. The diaphragm was considered the key; and each new muscle relaxant that was introduced was loudly acclaimed as a diaphragm-sparing drug.

Aiding and abetting the confusion was the fact that, in the many instances in which ventilation was not assisted, most patients could indeed produce sufficient respiratory exchange to maintain life, despite the use of the relaxant.

The day of reckoning could not be postponed indefinitely, however. Certain patients involved were anesthetized with agents that sensitized the myocardium to catecholamines, which the inevitable hypercarbia produced in abundance; and certain other patients suffered from cardiopulmonary disease which accentuated the unpleasant effects of the relaxant's ventilatory depression and subsequent carbon dioxide accumulation and hypoxia. These combinations could be lethal.

In time, the morbidity and mortality became of vital concern. Ten of the major University Departments—The Massachusetts General Hospital (Harvard University); The Presbyterian Hospital of New York (Columbia University College of Physicians and Surgeons); The Hospital of the University of Pennsylvania (University of Pennsylvania); The George Washington University Hospital and the Gallinger Municipal Hospital (George Washington University); The Duke University Hospital (Duke University); The Vanderbilt University Hospital (Vanderbilt University); The Charity Hospital of Louisiana (Tulane University); The University of Minnesota Hospitals (University of Minnesota); The Salt Lake County Hospital (University of Utah); and the Stanford University Hospitals (Stanford University—undertook a comprehensive, retrospective study of the deaths associated with anesthesia and surgery in a 5 year period that extended from January 1, 1948 to December 31, 1952.

It was a remarkably important investigation. It infuriated a great many anesthesiologists, but it also taught a number of significant lessons. The foreword to the report of the investigation explained the scope: "Anesthesia is an adjunct to the care of the patient; hardly ever is it an end in itself, except where it is the principal physician tool used in the study and treatment of paresthesias or circulatory disorders. In such limited cases, anesthesia is perhaps an end in itself. This study, however, is concerned with anesthesia as a part of the total surgical care of the patient. Anesthesia in this role is not of itself the therapeutic act which makes possible the correction of deformity, the restoration of health, or the staying of death. It merely makes possible the acts which can accomplish these things. We set down these truisms here, for it is our belief that one of the principal accomplishments of this survey is to show, within the precise framework to be described, the extent of the responsibility which must be borne by anesthesia for failure in the total care of the surgical patient."

The results of the study were startling, to say the least. They showed that, in the 10 institutions in which the study was conducted, the use of curare increased the mortality rate 6-fold in comparison with those patients who did not receive a muscle relaxant drug. The conclusion drawn— that curare was inherently cardiotoxic— was patently in error; almost certainly the technique of using curare to provide some relaxation, while at the same time ignoring its respiratory effects, was the major factor.

This conclusion was borne out by the experience with curare across the Atlantic. The method of use of muscle relaxants in Europe was rather different from that practiced in most North American centers at that time. The group in Liverpool pioneered the so-called "pure" technique, employing large and paralyzing doses of curare with nitrous oxide-oxygen anesthesia and controlled respirations, usually to the extent of hyperventilation. Not only did the European method not show the same increase in mortality noted in this country, but in fact the mortality was lower in those receiving relaxants. The European technique which led to these more favorable results was reported by Gray and Halton in an article entitled, "A Milestone in Anaesthesia? (*d*-Tubocurarine Chloride)," which was published in the Proceedings of the Royal Society of Medicine in 1946 (Gray, T. C. and Halton, J.: *Proc. R. Soc. Med., 39:* 400–410, 1946) and is reprinted below with the kind permission of the authors and the publisher.

[*March* 1, 1946]
A MILESTONE IN ANAESTHESIA? (D-TUBOCURARINE CHLORIDE)

T. Cecil Gray, M. B., Ch.B., D.A.
AND
John Halton, M. B., Ch.B.

Proc. Royal Soc. Med., 39: 400–410, 1946

*   *   *   *

"Three main techniques have been employed:

"(1) The single dose method, for the induction of anaesthesia, short operations and endoscopies, oral and anal.

"Employed in this way a mixture of 15 mg. of tubocurarine with 0.5 gramme of pentothal is injected fairly rapidly. After two or three minutes respiration becomes very shallow or ceases altogether, the jaw is completely relaxed and there is no spasm or cough when an airway is inserted or an endotracheal tube is passed. Furthermore, the patient is able to tolerate straight away, without distress, an anaesthetic vapour strong enough to maintain the anaesthesia should this be desired. Induction time is thus tremendously shortened.

"With this dose bronchoscopy is easily performed, and because of the relaxation of the pharyngeal and anal sphincters, oesophagoscopy or sigmoidoscopy can be carried out with ease.

"Patients recover quickly after this form of administration.

"(2) For longer procedures in conjunction with the intermittent injection of an intravenous barbiturate. A remote control tap has been devised which facilitates this technique. Its use overcomes two difficul-

ties of administration, namely, the arm can be placed in any position during the operation without fear of the intravenous needle becoming displaced, and precipitation of the barbiturate by the curare is prevented.

*   *   *   *

"After an induction as described above, small increments of barbiturate and curare are made. 0.1 gramme of pentothal and 2 to 4 mg. of curare are given from time to time as the reaction of the patient to stimuli and the demands of the surgeon dictate. If the length of the operation is such that a dose of more than 1.5 grammes of pentothal or 3 to 4 grammes of kemithal has to be exceeded, which occurs very rarely, we prefer to continue the anaesthesia with minimal amounts of cyclopropane or ether.

"(3) As an adjuvant to inhalational anaesthesia. The intermittent fractional injection of a total dose of 15 to 30 mg. of curare is utilized to produce relaxation while still keeping the patient in a light plane of anaesthesia.

"Whichever of these three methods is used, oxygen may be supplied in abundance, and preferably by means of a closed circuit, for by this means adequate and complete ventilation of the lungs can be ensured."

*   *   *   *

"There are two signs of curarinization which must be mentioned. The first is the typical respiration characterized by a pushing-out of the lower part of the chest and of the abdomen with each diaphragmatic contraction, and accompanied by a jaw and tracheal tug. This is not the same as the gasping respiration seen in deep ether anaesthesia, when a partially paralysed respiratory centre is endeavouring to cope with the situation. It is at this point that all effort should be concentrated on ensuring full ventilation of the lungs. Should this not be maintained, the condition will deteriorate, and the surgeon will be embarrassed by the exaggerated diaphragmatic excursion. In this event control of the respiration with the rebreathing bag is easily attained.

"The second sign, and a most valuable one, is the ease with which the lungs may be inflated by pressure on the rebreathing bag (Morton, 1945). The absolute intercostal and abdominal relaxation, with the complete absence of laryngeal spasm, makes this manoeuvre easy and satisfying.

*　　*　　*　　*

Published April, 1969

From the very first moment of surgery—at the time that the first Mesopotamian trephined the skull of a fellow man—bleeding has been a surgical problem, and attempts to control it have been a primary concern of the surgeon. In the main, these techniques have recognized what few surgeons themselves ever discuss: *i.e.*, that the cause of bleeding during surgery is that blood vessels have been cut, since the normal blood vessel does not allow blood to escape its confines during operation unless it is severed by a scalpel or scissors. Everything imaginable—from the weather down through to the circulating nurse's misdirection of the light—has, at one time or another, been the surgical explanation for either ooze or frank hemorrhage; but over the years, the anesthesiologist and his drugs have probably been the major targets of surgical implorations and entreaties concerning bleeding. Indeed, beginning a bit after 1930, probably the most common surgical response to undue bleeding was a scathing, "You're using cyclopropane, aren't you?" And then in the 1940's, when the surgeon finally divorced himself from the barber's pole, began reading the physiologic literature, and recognized the effect of carbon dioxide accumulation upon bleeding, the remark became a thunderous, "You're not ventilating him!"

The attempts to actually *stop* the bleeding, however, have all tacitly acknowledged that the cut vessel was the problem and have been specifically directed toward sealing off the opened moat. Direct pressure over the bleeding area or vessel is both the most naturally obvious and oldest method for the achievement of hemostasis, and the

CONCLUSION

"The road lies open before us, and with a grave and insistent warning to the inexperienced that we are dealing with one of the most potent poisons known, we venture to say that we have passed yet another milestone, and the distance to our goal is considerably shortened."

use of tourniquets and Esmarch bandages for operations upon the extremities has been a well known maneuver for a long time. The application of vasoconstrictor substances to the tissues of the operative site has also been employed to provide hemostasis, but the usefulness of this technique has been restricted somewhat, both because of the danger of toxic absorption and the problem of reactive vasodilation and therefore reactionary hemorrhage. More direct procedures have included the application of hemostats or clamps to bleeding vessels with subsequent tying of the vessels or the insertion of mattress sutures which incorporate them. Cautery, chemical agents of an escharotic nature, and, more recently, hemostatic sponges or packs, have proven useful in controlling vascular ooze in limited areas of the operative site. The application of both heat and cold have been used for the achievement of hemostasis in the past, and more recently hypothermia has been employed as a generalized rather than a local measure—and for a quite different rationale.

A different approach to the control of bleeding during surgery has been inherent in the techniques which have been variously called "controlled hypotension," "induced hypotension", and "intentional hypotension". The concept in these techniques has not been to seal off the moat, but to lower the amount of flow within the moat to the point at which it would no longer seek exit. It should be emphasized, however, that this method does not imply that the flow of blood through small vessels can be considered as though the latter were simply rigid tubes, with a linear relationship between flow and pressure, and a cessation of flow when the pressure is zero; rather, the relationship must be considered to be non-linear, with flow ceasing at a critical closing pressure. Furthermore, an integral part of the techniques of "controlled hypotension" is the proper positioning of the patient upon the operating table so that the operative site is superior and "postural ischemia" is produced. The promotion of venous drainage is, of course, the most important factor in this regard: if the surgical wound is dependent in relation to all or much of the body, the venous blood, in order to leave the wound, must oppose the hydrostatic force of the weight of the column of blood, in addition to having to exert an antigravitational force. Furthermore, it is also necessary to consider the effect of posture upon arterial pressure in relation to "postural ischemia": the *local* blood pressure in the wound is reduced 30 mm. Hg for every 15 inches of vertical height of the operative site above the level of the heart, and therefore gravity opposes the hydrodynamic factor in the arteries; whereas, conversely, when the operative site is below heart level, the hydrostatic and hydrodynamic factors are additive insofar as arterial flow is concerned.

Without doubt, the most common method of inducing intentional hypotension during operation today is a careful combination of halothane anesthesia and positive pressure respiration. Halothane lowers blood pressure by a combination of pharmacologic effects which include depression of the central vasomotor mechanism, myocardial depression, ganglion blockade, direct depression of the muscles of the vessel walls, and an inhibition of the sympathoadrenal system. Positive intrapulmonary pressure reduces venous return to the heart on a fairly mechanical basis, and therefore also lowers blood pressure by lowering cardiac output. The combination is a pretty one from the clinical point of view since it is extremely controllable, but it is one which would give a physiologist the shudders.

A decade ago, the most common method of producing "controlled hypotension" was by the reduction of peripheral resistance. The peripheral resistance resides largely in the variably-contractile arterioles and is maintained by the continuous stream of vasoconstrictor impulses arising from the brain stem and carried via the sympathetic nerves to the vessel walls themselves. Interruption of this efferent sympathetic outflow results in arteriolar dilation and thus effects a reduction of peripheral resistance: the capacity of the vascular bed is increased thereby relative to the total circulating blood volume, and this disruption of the finely-adjusted balance between the two produces hypotension. A number of ganglion blocking drugs were employed—and to some extent still are—to reduce peripheral resistance and so lower blood pressure during surgery: the hexamethonium salts, pentamethonium (C5) and hexamethonium (C6); pentolinium tartrate (Ansolysen); trimethaphan camphorsulphonate (Arfonad); and phenactropinium chloride (Trophenium). Less widely used, but a most effective method of inducing intentional hypotension, was total spinal block, which also reduces peripheral resistance by the interruption of sympathetic outflow from the cord, but has the advantage over ganglion block that it also provides anesthesia for the surgical procedure itself in many instances (depending, of course, upon the site of that surgery), and does not produce parasympathetic block concurrently.

The forerunner of all of these techniques was the brainchild of a neurosurgeon who noted that, when the patient was partially exsanguinated, the bleeding stopped and the tumor could be removed. The method was described in a paper entitled, "The Control of Bleeding during Operation by Induced Hypotension" (Gardner, W. J.: *J.A.M.A., 132:* 572, 1946), and is reprinted below with the kind permission of the author and the publishers.

THE CONTROL OF BLEEDING DURING OPERATION BY INDUCED HYPOTENSION

GARDNER, W. J.

J.A.M.A., 132: 572, 1946

Gardner reports his successful removal of a meningioma from an obese hypertensive female with minimal bleeding because of his use of a technique now known as autotransfusion. He cannulated a dorsalis pedis artery and during the scalp incision allowed 1600 ml. of blood to collect in a bottle containing heparin, decreasing systolic blood pressure from 140 to 100 mm Hg. After removal of the tumor, most of the blood was returned intraarterially and additional hemostasis carried out. Operative time was decreased and no homologous transfusion was necessary. In a footnote, he reports that six additional patients had been operated upon in this manner with "similar gratifying results."

Published December, 1967

Otto Loewi's brilliant researches, which were republished in "Classical File" 2 months ago, earned him a Nobel Prize for establishing the first real proof of neurohumoral transmission. He strongly suspected that his *Vagusstoff* might be a choline ester: he compared its properties with acetylcholine and showed that there was choline in the perfusion fluid from his classic experiment—but this choline was relatively inactive and therefore was not *Vagusstoff* itself. In 1926, Loewi and Navritil compared the rate of destruction of acetylcholine with that of *Vagusstoff* and demonstrated the inhibition of the destructive mechanism by eserine. Four years later, in collaboration with Englehart, Loewi established that the action of eserine served to inhibit the enzyme that destroys acetylcholine, and that it did so even when it was greatly diluted. One link in the chain of evidence was lacking, however; for while epinephrine had been shown to be a natural product of the body, acetylcholine had never been identified as such. Dale and Dudley settled this question when they isolated acetylcholine from the spleen of an ox and thereby established it as a normally occurring substance, in all likelihood identical with *Vagusstoff*.

Meanwhile, over on the other side of the autonomic nervous sytem, there was considerable investigative activity on the mechanism of sympathetic, or rather adrenergic, nerve action. Loewi's classic experiments, in addition to revealing the liberation of *Vagusstoff* upon stimulation of the vagus nerve, had of course also demonstrated that an accelerator substance similar to epinephrine was liberated into the perfusion fluid when the action of the sympathetic fibers in the frog's vagus predominated over that of the inhibitory fibers (the cardiac nerve from the vagus in the frog is a mixed nerve). The great Walter Cannon had also established that stimulation of adrenergic nerves was accompanied by the liberation of some active principle with sympathomimetic properties. It was widely assumed that this neurohumoral agent was identical with epinephrine, but this view had to be modified when Cannon and Rosenblueth subsequently demonstrated that stimulation of sympathetic nerves elicited remote actions which did not wholly conform with those of epinephrine. In order to reconcile the seemingly conflicting evidence, Cannon and Rosenblueth put forth the hypothesis that a primary mediator substance is released from adrenergic nerve endings, and that this primary liberation then combines with some constituent(s) within the effector cells to form the final active substances which, on account of their supposed actions, were termed sympathin E (excitatory) and sympathin I (inhibitory). They assumed that the primary mediator substance was epinephrine. The problem was, however, that substances with the properties of the postulated sympathin E or sympathin I could not be isolated or prepared from tissues or organs.

The riddle was solved when Ulf Svante von Euler proposed that the sympathetic transmitter is in fact norepinephrine, but that sympathetic nerve stimulation on some occasions may, in addition, liberate small quantities of epinephrine itself. One of his first and most important papers in support of this concept demonstrated a substance very similar—if, not indeed, identical—to norepinephrine in the spleen of cattle (the same organ from which Dale and Dudley, it will be recalled, had isolated acetylcholine). Von Euler's report was entitled "The Presence of a Substance with Sympathin E Properties in Spleen Extracts" (*Acta physiologica Scandinavica, 11:* 168–186, 1946), and it is reprinted below with the kind permissions of the author and the publishers.

THE PRESENCE OF A SUBSTANCE WITH SYMPATHIN E PROPERTIES IN SPLEEN EXTRACTS

U. S. v. EULER

Received 27 November 1945

From The Physiological Department, Karolinska Institutet, Stockholm, Sweden

Acta Physiolog. Scand., 11: 168–186, 1946

*   *   *   *

SUMMARY

"1. Extracts of fresh cattle spleen possess a pressor activity equivalent to some 10 μg adrenaline per g of tissue.

2. The purified substance increases the heart rate and raises the blood pressure of the cat in chloralose anaesthesia.

3. The pressor action is enhanced by cocaine.

4. Ergotamine in doses which annul or reverse the pressor action of adrenaline is less active in depressing the action of purified spleen extracts, which in this respect resembles certain catechol amino-bases, such as nor-adrenaline or 3:4-dihydroxy-nor-ephedrine (D. N. E.).

5. Adrenaline inhibits the isolated rabbit's intestine and the non-pregnant cat's uterus more powerfully than equipressor doses of spleen extracts of D. N. E.

6. Purified spleen extracts, like D. N. E., are less active in stimulating the rabbit's uterus than equipressor doses of adrenaline.

7. Purified spleen extracts and D. N. E. have a weaker pupil dilating action than equipressor doses of adrenaline.

8. Purified spleen extracts stimulate the isolated heart in much the same way as equipressor doses of adrenaline and D. N. E.

9. Purified spleen extracts and D. N. E. do not give the fluorescence reaction characteristic of adrenaline in equipressor concentrations.

10. Purified spleen extracts and D. N. E. give the $FeCl_3$ colour reaction to about the same strength as equipressor concentrations of adrenaline.

11. The biological tests, colour and fluorescence reactions of purified spleen extracts thus bear a good resemblance to those of nor-adrenaline or D. N. E. and differ from those of adrenaline.

12. The similarity between the action of the purified spleen extracts and the postulated sympathin E on the one hand and nor-adrenaline or D. N. E. on the other is pointed out."

1947

Published June, 1958

The earliest professional anesthetists were all aware of the importance of cyanosis as a warning of dire maladministration, and Snow advised discontinuing administration of the anesthetic by removing the facepiece for half a minute if cyanosis appeared at any stage. Nevertheless, for a very great number of years following the introduction of clinical anesthesia, cyanosis during etherization was, if not disregarded, at least accepted as inevitable. C. S. Tomes, an English dentist of some standing, wrote the following account of the anesthetic procedure prevalent in the United States in 1873:

"It was at the Massachusetts General Hospital, Boston, that ether was first administered . . . and I cannot do better than describe the course of the procedure at this institution which . . . unquestionably takes the first place among the hospitals of this country.

"The patients are etherized in small anterooms adjoining the operating theatre, the ether being administered by one of the junior house officers, who is, in nine cases out of ten, not yet qualified. Two or three ounces of pure anhydrous ether are poured upon a conical sponge which has been previously moistened with water; this is at once placed over the patient's mouth and nose. If he struggles, which he generally does, as he experiences the suffocating sensation produced by the pungent vapour, he is held down by main force till he succumbs to its influence. Ether is lavishly poured upon the sponge, so that it often runs down the patient's face and neck, and half a pound is not rarely used for a single administration.

"Not uncommonly there is a good deal of spasm of the expiratory muscles, stridulous breathing, and laryngeal spasm, and I have several times seen a degree of asphyxial lividity transcending that which I have ever observed during the administration of nitrous oxide. Though these asphyxial symptoms are strongly pronounced, not the slightest anxiety is felt; the sponge is merely removed for half-a-minute, or a minute, the blood at once recovers its colour, and the administration is proceeded with . . . I do not remember to have ever seen the administrator feel the patient's pulse."

But it was the widespread popularity and utilization of nitrous oxide anesthesia which gave the development of cyanosis during operation its full acceptance, and the technique of secondary saturation was, of course, the epitome of such acceptance:

"A secondary saturation requires an intimate knowledge of the signs of anesthesia, a disregard of cyanosis, and an apparatus capable of delivering oxygen under pressure for resuscitation if necessary."

Indeed, Clement, one of the world's outstanding authorities on nitrous oxide anesthesia, has written:

"Cyanosis is too often confused with the really dangerous condition of extreme hypoxia. Cyanosis results when the amount of oxygen in the blood is insufficient to saturate the greater part of the hemoglobin present. Hypoxia, on the other hand, indicates a reduction of the free and essential oxygen in the tissues. Cyanosis and hypoxia may be present at the same time or either condition may be present alone. A patient may be cyanotic during nitrous oxide-oxygen anesthesia without the respiratory and circulatory reactions which indicate depression from hypoxia."

Despite these firm convictions of the proponents of nitrous oxide anesthesia on the innocuousness of cyanosis, there developed a progressive inclination amongst most anesthetists to correlate cyanosis with hypoxia. The difficulties of recognizing cyanosis in dark-skinned or anemic patients were well understood, but the fact that its absence in anemic, white patients was no indication of safety was slow to be realized. The July, 1947, issue of *The American Journal of Medical Sciences* contained the article by Comroe and Botelho on "The Unreliability of Cyanosis in the Recognition of Arterial Anoxemia" which showed beyond doubt that the clinician's failure to observe cyanosis was no guarantee of normal oxygenation.

THE UNRELIABILITY OF CYANOSIS IN THE RECOGNITION OF ARTERIAL ANOXEMIA

COMROE, J. H., JR. AND BOTELHO, S.

Am. J. Med. Sci., 214: 1–6, July, 1947

"SUMMARY AND CONCLUSIONS

1. The ability of observers to detect cyanosis was evaluated by comparing their color estimations with known arterial oxygen saturations (oximeter).

2. The majority of 127 observers were unable to detect the presence of definite cyanosis until the arterial oxygen saturation fell to approximately 80%; 25% of observers did not note definite cyanosis even at arterial saturation levels of 71 to 75%.

3. There were marked variations in the ability of an observer to note cyanosis in different subjects or even in the same subject at different times. There were wide variations in color estimations when 5 to 10 observers watched cyanosis develop in the same subject at the same time.

4. The detection of cyanosis is dependent not only upon variable factors in the patient but also upon the ability of individual observers to note color changes.

5. Visual impressions of cyanosis are unreliable. Serious grades of arterial anoxemia may be unrecognized by many physicians unless arterial blood is obtained and analyzed for oxygen content and capacity."

Published December, 1959

The introduction of new therapeutic measures in medicine leads inevitably to human experimentation; for however carefully a drug is screened, or an operation perfected, or a regimen tested in the laboratory animal, the day must come when a clinical trial is conducted. No matter what may be said of human experimentation—and much has been said, both loud and often—it is an inexorable step of investigation in medicine. The patent ductus arteriosus was closed again and again in animals; the heart-lung machine was designed and redesigned for years; the Salk vaccine was screened over and over; but in each instance there had to be a first clinical trial.

Excluding the public's present emotional and litigious reaction to human experimentation, it must be emphasized that since the time of Hippocrates ("I swear . . . so far as power and discernment shall be mine, I will carry out regimen for the benefit of the sick and will keep them from harm and wrong. To none will I give a deadly drug even if solicited. . . . ") physicians have been concerned with the moral and ethical rectitude of their "clinical trials". Volunteers (both paid, such as medical students and interns, or unpaid, such as conscientious objectors in times of war or civilian prisoners in times of peace) are a significant source of material for such trials. Frequently employed, too, has been the application of the new drug, technique, or regimen to the "hopeless" case, with the blessing of both patient and the patient's family, when the new therapy offers some possibility for improvement, amelioration, or cure. But when the really unlikely idea strikes, albeit flinted on a concept of reason and logic, it is to himself that the physician turns for the clinical trial.

The physician's use of his own body as the subject for his experiments goes back through the ages, and perhaps in no field has self-experimentation been so assiduous and so rewarding as in anesthesia. Indeed, among the very earliest investigations into what was to become inhalation anesthesia were the experiments carried out by Humphry Davy upon himself in 1799 at Beddoe's Pneumatic Institution. Davy had succeeded in producing nitrous oxide in a pure state and in his classic, *Researches, Chemical and Philosphical, Chiefly Concerning Nitrous Oxide,* are described the results of numerous studies when he inhaled the gas: "It passed through the bronchia without stimulating the glottis and produced no uneasy feeling in the lungs . . . I found that I could breathe nine quarts of nitrous oxide for three minutes (from and into a silk bag, the lung being previously exhausted and the nostrils closed) and twelve quarts for rather more than four. I could never breathe it in any quantity so long as five minutes. . . . Whenever its operation was carried to the highest extent, the pleasurable thrilling at its height about the middle of the experiment, gradually diminished, the sense of pressure on the muscles was lost, impressions ceased to be perceived: vivid ideas passed rapidly through the mind, and voluntary power was altogether destroyed, so that the mouthpiece generally dropt from my unclosed lips". Davy's self-experimentation clearly led him to the concept of anesthesia: "As nitrous oxide in its extensive operation appears capable of destroying physical pain, it may probably be used with advantage during surgical operations. . . .".

Almost half a century was to elapse before the prophecy was fulfilled, and when it was, self-experimentation again provided the fulfillment. The Hartford dentist, Horace Wells, was present in Union Hall in Hartford on the evening of Tuesday, December 10, 1844, to witness the public entertainment by Gardner Quincy Colton, "A Grand Exhibition of the Effects Produced by Inhaling Nitrous Oxid, Exhilarating or Laughing Gas!" One of the young volunteers who inhaled the gas barked his shins to the extent that the bruises were bleeding as he left the stage, and yet injuries that should have had him literally hopping with anguish left the young man totally unperturbed. Wells questioned the man closely on this point, for he instantly perceived the possibility of employing nitrous oxide to lessen the terror that the dental chair held for his own patients. At the end of the evening's entertainment, Wells prevailed upon Colton to agree to a trial of laughing gas the very next morning, as Colton's traveling show was due to move to other cities. Seeking a suitable subject

for the "trial", Wells settled upon a troublesome wisdom tooth of his own, for not only was time short, but there were also disquieting rumors that persons had succumbed to an excess of nitrous oxide— such as would be necessary "to make a patient insensible to the wrenching of a tooth from live bone". So it was that the next morning Wells seated himself in his own dental chair, took into his mouth the rubber tube that Colton handed him, breathed deeply until quiescent, and moved not a muscle while his assistant gripped the root of the tooth, rocking it to break it loose, and pulled. "He held the bloody molar in the air while Wells did not even stir in his seat". When Wells tranquilly regained consciousness and saw the tooth still gripped in the forceps, he exclaimed, "It is the greatest discovery ever made; I did not feel it so much as the prick of a pin."

From those early times of Davy and Wells to the present day there have been innumerable instances of self-experimentation by those interested in anesthesia. Perhaps none, however, surpassed in courage and imagination the investigations into the cerebral effects of curare conducted by Scott Smith upon himself. These astonishing studies were published in the January, 1947, issue of *Anesthesiology* under the title, "The Lack of Cerebral Effects of *d*-Tubocurarine".

THE LACK OF CEREBRAL EFFECTS OF *d*-TUBOCURARINE

SCOTT M. SMITH, M.D.,
HUGH O. BROWN, M.D.,
JAMES E. P. TOMAN, PH.D.
AND LOUIS S. GOODMAN, M.D.

Salt Lake City, Utah

Anesthesiology, 8:1–10 Jan., 1947

*   *   *   *

"The subject was a healthy male adult, 34 years of age, weighing 80 Kg. To facilitate administration of *d*-tubocurarine and subsequently neostigmine, an intravenous infusion of sterile 0.9 per cent sodium chloride solution was instituted, and the appropriate agents injected via the rubber tubing. Continuous recordings of the electro-encephalogram (standard leads) and the electrocardiogram (lead 2) were obtained throughout the control period, experimental procedures, and postexperimental period. Pulse rate, blood pressure, respiratory rate and character, neurologic signs, psychologic indexes, and sensorium were followed and recorded almost continuously. When verbal contact with the subject was lost, communication was continued as long as possible by means of prearranged signals involving voluntary contraction of such muscles as were not yet completely paralyzed. When paralysis was complete, the subject was instructed to make mental notes of all experiences, and these were dictated to a stenographer immediately upon recovery of intelligible speech. The only objective index of cerebral function which could be followed during complete skeletal muscle paralysis was the character of the electro-encephalogram and its response to pattern vision.

"Oxygen was administered early, and shortly thereafter, when the first evidence of respiratory embarrassment was noted, artificial respiration with oxygen was instituted by means of a rebreathing bag, face mask, and carbon dioxide absorbing unit. Adequate pulmonary exchange was maintained at all times. Tracheal intubation was performed for a six-minute period at the height of paralysis in order to obtain evidence on visceral pain. Nasal and oropharyngeal suction was performed as needed. Neostigmine methylsulfate was injected to facilitate emergence from curare-induced paralysis."

*   *   *   *

SUMMARY

"A dose of *d*-tubocurarine chloride two and one-half times that necessary for complete respiratory paralysis and adequate for complete skeletal muscular paralysis was given intravenously over a period of thirty-three minutes to a healthy trained adult observer not undergoing operation. Inasmuch as no changes occurred in the electro-encephalogram, consciousness and sensorium, or in any aspect of higher central nervous system function, it is concluded that *d*-tubocurarine chloride has no significant central stimulant, depressant or analgesic action. Attention is called to the importance of this observation for the proper use of curare as an adjuvant in anesthesia."

Published August, 1966

"No time was wasted on recriminations. The 39 year old man's suffering at this time was intense. His hands were cold, his skin clammy, his face pale, the lips compressed and bloodless, and pulse rapid, weak, and thready. Not a groan escaped him, not a sign of suffering except the slight corrugation of his brow, the fixed rigid face and the thin lips so tightly compressed that the impression of his teeth could be seen through them." So runs the description of one of the more famous examples of shock, that of "Stonewall" Jackson. General Jackson, after making his brilliant countermarch around Hooker's Union Army at Chancellorsville, went out ahead of his troops to reconnoiter at night and was shot by his own pickets. Falling off his horse, he staggered back with a broken arm and a severed brachial artery. He was in a state of profound shock; since he continued to bleed and it was recognized that the shock could not be dealt with unless the bleeding could be stopped, the arm was amputated (under chloroform anesthesia, incidentally). He lived 3 more days. The Confederate Army won the batle in which Jackson fell, but his death more than offset the victory over the Union forces.

Jackson's wound produced a state which is almost a classical description of shock, yet one which defies precise definition. Each generation of physicians has added its own several definitions of the term "shock" to the ample supply already available. Dr. John Remington, of the University of Georgia School of Medicine, has stated the problem of a definition of shock in the following manner: "There have been many animals killed by a great variety of techniques, and each worker carries in his mind a picture, unexpressed in words, of the pattern of signs that preceded death. There has been a constant stream of definitions of shock, none widely accepted, either because they were so vaguely termed as to be rather meaningless or because they did not frame the picture that someone else had. And so we go blithely on talking about shock, whether we are working with dogs, cats, rats, guinea pigs, goats, or humans, as though it were always the same thing but we are not really talking each other's language." And Dr. Remington is quite correct. It is true that, in its most typical form, shock is characterized by a slightly cyanotic pallor, sweating, cool skin, restlessness, weakness, a rapid, thready pulse, and hypotension. But it is quite possible for shock to be present in the face of many deviations from this accepted pattern of symptoms and signs; the pulse may be slow and full; the skin may be flushed, warm, or dry; hypotension may be present primarily, without the concomitant appearance of any other signs; or the blood pressure may be perfectly normal despite the undoubted existence of the shock syndrome. Thus, one group of workers has described 6 main disturbances of the normal circulatory pattern during shock. (1) *Cold tachycardia* in which there is a normal blood pressure, a fast pulse rate, cold extremities, and usually a pale face. It occurs during the first 2 hours after injury and is commonly associated with a moderate blood loss and a blood volume reduced to between 70 and 80 per cent of the normal. (2) *Warm tachycardia* in which there is a normal blood pressure, a fast and bounding pulse, warm extremities, and usually a well colored face. It is associated with a blood volume of 70 per cent of normal or over and occurs in injured patients in whom hemoglobin has fallen to a very low level. (3) *The hypertensive* pattern which consists of a raised blood pressure and a normal or slow pulse rate. The extremities may be either warm or cold, and the face may be either well colored or pale. It is associated with a small blood loss and a blood volume of 80 per cent or more. It

occurs soon after an injury and is usually transient, but it may also occur before and during operation if suitable stimuli are applied, usually either sensory or emotional stimuli. (4) *The vasovagal pattern* which consists of a low blood pressure, a slow pulse rate, cold extremities, and a pale face. To these may be added sighing respirations, sweating, nausea and vomiting. It is also commonly met with soon after injury, is transient, and is due to sensory and emotional stimuli rather than to blood loss. On rare occasions it occurs both before and during operation when suitable stimuli are applied. Even more rarely it is the result of a great deal of blood loss and is seen as a terminal pattern in patients dying from hemorrhage. (5) *Cold hypotension* which consists of a low blood pressure, a fast pulse rate, cold extremities, and a pale face. It is generally seen in patients with a great deal of blood loss and a blood volume reduced below 60 per cent of the normal. In such instances, there is also restlessness, dyspnea, and sweating. In this form, there is immediate need for voluminous and rapid transfusions if life is to be saved. A less intense form of cold hypotension is also encountered in patients suffering from a heavy infection, such as advanced peritonitis, and in these patients it may be associated with a normal blood volume and is not abolished by transfusion. (6) *Warm hypotension* which consists of a low blood pressure, a fast pulse rate, and warm extremities. The face may be either pale or well colored. Blood volume is generally reduced, but not below 70 per cent of normal. This state is generally, but not always, transient, and the factors provoking it are little understood. It is usually met with in warm surroundings, often after operation, when it is thought to be due to a combination of factors such as the anesthetic drug (ether or cyclopropane), body warming, and previous transfusion. All of these patterns, it should be understood, are merely variations of the shock state due to wounding or hemorrhage; it is little wonder, in view of the numerous other etiologic factors involved in the production of the shock state, that precise definition of the shock syndrome is impossible. To quote Dr.

Remington again: "Perhaps we should forget that the term 'shock' was ever coined and admit only that we are students of the death process."

It is sufficient for the purposes of this discussion, although perhaps not quite precise on a semantic basis, to recognize shock as simply a type of circulatory failure which does not provide the tissues with an adequate blood flow and is therefore a threat to life. Such a definition allows for the numerous variations and guises of the shocklike state which arise as a result of the two fundamental factors already enumerated: first, the fact that shock is not a stable entity, but is a dynamic and rapidly changing process which has several different phases and which may take any one of several different directions. The second is the fact that shock is not a *single* entity, but occurs in response to a number of different etiologic factors of diverse origins. Thus the patterns, the mechanisms, and the factors involved in the production of the shock syndrome may vary from patient to patient; it is the derangement of circulatory homeostasis that is the common denominator.

It has been said that "shock is hemorrhage, and hemorrhage is shock," but the shock state can occur, of course, in the absence of true hemorrhage as such. *Neurogenic shock* occurs as a sudden increase in the capacity of the vascular bed, to the extent that the normal blood volume is no longer sufficient to fill the vessels; it is due primarily to an inactivation of the vasomotor center brought about by the actions of pain, emotion, fright, excessive heat, sedatives, narcotics, drugs, or increased intracranial pressure. *Cardiac shock*, as the term is applied in relation to myocardial infarction, is often described as a separate entity since the myocardial depression is so much more important as a precipitating factor than vasodepresser impulses. *Anaphylactic shock* occurs as an allergic manifestation resulting from chemical reactions between antigens and antibodies within the tissue cells which release a vasodilator substance, presumably histamine. *Traumatic shock* is partly neurogenic in origin, in that the pain produced by injury may inhibit the sympathetic centers of the medulla and result in vasodilation; but there is also another element present, which research workers have pursued for years, in the form of a toxic substance or substances released from the traumatized tissues and then spread throughout the body to cause vasodilation and/or increased capillary permeability.

The administration of anesthesia and the performance of surgical operations also may be accompanied by the occurrence of shock, and for many years this type of shock was called *anesthetic shock* by surgeons and *surgical shock* by anesthetists. Both of these were wastebasket terms, catch-alls which served as repositories for many different types of shock which occurred during or after operation but could not be diagnosed as specific entities. Within recent years this attitude has changed; and it is now possible, in an increasing number of instances, to define the mechanism by which the shock occurring in conjunction with anesthesia and surgery is produced. One of these is "cyclo shock". This was elucidated by Dripps in an article entitled, "The Immediate Decrease in Blood Pressure Seen at the Conclusion of Cyclopropane Anesthesia: 'Cyclopropane Shock'." (Dripps, *R. D. Anesthesiology,* 8: 15–35, January, 1947), which is reprinted below with the kind permission of the author and publisher.

THE IMMEDIATE DECREASE IN BLOOD PRESSURE SEEN AT THE CONCLUSION OF CYCLOPROPANE ANESTHESIA: "CYCLOPROPANE SHOCK"

ROBERT D. DRIPPS, M.D.

With the Technical Assistance of Patricia K. Walker

Philadelphia, Pa.

Anesthesiology, 8:15–35, Jan., 1947

*　　*　　*　　*

SUMMARY

"The etiology of the decrease in blood pressure not infrequently noted at the conclusion of cyclopropane anesthesia has been investigated. Evidence is presented to suggest that this hypotension is related in part at least to an abnormally high level of carbon dioxide in the arterial blood during anesthesia. This increase in arterial carbon dioxide tension results from the respiratory depressant action of cyclopropane. With increasing respiratory efficiency in the immediate postoperative period the respiratory acidosis is corrected and blood pressure falls as the stimulant action of carbon dioxide is removed. The possibility has been considered that other physiologic imbalances secondary to the closed system method of administration may be concerned in the postoperative decrease in blood pressure."

Published April, 1973

A recent presentation title, "Balanced Anesthesia Revisiting," documents today's extensive use of nitrous oxide-relaxant-narcotic anesthesia in vivid detail. The reblossoming of this technique after a decade of halogenated hydrocarbon anesthesia can unquestionably be traced to 2 major developments; the fantastic growth of cardiovascular surgery, and the recent studies which have elucidated the true pharmacology of morphine.

To consider the former first, it was apparent, as open heart surgery became more commonplace, that the anesthetic regimens employed for such major cardiac and vascular surgery in the gravely ill patient did not always produce satisfactory results. Prolonged periods of general anesthesia were required, of course, which frequently resulted in deleterious alterations of cardiovascular hemodynamics in the poor risk patient with severe cardiopulmonary disease. Many of these anesthetic administrations provided more actual anesthesia than was necessary—and therefore more depression of cardiovascular hemodynamics than was desirable—whereas the true requirements were simply for sedation, analgesia, and amnesia. The need for some other method of anesthetic management was therefore obvious.

At first glance, morphine appeared to be an unlikely candidate for this purpose for, despite the fact that the drug has been used for many years in the treatment of patients with heart disease, heart failure and pulmonary edema, and the further fact that it is one of the best pain relieving and sedative drugs employed clinically, the earlier pharmacologic studies appeared to suggest that it was not suitable—indeed, was even dangerous—for use during anesthesia. Hanzlic in 1921 first demonstrated direct depression of the isolated heart by morphine, a fact which was subsequently confirmed by Gruber in 1929, by Schmidt and Livingstone in 1933, and—using the isolated rat trabeculae carnae muscle preparation—by Goldberg and Padget just 3 years ago.

However, all of these preparations were nourished by saline solutions; and in contrast to these findings, Flacke could demonstrate no depressant effect from doses as high as 30 mg. per kg. in the blood-perfused dog or cat heart-lung preparation. Furthermore, myocardial depression has not been convincingly demonstrated in the intact experimental animal. Schmidt and Livingstone, in another set of investigations, and using intact dogs on this occasion, found no cardiac depression with doses up to 100 mg. per kg.; and Vasco and his associates, using the dog right heart bypass preparation, actually demonstrated a positive inotropic effect from morphine.

The effect of morphine in the intact human being depends on a variety of factors, including posture, the blood volume, the condition of the heart, and the state of the sympathetic nervous system. When the drug is administered intravenously to supine, normal man, only minor and transient hemodynamic changes are observed; and in the patient with cardiac disease, but not in congestive failure, only slight decrease in cardiac output is noted when the drug is administered in the supine position. However, even in the normal subject, tilting after a therapeutic dose of morphine will produce severe orthostatic hypotension, presumably due to venous pooling in the dependent portions acting as an "internal phlebotomy." Likewise, administration of morphine to hypovolemic individuals, even though they are supine and remain so (*i.e.*, are not tilted or moved), may cause severe hypotension.

Lowenstein and his colleagues have administered morphine intravenously in a dose of 1 mg. per kg. both to subjects with aortic valve disease severe enough to require open-heart surgery and to control subjects without major cardiac or lung disease. The patients with cardiac disease had higher initial pulse rates and lower stroke indices than the normal subjects; but in contrast to the latter, developed significant increases in cardiac index, stroke index, central venous pressure, and pulmonary artery pressure, and a significant decrease in systemic vascular resistance. These findings were in line with experimental studies in animals, noted above, which have demonstrated that morphine causes relaxation of the peripheral vascular bed but has no direct cardiac effects, all of which suggests that large doses of morphine may be used with safety in patients with minimal circulatory reserve.

These findings, plus the important observation that doses of morphine sufficient to suppress respiration during treatment of patients requiring mechanical ventilation for respiratory failure usually did not have discernible hemodynamic effects, despite the large doses employed, led to the use of morphine as an anesthetic agent in patients with minimal circulatory reserve undergoing major cardiac surgery. Indeed, morphine, administered intravenously in doses ranging from 0.5 to 3.0 mg. per kg., has now been administered to many thousands of patients for major cardiac and vascular surgery in the nitrous oxide-relaxant-morphine technique. The drug stands in striking contrast to the other anesthetic agents, which can produce considerable cardiac depressant effect. When hypotension has developed during morphine anesthesia, it has been readily reversed by blood volume expansion or the administration of vasoactive agents.

In spite of today's surge of enthusiasm for the use of nitrous oxide-relaxant-narcotic anesthesia, however, it is scarcely a new technique—it is, as the recent presentation suggests, "revisiting." What is new is the substitution of morphine in the technique for meperidine, alphaprodine, and other narcotics. The original technique, in point of fact, employed meperidine, and the first formal description was that by Neff and his colleagues in the February, 1947, issue of *California Medicine* (Neff, W., Mayer, E. C., and de la Luz Peralez, M.: Nitrous oxide and oxygen anesthesia with curare relaxation. *Calif. Med.*, 66: 67, 1947), which is reprinted below with the kind permission of the authors and the publisher.

NITROUS OXIDE AND OXYGEN ANESTHESIA WITH CURARE RELAXATION

WILLIAM NEFF, M.D.,
EDWARD C. MAYER, M.D.,
AND MARIA DE LA LUZ PERALES, M.D.

San Francisco

Calif. Med., 66:67, 1947

*　　*　　*　　*

SUMMARY

"1. A method of rendering nitrous oxide anesthesia more flexible by the use of curare for obtaining muscular relaxation has been outlined based on experience in 160 clinical cases.

"2. The importance of first securing adequate pain relief before the administration of curare has been stressed. The intravenous injection of Demerol to fortify the anesthetic properties of nitrous oxide has been suggested.

"3. The problems of altered respiratory physiology consequent upon the employment of the nitrous oxide-Demerol-curare combination have been discussed.

"4. Satisfactory anesthesia for major abdominal operations may be provided by nitrous oxide and oxygen when the skeletal musculature has been relaxed with curare.

"5. The toxicity of nitrous oxide and curare are low and the safety of the method depends on the ability of the anesthetist to apply his physiological knowledge to a clinical procedure."

1948

Published October, 1980

In 1943, Kohlstaedt and Page, at the Cleveland Clinic, described an ingenious approach for the study of shock by a technique of arterial bleeding and infusion. The method consisted of introducing a cannula into the femoral artery of the dog and connecting it to a closed reservoir into which the dog was bled until the systolic blood pressure had been lowered to 30 mm. Hg. Anticoagulant was added to the withdrawn blood during the bleed, so that the blood pressure could be raised again to any desired level by the simple expedient of returning the withdrawn blood from the closed reservoir through the arterial cannula, i.e., by arterial reinfusion. The technique therefore permitted the investigator to reduce the blood pressure to any desired level, hold it at that level for as long as the investigative protocol might require, and then restore it to normal levels (provided that the animal had not been permitted to go into irreversible shock) by the simple process of arterial reinfusion.

Gardner, a neurosurgeon and also from the Cleveland Clinic, seized upon this experimental technique and transported the concept to the clinical setting of the operating room:

"The olfactory groove meningioma is a benign tumor which arises from the midline of the floor of the anterior fossa of the skull, and its removal is beset with difficulties for the following reasons: first, the location of the tumor renders it relatively inaccessible; second, it is a large and vascular growth; third, its nutrient vessels come up through the base of the skull so that they are difficult to control until after the tumor is removed.

"The best method of dealing with these tumors is to perform a right frontal craniotomy and to excise the portion of the right frontal lobe overlying the lateral aspect of the growth. With the electrosurgical unit the tumor is then removed in fragmentary fashion, after which the nutrient vessels in the floor of the skull at its area of attachment are treated by application of the cautery and bone wax. The loss of blood during the operation may be severe. In many cases the surgeon makes extremely slow progress with the removal of the tumor until the patient's blood pressure falls as the result of loss of blood. After this occurs, bleeding from the cut surface of the tumor can be readily controlled, and the removal of the tumor goes on apace.

"This was well illustrated by a patient who was operated on recently. The operation required three hours. In the first two hours less than one third of the growth had been removed. At this point the blood pressure fell from 130 to 80 because of loss of blood. Thereafter hemostasis was more readily effected, and the remainder of the tumor was quickly removed. Bleeding from the nutrient vessels coming up through the floor of the skull was then easily controlled by electrocautery, bone wax and pledgets of cotton soaked in thrombin solution. The patient received 1,500 cc. of blood during the operation, despite which the hemoglobin fell from a preoperative level of 12 Gm. to 8.9 Gm. forty-eight hours later.

"For some years I have entertained the idea of lowering the patient's blood pressure by venipuncture during the first stage of these operations in order that bleeding from the tumor might be more readily controlled. Afterward the patient's own blood could be returned instead of transfusing blood from a donor. This method, however, has not been actually employed."

Gardner used the dorsalis pedis artery and connected the cannula to a reservoir flask. While the scalp incision was being made, 1600 ml. of blood was allowed to flow rapidly into the reservoir, with a resultant fall in intraarterial pressure and rise in pulse rate. When the tumor had been removed, the collected blood was reinfused from the reservoir into the dorsalis pedis artery until about two-thirds of the withdrawn blood had been replaced. This allowed bleeders in the scalp incision to be identified, and the wound was then closed.

Arteriotomy thus became the first of the techniques which have been variously called "controlled hypotension," "induced hypotension," and "intentional hypotension." A number of other workers added certain refinements to the technique of arteriotomy, the use of which was confined almost entirely to neurosurgical procedures (i.e., craniotomy) and the fenestration operation. It offers certain well-defined advantages as compared to other techniques of "controlled hypotension." First, and most importantly, there is the obvious hemostatic effect due to the generalized vasoconstriction, neurogenic in origin, which is the initial response to bloodletting. As the blood volume is reduced further, there is a fall in blood pressure, which then also contributes to the hemostatic effect. A second great advantage of arteriotomy is the fact that repeated small bleedings and reinfusions permit a degree of controllability, both of the arterial pressure as well as the total blood volume, that is not possible with most of the other techniques of "controlled hypotension." When reinfusion is necessary, the intraarterial route provides an efficient method of raising the blood pressure rapidly, particularly in the presence of shock and myocardial ischemia due to decreased aortic pressure. Finally, the reduction of both the total blood volume and the arterial pressure was thought to have an important advantage for intracranial surgery: the tension of the brain was greatly reduced, which facilitated retraction during difficult exposures and increased the ease with which congenital aneurysms and other deep-seated lesions could be approached.

Despite these advantages, however, there are several disadvantages to the use of ar-

teriotomy. The major disadvantage, of course, stems from the vasoconstriction which is produced, since the combination of both a reduction of total circulating blood volume and the vasoconstriction which this induces approximates a state of hemorrhagic shock. During such hypovolemic hypotension, the ability to withstand even a minute blood loss is obtunded, and the danger of circulatory depression passing into an irreversible stage is constant. Furthermore, the equipment is cumbersome, and the technique itself is time-consuming to initiate; the dangers of infection and air embolism both exist and have been encountered during the clinical use of the method; and the possibility of clot formation within the apparatus is ever present.

A different approach to the problem of control of bleeding during operation than the reduction of blood volume and the production of vasoconstriction was by the reduction of peripheral resistance. The peripheral resistance resides largely in the variably contractile arterioles and is maintained by the continuous stream of vasoconstrictor impulses arising from the brain stem and carried via the sympathetic nerves to the vessel walls themselves. Interruption of this efferent sympathetic outflow results in arteriolar dilation and thus effects a reduction of peripheral resistance: the capacity of the vascular bed is increased thereby, relative to the total circulating blood volume, and this disruption of the finely adjusted balance between the two produces hypotension.

A considerable number of methods of producing a reduction of peripheral resistance have become the basis of techniques of "controlled hypotension." One of the first of these to be used clinically was that of total spinal block, which was reported by Griffiths and Gillies in a paper entitled, "Thoraco-Lumbar Splanchnicectomy and Sympathectomy: Anaesthetic Procedure," which was published in the July, 1948 issue of *Anaesthesia* (Griffiths, H. W. C. and Gillies, J.: *Anaesthesia*, *3*: 134, 1948), and is reprinted below with the kind permission of the publishers.

THORACO-LUMBAR SPLANCHNICECTOMY AND SYMPATHECTOMY. ANAESTHETIC PROCEDURE.

H. W. C. Griffiths

AND

John Gillies

Department of Anaesthetics,
University of Edinburgh,
Scotland

Anaesthesia, 3: 134, 1948

To adequately control bleeding in this operation, a total spinal block was evaluated in 84 operations involving 44 patients, the second operation usually being done within 14 days of the first. The term, total spinal block, implies a total sympathetic block with lesser degrees of sensory and motor paralysis, designed to effect the maximal fall in pressure, leaving the muscles of respiration and medullary centers unaffected.

Following Omnopon and scopolamine premedication, the patient received in the anesthetic room thiopental i.v., usually 1,000 mg. Lumbar puncture was then performed and procaine 150 to 250 mg. dissolved in 3 to 4 ml. of cerebrospinal fluid was injected. The patient was turned on his back and placed immediately in a steep Trendelenberg position until an appreciable fall in blood pressure occurred. An airway was inserted and 100 per cent oxygen given. Fractional doses of thiopental were often given during operation to maintain narcosis.

Blood pressure fell rapidly to a low level: within 10 to 20 minutes no pressure could be recorded from the brachial artery and no pulse was palpable at the wrist. However, the apex beat was easily palpable, usually at a rate of 40 to 50 beats per minute. The patient's color was usually good and the skin dry. Respiration was slow, usually 12 per minute, and largely diaphragmatic. This clinical state lasted an average of 20 to 30 minutes, after which the cardiorespiratory functions began to return towards normal.

Four patients developed cyanosis, probably the result of inadequate active or passive oxygenation. Respiratory arrest occurred on two occasions necessitating passive ventilation. One death occurred on the operating table due to failure to maintain oxygenation because of a large pleural effusion on the side operated on 13 days earlier.

No permanent dysfunction of the central nervous system was seen in this series. In three patients drowsiness and delayed response to stimuli were present postoperatively, but these signs disappeared when the blood pressure improved. No cardiac complications such as anginal attacks developed after operation, and there were no episodes of cerebral thrombosis.

Published April, 1961

Until about the turn of the century, almost all general anesthesia was achieved by the administration of but three anesthetic agents (ether, chloroform, or nitrous oxide) and almost all regional anesthesia by the injection of but a single local anesthetic drug (cocaine). There were, of course, a number of exceptions to the rule—the use of morphine or chloral hydrate intravenously to induce general anesthesia; the employment of rectal anesthesia; and the use of an ethyl chloride spray to produce either general or local anesthesia—but the vast majority of general anesthesia was by the administration of ether, chloroform, or nitrous oxide (or mixtures of the three: *i.e.,* G.O.E., A.C.E.), and the vast majority of regional anesthesia was by the injection of cocaine.

During the course of the last 50 years, the number of drugs in the anesthetist's armamentarium has increased many-fold, so that now scarcely a month goes by without at least one panacean anodyne being offered to the unwary anesthetist by the pharmaceutical houses. In many instances, the anesthetic uses of these new drugs have been either stumbled upon quite inadvertently or have been revealed as the result of mass screening. With increasing frequency, however, they have been developed as the result of what Leake has called, "biochemorphology," a process representing the highest form of intellectual cooperation between the pharmacologist and the chemist. To quote Leake himself, "scientifically, such an effort is usually based on some phase of what may be called biochemorphology, *i.e.*, the relation between chemical constitution and biologic action. A chemist, after considering, for instance, the biochemorphic aspects of hypnotics, synthesizes a new substance, which is found to have hypnotic action." The chemist is pleased, but not particularly surprised: his study of the chemical structure of numerous hypnotic drugs and his frequent consultations with the pharmacologist had convinced him that hypnotic activity was associated with a given chemical configuration, and he had every reason to believe and hope that synthesis which included that chemical configuration would produce a substance that possessed hypnotic activity.

The introduction of divinyl ether into anesthesia was the result of Leake's own application of biochemorphology to the problem of general anesthetic drugs: "A consideration of the biochemorphic aspects of general anesthetics led to the prediction that a compound incorporating the structural characteristics of ether (CH_3—CH_2—O—CH_2—CH_3) and ethylene (CH_2=CH_2) would be a general anesthetic, and further that this unsaturated ether

(CH_2=CH—O—CH=CH_2, divinyl oxide)

would be better than any unsaturated ether with a greater number of carbon atoms in the side chains. When this prediction was made, divinyl oxide, although theoretically known to chemists, did not exist. When I requested this specific compound with other unsaturated ethers from Prof. Lauder Jones of Princeton University, his associates, Drs. Randolph Major and W. T.

Ruigh, sent me an impure sample, which was found, however, to have the properties predicted of it. Later Drs. Major and Ruigh became associated with the Laboratory of Pure Research of Merck & Company and prepared for the first time pure divinyl oxide, which they were kind enough to furnish in amounts large enough for pharmacologic study and later for clinical trial when its advantages had been demonstrated. Pure divinyl oxide, although explosive like ether and ethylene, is more powerful and rapid in its anesthetic action. It is more volatile than ether (boiling point 28.3°C.) and less irritating locally, and its general physiologic effects are less severe. It has no significant pathologic effect when administered without anoxemia. Its minimal certain anesthetic concentration, like ether, is about one-third its minimal toxic concentration when allowed to act for ten minutes, but greater circulatory reserve remains when respiration fails. Recovery is more prompt than from ether or ethylene and less attended with nausea or other complications . . . . Following our pharmacologic studies, Gelfan and Bell of the University of Alberta demonstrated its safety in anesthetic concentrations for man. At its first surgical use with Dr. Dorothy Wood as anesthetist at the University of California Hospital, San Francisco, in an operation on an obese patient for removal of the gallbladder, its practical advantages were clearly evident. These have now been independently confirmed." (Leake, C. D.: The role of pharmacology in the development of ideal anesthesia. *J. A. M. A.*, *102:* 1–4, 1934).

A more recent anesthetic example of biochemorphology was contained in the development of the muscle relaxant drug, decamethonium, which was reported by R. B. Barlow and H. R. Ing in the *British Journal of Pharmacology*, *3:* 298–304, 1948, under the title of "Curare-like Action of Polymethylene Bisquaternary Ammonium Salts," and which is reprinted below.

CURARE-LIKE ACTION OF POLYMETHYLENE BIS-QUARTERNARY AMMONIUM SALTS

R. B. BARLOW

AND

H. R. ING

From the
Department of Pharmacology, Oxford

Br. J. Pharmacol., 3: 298–304, 1948

*   *   *   *

SUMMARY

"(1) The following series of polymethylene bis-quarternary ammonium dibromides have been prepared and tested for curare-like activity on the phrenic nerve-diaphragm preparation of the rat (n = number of carbon atoms in the polymethylene chain):—bis-trimethylammonium series, n = 2, 3, 4, 5, 7, 8, 9, 10, 11, 12, and 13; bis-triethylammonium series, n = 2, 3, 4, 5, 7, 8, 9, 10, and 13; bis-strychninium series, n = 2, 3, and 5; bis-quinolinium series, n = 3, 5, and 10; bis-(phenyldimethylammonium) series, n = 3 and 5.

"(2) In the bis-trimethyl series, the salt with n = 2 is about twice as active as tetramethylammonium iodide; salts with n = 3, 4, or 5 are only feebly active; activity increases from n = 7 to n = 9; salts with n = 9, 10, 11, and 12 are all about 5–6 times as active as tetramethylammonium.

"(3) In the bis-triethyl series, salts with n = 2 or 3 are relatively inactive; activity increases from n = 4 to n = 13, the last member being somewhat more active than the bis-trimethyl members in which n = 9.

"(4) None of the members of the other three series was so active as the most active members of the bis-trimethyl series.

"(5) In the rabbit head-drop test the bis-trimethyl member with n = 9 was nearly as active as tubocurarine chloride; the member with n = 10 was about three times as active. The bis-triethyl member with n = 13 was about two-fifths as active as tubocurarine chloride.

"(6) Some bis-onium salts, particularly bis-triethylammonium, bis-strychninium, and bis-quinolinium, augment the response of the rat diaphragm to maximal stimuli and inhibit the cholinesterase of caudate nucleus (dog)."

Published February, 1974

Ralph Milton Waters is one of the truly great pioneers of anesthesiology in the United States.

He was born on a farm in the tiny village of North Bloomfield, Ohio, on October 9, 1883, and he has never lost his love for, and interest in, farming. In fact, he spent the first 15 summers of his life farming; and more recently has described his spare time interests as "golf and fishing until 1927. Too busy after that. Farming and loafing from 1948" at his retirement home in Orlando, Florida. (During his high school years at Grand River Institute, from which he graduated in 1901, he spent his summers as a cement shoveler and finisher!) He attended Adelbert College of Western Reserve University and graduated with a B.A. degree in 1907; and he graduated from Western Reserve University Medical School with the M.D. degree in 1912. He interned at the German Hospital in Cleveland, Ohio, from 1910 to 1912, and following this had a residency (in what would today be called Family Practice) at the same hospital. In 1913 he married Louise Diehl, and they had 4 children: Elva Jane, Barbara, Darwin Diehl (a Board certified Anesthesiologist with an active practice in Madison, Wisconsin), and John Calvin. In 1914 he began general practice in Sioux City, Iowa, where he practiced until 1923, when he moved to the Research and Children's Hospital in Kansas City, Missouri. During World War I, he was in the Iowa National Guard, and spent part of 1916 as "Army US lst Lieut Ambulance Co. Mexican Border." He says his major duties were "overseeing enlisted personnel and intelligent government mules." In 1927 he left Kansas City to accept a post on the medical faculty of the University of Wisconsin; and there,

6 years later, in 1933, he became the first University Professor of Anesthesiology in the United States.

Dr. Waters is perhaps best known for his clinical introductions of both soda lime for the removal of carbon dioxide (1924) and of cyclopropane (1933), but his anesthetic interests and writings have been catholic: "Effects of Anesthetics on Osmotic Resistance of Erythrocytes"; "The Anesthetic Properties of Carbon Dioxide"; "Cerebral Stimulation"; "Tribromethanol Anesthesia"; "Respiratory and Circulatory Changes during Spinal Anesthesia"; "The Diffusion of Nitrous Oxide, Ethylene and Carbon Dioxide Through Human Skin during Anesthesia"; "Possible Influence of Rare Gases on Physiology"; "Sodium Ethyl (1-Methyl Butyl) Thiobarbituate"; "A Method for the Determination of Cyclopropane, Ethylene, and Nitrous Oxide in Blood with the Van Slyke-Neill Manometric Apparatus"; "Respiratory Alkalosis During Anesthesia"; "Trichlorethylene Anesthesia and Cardiac Rhythm"; "Toxic By-Products of the Atropine Group"; "Factors Influencing the Safety of Ether Anesthesia"; "Oxygen Therapy"; "Closed Endobronchial Anesthesia in Thoracic Surery"; "Procaine Toxicity"; "Leucocytosis following Inhalation Anesthesia"; "The Teaching Value of Records"; "John Snow, First Anesthetist"; "Artificial Respiration: Comparison of Manual Methods"; "Pain Relief for Children"; "A Study of Morphine, Scopolamine and Atropine and Their Relation to Preoperative Medication and Pain Relief"; "Factors Influencing the Safety of Pain Relief in Labor"; "Bronchopneumonia: The Anesthetist's Responsibility?"; "Anoxia"; "Morbidity Accompanying the Therapy of Pain: The Cost of Comfort"; "Explosion Jitters"; "Deaths in the Operating Room"; "Nitrous Oxide-Oxygen and Curare"; and "Drugs and Methods for the 'Occasional' Anesthetist," to mention but a few.

Dr. Waters' emphasis on the close relationship of physiology and pharmacology to progress in anesthesia practice was a major contribution, but another was the key role he played in the development of Anesthesiology as a specialty in this country. He was one of the original "Fellow in Anesthesiology" recipients of the New York Society of Anesthetists, which of course later became the American Society of Anesthesiologists. He was a Founder of the American Board of Anesthesiology (and holds Diploma # 7 of the more than 5500 which have been issued). He was on the original Editorial Board of the Journal, *Anesthesiology*. He was a founding member of The Anesthetists' Travel Club, which has since become the Academy of Anesthesiology, but which at the time was one of the few methods for the exchange of new ideas and information among the leaders of the specialty in this country. In short, he had a hand in almost every important venture in the organizational growth of the specialty.

Perhaps Dr. Waters' most important contribution, however, was in the area of education and teaching the future teachers of anesthesiology. The list of the residents whom he trained reads like a partial Who's Who of academic anesthesia of those decades: Frederick A. D. Alexander; Virginia Agpar; Howard M. Ausherman; Betty J. Bamforth; Ann Bardeen Henschel; Max Baumeister, Jr.; Willard Bennett; Dorothy M. Betlach; Luis G. Bouroncle; Norma B. Bowles; Simpson S. Burke, Jr.; William H. Cassels; W. Allen Conroy; William Francis Cormack; Milton Davis, Jr.; Karl-Gustav Dhuner; William H. L. Dornette; Franklin M. Dowiasch; Robert D. Dripps, Jr.; Richard Foregger; Olle F. Friberg; Gordon M. Garnett; Torsten Gordh; Jose Q. Guerra; Merel Harmel; Hubert R. Hathaway; Malcom H. Hawk; Larry H. Hogan; Ferdinand C. Jacobson; Donald R. Kindschi; Austin Lamont; Bruce V. Landry; M. Digby Leigh; Jose Adolfo de Basto Lima; Alexander M. Mackay; John A. Moffitt; Jane Moir; Lucien E. Morris; William B. Neff; Sven Eric Nilsson; Carlos P. Parsloe; Alfredo Pernin; Emery A. Rovenstine; J. Eugene Ruben; Adolph Shor; Karl L. Siebecker; Ronald A. Simpson; Barinda N. Sircar; Harvey C. Slocum; John A. Stiles; Ivan B. Taylor; David N. Treweek; Perry P. Volpitto; Clayton P. Wangerman; Darwin D. Waters; Rosaline L. Wilhelm; Albert J. Wineland; John J. Wu; and Robert M. Wylde.

In today's rush to produce more and more physicians and specialists—in the mistaken belief that increased numbers of physicians will somehow ameliorate their maldistribution—the leaders of American Medicine have supported a 3 year medical school curriculum, decreed the abolition of the free-standing internship, and urged a reduction in the length of residency training. Many thoughtful anesthesiologists find it difficult to believe that a 3 year medical school training, no internship, and a 2 year residency program can combine to produce anything but anesthetic technicians. In fact, they are convinced of it; and they base their convictions on what Dr. Waters preached many years ago about the making of an anesthesiologist. Fundamental to Dr. Waters' philosophy of the education of the anesthesiologist was his firm conviction that the anesthesiologist must be, first and foremost, a competent clinical physician. It is refreshing in these days of deteriorating medical education to republish his article expounding that philosophy, which was entitled "Pioneering in Anesthesiology." It has been called his biography, which in a way it was. But even more importantly, it was a credo of the education of the anesthesiologist, and it emphasizes the fatuity of today's approach to the matter. It was published in the September, 1948 issue of *Postgraduate Medicine* (4: 265, 1948), and is reprinted below with the kind permission of the author and the publishers.

PIONEERING IN ANESTHESIOLOGY

RALPH M. WATERS*

Madison, Wisconsin

Postgrad. Med., 4: 265, 1948

On a cold, windy day in the winter of 1912–13, a medical practitioner in a small city in our Missouri River Valley turned over to me his office, whatever I could retain of his practice, and his bull terrier. He was bound for Vienna, postgraduate study, and, I suspect, specialization in the

* Professor of Anesthesiology, University of Wisconsin Medical School, Madison.

future. The office was spacious and "well located" over a drug store. The practice which came to me, largely referred by the pharmacists downstairs, most often proved to be drug addicts seeking relief in those days before the Harrison antinarcotic law. The dog, a very unsatisfactory companion for a bachelor, would not eat in the presence of human observers and caused me much inconvenience. I collected $144 in fees the first month without accepting the largest roll of bills I had ever seen up to that time; it was offered by an addict if I would inject a syringeful of cocaine solution into his vein.

One of my duties in conducting the practice was occasionally to administer somnoform (a then popular mixture of ethyl and methyl chloride and ethyl bromide) to the patients of a neighboring dentist. I was permitted to join the informal and unorganized staff of my predecessor's hospital. A surgeon there possessed an apparatus for the administration of nitrous oxide, but no one, except the advertising "painless" dentists, knew how to use this agent. I volunteered, and thus the foundation for my career of specialization was laid.

In general, the line drawn between specialists and general practitioners was at that time neither very straight nor very distinct. For instance, I am sure that 75 per cent of the members of the county medical society attempted, at least occasionally, to perform major surgical operations. I was not without guilt myself in those days. In a then recognized hospital, I once anesthetized a woman while a man removed her uterus without benefit of ligature or suture. Clamps were applied to the vessels *after* the bleeding had become "less active" and the wound was closed with the clamps. Believe it or not, she lived long enough to regain consciousness. In the good old days a suction tip in the anesthetist's hand often supplemented the skill of the surgeon's dissection of numerous pairs of tonsils.

The requirements for specialization in many midwestern hospitals consisted of the possession of sufficient audacity to attempt a procedure and persuasive power adequate to gain the consent of the patient or his family.

With native intelligence and periodic visits to centers of medical learning in this country and abroad, a creditable specialist often eventually resulted. Technics were not so intricate nor was the breadth of knowledge so extensive as at present. Frequently a "half-baked" specialist designated himself as paying "special attention to" this or that. A practitioner especially interested in gynecology for instance, had printed on the door of his office and on his professional cards and stationery, "John Doe, M.D., Special Attention to Diseases of Women." The first formal recognition of limitation in my own practice was upon professional cards carrying the notation "Practice Limited to Obstetrics and Anesthesia." This was solely because I liked to do such work and had no thought of the impossible conflicts in appointment that were bound to occur.

After three years of mixed experience and a month's visit with an eastern anesthetist, my practice in the small midwestern city became "limited to anesthesia." I was a specialist. Many a fellow practitioner in the Mississippi Valley and its tributaries became a specialist in similar fashion in the years before the first World War. To be sure, residencies in some of the specialties were available in hospitals associated with the better medical schools. Occasionally a man studied a specialty for several years in European clinics. On their return these men usually settled in the large centers on the seaboard. Some became specialists by associating themselves with an older preceptor in the specialty. In the main, however, specialists as I saw them in the midwest originated as I have described.

Generally, incomes depended more upon the boldness of the man and his economic acumen than upon his professional proficiency. Then, even more than now, the color of man's necktie, the length of his waistline, his glibness of tongue, or his cheery manner had much to do with his success. I once had the unpleasant duty of anesthetizing a woman for the removal of her kidney by a "surgeon" who had tied off the ureter at a previous simple hysterectomy. When I returned the patient to her room, the husband detained me for some time with a recitation of the virtues and skill of the operator.

From what I have said, it should be obvious that financial success and even professional recognition in a specialty could be gained without a great outlay of time and study. It was quite another matter regarding one's own self-respect and personal satisfaction. Within a few months of the beginning of my special interest it became evident to me that (1) interest in anesthesia was superficial when it existed at all in this country; (2) opportunities were scarce; and (3) such contributions as were being made came largely from those whose primary interest was surgical or that of the laboratory. Real specialists in anesthesia were rare indeed.

In certain centers a very few physicians had interested themselves in the practical and technical aspects of the subject. I found that the source of this interest was Great Britain and that the first scientific specialist in anesthesia (I had almost said the only one) began his practice and his investigations almost with the first public demonstration of surgical anesthesia.

It was on October 16, 1846, that Morton first administered ether at Massachusetts General Hospital in Boston. A month later, John Snow began the study and the administration of ether.[1] Dating from January 28, 1847, he reported that "the ether produced the desired effects in every operation performed in St. George's Hospital." Snow's biographer says, "What had been a mere accidental discovery, I had almost said a lucky adventure, was turned by the touch of the master [Snow] into a veritable science." Although Snow died eleven years later, his influence remained. His scientific study and application explains much of our present knowledge and skill at the end of the first century in the use of anesthesia. The respect in which Snow was held by the profession in Great Britain influenced high-caliber men throughout the British Empire to follow in his footsteps. The few men such as Bennett, Gwathmey, and others who specialized in anesthesia in this country received their inspiration not from New England but from Snow and his followers in Great Britain. To this day, in the British Empire, the administration of anesthetic agents has never been entrusted to those who do not have a medical degree.

I have written elsewhere of the influence of publications and organizations upon the development of this specialty during the present century.[2] Others will record the development of the recent war. My own effort has been along lines of undergraduate and graduate teaching and investigation; in other words the contribution of the medical school. After ten years of private practice "limited to anesthesia," two things seemed obvious to me. First, improvements in our knowledge of the subject, the whys and hows of both the science and the art, depended upon close cooperation of those who administered drugs in the operating room with those who worked in the laboratories. Only in the medical school can such cooperation be established. Second, so long as the majority of physicians had little or no understanding of the dangers, the importance, and the possible contributions to the welfare of patients which anesthesiology can offer, no improvement or recognition could be expected. Again the medical school was the answer. Only when every medical college is teaching those whom it graduates the real foundations upon which administration of narcotic drugs must be based, can we expect the profession to appreciate and demand legitimate service for its patients.

In early days the deplorable belief was common, and still lingers in the minds of some of the profession, that the best in anesthesia lay in the "choice of agent," the selection of a particular drug with some occult fitness for administration in a given case. Little consideration was given to the all-important fact that all known anesthetic drugs and methods of using them often produce dangerous side effects. We were long in recognizing that it is the anticipation and recognition of these undesirable physiologic disturbances accompanying anesthesia and their management and control which constitute wise and safe anesthesia.

In 1927, I was glad to accept a place on the medical faculty at Wisconsin. Objectives of that position from the beginning have been fourfold. In order of their importance they still remain: (1) to provide the best possible service to patients of the institution; (2) to teach what is known of the principles of anesthesiology to all candidates for the medical degree; (3) to help long-term graduate students not only to gain a fundamental knowledge of the subject and to master the art of administration, but also to learn as much as possible of effective methods of teaching; and (4) to accompany these efforts with the encouragement of as much cooperative investigation as is consistent with achieving the first three objectives.

Some of the details of our attempts to carry out these objectives have been published in previous papers.[3,4,5,6] It will be sufficient to say here that we believe our undergraduates have acquired only what is essential by a didactic period once a week during the second half of their third year (junior) and a service of two weeks in the operating room during their senior year. This we feel gives only the minimum of information and experience in anesthesiology necessary for any well-informed physician. If anesthesiology as a specialty is contemplated, a residency of at least three years' duration seems to be advisable. To review our experiences and personal conclusions regarding these residencies at Wisconsin after twenty years may be of interest to others. Some of the conclusions apply to the specialty of anesthesiology only. Others seem to me of general application to graduate instruction in all the specialties.

Possibly by accident, and certainly for selfish reasons at first, resident graduate students in the specialty were chosen who had some experience in anesthesia as a special interest during a period of general practice. Compared with individuals who come right to specialization from a rotating internship, such residents seemed to have definite advantages. It has been my practice, almost without exception, to urge, if not require, that every applicant for an appointment on our service finish a period of two or three years in general practice before he makes a final decision as to what specialty he desires to enter.

After observing individuals for twenty years, both during their training period and following it, I feel quite sure that an interval in general practice before specialization is highly desirable. I believe that the younger doctor who follows the plan of internship, general practice, final decision as to his specialty, and then a long-term residency will be more successful and more satisfied ten years after graduation than would the same individual if he went into a specialty directly following his internship. This statement, I realize, demands some defense.

From the young man's standpoint it may be argued that a period of general practice before specialization delays the beginning of one's real life work until the individual is too old for real enthusiasm. Economic security may be delayed, and the early establishment of a family and a permanent home of one's own may be impossible. However, as I look back upon those who have been associated with me in the study of anesthesiology in the long past, these two objections seem to be overbalanced by numerous advantages. At least some of these men who became specialists married, had families, and yet were economically stable and happy.

The hospital staff and management may argue that the resident with previous experience in general practice is intractable, less cooperative, less studious, and more demanding. Some of these objections depend upon the point of view. If, as a primary function, the hospital expects its residents in the specialties to care for its patients, and to do the work of the hospital and the visiting staff, then the younger and less experienced in life they are, the better. For instance, I know of hospitals that have "modernized" their service in my own specialty by replacing former technicians in anesthesia—the so-called "anesthetic nurses" who got a salary of $150 or more a month—with "residents" in anesthesia, young doctors at 25 dollars a month. These "residents" have been allowed to anesthetize patients, private and others, without proper supervision or instruction while the hospital budget is balanced by the fees which it collects for their services.

If, as I believe, residencies or fellowships in the specialties are maintained primarily for the purpose of creating capable specialists who will contribute the maximum in efficient service to the public in the future,

it is the responsibility of the hospital to provide time, opportunity, and instructors necessary to prepare them. An immature youngster just finishing his internship may be happy with the opportunity to care for patients independently, to operate upon them, or to anesthetize them, and to permit such experience to be called "training for a specialty." The man with experience in general practice does not accept such conditions as "graduate training for a specialty." We, as staff members and hospital administrators, must guard against having opinions or supporting practices which contribute to the convenience of the visiting staff and the economic security of the hospital at the expense of the quality of special training offered. I am suggesting that the maturity of the man who begins to specialize after a brief experience in general practice will prevent us—teachers, visiting staff, and hospital administrators—from exploiting, however unconsciously, the graduate student.

But, you say, common honesty and understanding on our part will prevent exploitation of the graduate student. Agreed. What then are the real advantages of the plan I am proposing? They extend in two directions—to the community and to the young doctor. One of our unsolved problems in recent years has been the deficiency of available family practitioners to serve our smaller communities. If every medical graduate, on finishing his internship, were to undertake a short period of general practice, this shortage would not exist. A few months or years of such experience gives the young doctor an opportunity to learn how to collect and spend money, how to conduct himself in his relations with the community in which he lives, with patients and their families, and with other physicians. It is so easy to acquire a critical and unsympathetic attitude in a specialty. It is less easy when one has lived "on the other side of the fence." But more especially the young doctor during general experience will see all sides of the practice of medicine; he will refer cases to specialists; he will learn that no patient is the problem of a single specialty. While making these observations, he will be in a position to decide just what specialty he will really enjoy and where his inclinations and skills will fit.

What about the community when he leaves to join his special residency or his fellowship? Once the custom becomes established, will not an inheritance develop much as it operates now regarding internships? Certain schools establish the custom of sending a man to this hospital, another to that, each year. As long as the hospital is satisfied, the habit continues. Sometimes it is a fraternity or some other small group which determines what hospital a particular senior will choose for his internship. Would not the same habit develop in determining where he would enter general practice the next year? The office, equipment, even the motor car and living quarters, might be handed down in a similar manner. If, as I am sure would happen, an occasional young doctor decided that he likes general practice and did not return for training in a specialty, I believe both the community and the profession would benefit by the doctor's decision.

To implement such a plan as I am advocating, a slight change is necessary in customs among administrators. Interns have said to me, "I like the idea of having experience in general practice before I decide what specialty I shall enter. But I get the impression that it will be next to impossible for me to secure a desirable appointment in a first-class department unless I arrange for it while I am an intern." Obviously, if the intern waits to avail himself of experience and maturity before choosing his life work, he must not be penalized for it. If more mature individuals are appointed, it is my firm conviction that the hospital superintendent and the director of training in any specialty will observe benefit not only to the graduate student but also to the service.

Even when a person has the advantage of a period of general practice during which he decides upon a specialty, he may be mistaken regarding his preference. Actual experience may prove that his aptitudes lie elsewhere. Both the candidate and our department always look upon the first six months of a resident's service as a trial period. If either side decides that a mistake

has been made, we try to rectify it as soon as possible. Although these methods of deliberation in planning one's future may seem like waste of time, they make for satisfaction and success in later life. Everyone is not intrinsically equipped to be a surgeon, an obstetrician, an internist, or an anesthetist. May it not be advantageous to spend a reasonable time in deliberation and experimentation? Certainly there should be no disgrace attached to changing one's mind about the choice of his future life work. If the choice has been right, life is a joy forever after. Uncongenial work is drudgery.

What does the evidence show in the later experience of our own men who have gone out as specialists in anesthesiology? I am quite willing to admit that the number has been altogether too small to have the slightest statistical significance. We have had with us residents of three categories: (1) those who came to the specialty from their internships; (2) those who have had an interval of two or three years in general practice; and (3) a few who have come to us late in life, sometimes after part-time specialization for some years. What can we say of their comparative accomplishments?

Those in the first group acquire knowledge and technical facility as readily as the others. On the other hand, as a group while in residency they show less good judgment, less independence of thought, and less self-reliance. They are more, rather than less, likely to give evidence of brashness or foolhardy conduct. After leaving us, when "out on their own" the first group have had more difficulty in building a place for themselves in the world. Their relations with hospital staff or medical school faculty, with hospital administrators, and with the community at large, have been more difficult at first and satisfactory adjustments have been made much more slowly.

The second group who have returned after an experience of two or three years in general practice, have, in our experience, shown little or no tendency to resist the necessary routine of a department, record-keeping, cooperation, and the like. They have adjusted to institutional life without difficulty. As a group, they offer more original ideas, good and bad, which not only prove a healthy stimulus to discussion in the department and to investigative effort, but also at times result in change of conviction in the department. The advantage to us and to our institution deriving from this second group over the first, though noticeable, may not have been great. The advantages to the resident himself, however, both during his training and in later life, seem to us considerable. He comes to us after a mature choice of what he wants to do. He works harder and grasps his opportunities with more vigor. Possibly the fact that he is older and more mature when he begins to practice "on his own" explains some of his advantage. However, I do not believe that age and maturity are the only factors. The broad viewpoint acquired as a general practitioner remains with him as a specialist. Experience in economic and social relations does not have to be acquired at a time when he is trying to establish himself as a specialist.

Finally, what of those in the third category who have been out in the world for a good many years either as part-time specialists or as general practitioners? Some of these are merely men who, through failing health, deficient professional background, or desire for change, wish to specialize. These must be discouraged at once. An old dog doesn't learn new tricks very easily. As a rule, those in the third class do not fit into a residency program nor do they benefit themselves thereby. We have met a few exceptions to the rule, but these are rare indeed.

Personal acquaintance with candidates through long correspondence and at least one protracted personal interview is necessary if the director of a training program is to fulfill all his obligations. These extend not only to the applicant but to the applicant's prospective fellow students, to the specialty and last, but most important of all, to the medical profession as a whole and the service it will render to the public. If we cannot help young physicians to become specialists who will be a credit to our profession, if we do not put them in a position to perform a useful service in years to come, our efforts had better not be devoted to the "training of specialists."

SUMMARY

Specialization in medical practice has developed as knowledge and skills have extended with the years. Methods of preparation of specialists have varied widely. I have recited some personal experiences and observations both as student and as teacher. The very informal customs I have described as being characteristic of some parts of our midwest at the time I began practice in 1913 had certain advantages. Independence, self-reliance, and originality were developed; or at least these qualities, when naturally present, were not diminished. Sometimes, however, the freedom allowed led to boldness, rashness, and foolhardy practice, resulting, in certain cases, in disaster and death, if not murder. Certainly it was not the ideal manner of preparation. We have speculated as to how the advantages of the informal, individualistic method of learning to be a specialist can be combined with the advantages of the formal training that is customary at the present time.

I think we may conclude that familiarity with physiologic functions and the manner in which these are affected by therapeutic procedure is the essential background of specialization. Added to such familiarity, technical skills in diagnosis and treatment are not enough to produce a real specialist. He must also have a rational, well-rounded attitude toward the general problems involved in the practice of medicine and the care of the sick. If our training of specialists sacrifices one of these three factors, either scientific background, special skills, or a rational, well-rounded attitude, it is not very successful.

Having tried to select those candidates for special training in anesthesiology who have conducted a general practice after internship and having watched a fairly large number of these later as specialists, in comparison with others who began to specialize directly after internship, I cannot avoid certain definite impressions.

1. The former general practitioners are happier and are better satisfied with their specialty.

2. They are more successful and more convincing professionally as specialists.

3. They more easily and completely command the respect and the economic recognition of fellow physicians, hospital administrators, and the public.

It is my belief that a young person will act for his own and the communities' best interest if he delays decision as to specialization and his choice of a specialty until he has passed through at least a short period in the general practice of medicine or its equivalent.

REFERENCES

1. WATERS, R. M.: John Snow, first anesthetist. *Bios.*, 7: 25, March, 1936.
2. ———: The development of anesthesiology in the United States, in *Journal of History of Medicine and Allied Sciences*, Vol. I, No. 4, 1946.
3. ———: The teaching value of records. *J. Indiana M. A.*, 29: 110, March, 1936.
4. WATERS, R. M., HATHAWAY, H. R. AND CASSELS, W. H.: The relation of anesthesiology to medical education. *J.A.M.A.*, 112: 1667, April 29, 1939.
5. WATERS, R. M.: The evolution of anesthesia. *Proc. Staff Meet., Mayo Clin.*, 17: 428, No. 27, July 15, 1942.
6. ———: Anesthesiology in the hospital and in the medical school. *J.A.M.A.*, 130: 909, April 6, 1946.

Published October, 1978

It took, really, a long time to recognize that respiratory function and circulatory function are not distinct and separate but, rather, intimately interwoven, and that a primary, common task of both the heart and the lungs is the supply of O_2 to the tissues. The term, "cardiopulmonary," emerged in common medical parlance only during the past generation or so, and the development of the "cardiorespiratory" laboratory is well within the memory of a number of aging anesthesiologists. However, the concept that the cardiovascular system and the pulmonary system are discreet lingers on, and standard modern textbooks of physiology continue to have one section devoted to The Heart, another section devoted to The Circulation, and yet another section devoted to Respiration.

This separation is not so surprising when one considers that even the existence of the circulation was unknown to the Ancient World and the Dark Ages, but came only with the dawning of the Late Renaissance. In 1553, Miguel Serveto, searching for a connection between the right heart and the left, discovered the lesser circulation; and in 1569, Caesalpinus traced the path of the greater circulation. Recognition of the centripetal movement of the venous blood stream was deduced more or less concurrently by Jacobus Sylvius (1543), Canani

(1564), and Fabricius of Aquapendente (1574) on the basis of the structure and arrangement of the valves of the veins, the new concept replacing the previous belief that the blood always flowed outward, even in the veins. The great William Harvey (1578–1657), one of the most gifted pupils of Fabricius, combined all of these individual findings with the results of his own researches to form the general picture of what we today call the circulation of the blood. This he did in his monumental treatise, *De Motu Cordis* (as it is usually called; the complete title was actually *Exercitatio Anatomica de Motu Cordis et Sanguinis in Animalbius*), which was published in 1628. Harvey had already expressed his ideas on the circulation of the blood as early as 1616 in his lectures at the Royal College of Physicians of London, but he waited until further experiments provided complete proof before publication. The *De Motu Cordis* was surely one of the most important books in the whole history of medicine because it laid the foundation for modern physiology and medicine.

The final important link in the chain of proof of the circulation of the blood was the existence of capillaries. Harvey had postulated the capillary circulation, but the actual identification of capillaries had to await the development of microscopy by

Anton van Leewenhoek and the description of capillaries in the lungs of the frog by Marcello Malphigi in his 1661 publication, *De Pulmonibus Observationes Anatomicae.*

Thus, by the beginning of the eighteenth century, the essential anatomic facts concerning the circulation of the blood had been established and investigations of its physiology were beginning. The forerunner of the latter were carried out by an English parson, the Reverend Stephen Hales, a scientifically interested layman, who in 1710 performed the first catheterization of the heart of a living animal for a definite scientific purpose. The good parson bled a sheep to death and threaded a gun barrel through the neck vessels into the still-beating heart. Through this gun barrel, he filled the hollow chambers of the heart with molten wax and then, from the resultant cast, measured the volume of cardiac ejection and, by knowledge of the pulse rate, calculated the minute volume of the heart. Some years later, in 1727, to be exact, he also became the first to determine arterial pressure when he measured the rise of a column of blood in a glass tube which he had inserted into an artery.

The origins of modern trends in cardiovascular research, however, came from classic French experimental physiology, as exemplified by the technique employed by Claude Bernard (1813–1878), which he described in his *Physiologie Operative*; and particularly by the procedures developed by Chauveau and Marey in the late 1860's. These workers were the first to measure blood pressures within the heart and to record pressure curves from the interior of the heart in living animals. They achieved this with the use of manometers which were led through the neck vessels into both compartments of the right heart, as well as into the left heart chamber.

In 1812, Unger, Bleichroder and Loeb reported cannulation of the bifurcation of the aorta. Their objective was the introduction at this site of special chemotherapy for puerperal sepsis in order to achieve the highest possible concentration of the drug at the place where it would be most effective. After preliminary experiments in dogs, they carried out arterial cannulations in 4 humans in this trial of intra-arterial drug therapy. No ill effects were reported, but the placement of the catheters was not checked by X-ray. There was absolutely no consideration of the possible diagnostic or experimental cardiovascular aspects of the technique, but nevertheless the development of invasive cannulation of the arterial system of the human was a technical advance that was to become essential for diagnostic cardiology and the investigation of cardiopulmonary physiology.

The other essential, of course, was cardiac catheterization.

Werner Theodor Otto Forssmann was born in Berlin on August 19, 1904, the son of Julius Forssmann and Emmy Hindenberg. He was educated at the Askanische Gymnasium in Berlin; and in 1922 matriculated at the University of Berlin to study medicine, passing his State Examination in 1929. His clinical training was at the University Medical Clinic, working under Professor Georg Klemperer, and he studied anatomy under Professor Rudolph Fick. For clinical instruction in surgery he went, in 1929, to the August Victoria Home at Eberswalde near Berlin, and it was there that he was the first to develop a technique for the catheterization of the human heart. This he did by inserting, with the intrepidity of youth, a cannula into his own antecubital vein, through which he passed a catheter for 65 centimeters and then calmly walked to the X-ray Department, where a photograph was taken of the catheter lying in his right auricle.

This feat was obviously a remarkable advance, since it demonstrated that methods well known from animal experiments could also be adapted for studies in man. The technique was of paramount importance for a study of the pathologic changes in diseases of the heart and circulation, which could be reproduced with difficulty, or not at all, in animal experiments; but it also opened up the opportunities for roentgenologic examination of the right side of the heart and the pulmonary vessels after the injection of contrast medium directly into these organs. Forssmann also undertook experiments on himself for these purposes.

Forssmann was not unaware of the dangers of such self-experimentation; but in the end he was the victim, not of the invasions of his own body, but of the tragedy of attempting to introduce a new concept to the world. The world does not only dislike new ideas, it usually rejects them strenuously.

The situation at the time was that it was possible to record the pressure in the human peripheral arteries and superficial veins (values which reflect to some extent the conditions in the left ventricle and the right atrium), but measurements of the right ventricular pressure (which is of essential importance for knowledge of the work of the right side of the heart) could not be—or, at any rate, had not been—measured in man. Similarly, it was possible to determine the O_2 content of arterial blood in man but not of the mixed venous blood in the right side of the heart, a measurement which gives the average value for the body as a whole. Data concerning these measurements and determinations had long been available from animal experiments, of course, but in man it was necessary to resort to indirect methods, which not only yielded indirect results, but often required unavailable training and cooperation by the subject or the patient.

The world had adapted itself to this unsatisfactory state of affairs, and blithely accepted a roadblock that was preventing progress in cardiology and totally obstructing desirable developments in cardiorespiratory research. As late as 1928, therefore, a recognized textbook could state with equanimity and even smugness that data on cardiac pressures and mixed venous blood in man were "naturally" confined to those obtained by indirect methods. When Forssmann achieved his spectacular technical breakthrough, he not only was not applauded, but he was bitterly criticized in the most severe and exaggerated manner, on the basis of the preconceived opinion held by many of the unacceptable dangers inherent in such an invasive technique—which opinion, of course, he had already totally contradicted and negated by his own self-experimentation.

Forssmann's disappointment was immense, and the coals heaped upon the courageous young doctor's head robbed him of any further inclination to continue his work. His achievement lay essentially fallow (with the exception of isolated instances of its application in Prague and in Lisbon) because of the strong resistance by those who obstructed practical research work with threadbare ethical and moral objections.

But the triumph of intellectual bigotry over an essential and available scientific tool is necessarily self-limited, and within a decade the group of physiologists composed of Richards, Cournand, and their colleagues at Bellevue Hospital and Columbia University began the painstaking preparations and studies to make direct analyses of conditions in the right side of the heart. They proceeded with great hesitation and the beginning was not easy, for they too, like Forssmann, met strong and opinionated resistance; but in 1941 a turning point in the history of cardiology was achieved when they published a report of cardiac catheterization in man. They had made a few minor improvements in Forssmann's technique; but the main point was that a well known research group at a distinguished clinic had set their seal of approval on the method, which then made its triumphant entry into the world of clinical medicine.

In the course of the next 15 years, Cournand and Richards and their pupils used the technique for catheterization of the heart in studies of traumatic shock, the diagnosis of congenital heart diseases, the physiology of heart failure, measurement of the action of cardiac drugs, and various forms of dysfunction in chronic cardiac and pulmonary diseases and their treatment. The concept that the functions of the heart and the functions of the lungs were intimately interwoven, rather than separate and distinct, had finally arrived, and the terms, "cardiopulmonary" and "cardiorespiratory," were fully established as descriptions of the commonality and interdependence of the shared roles.

The investigations carried out by the Bellevue group, which were of perhaps the most practical interest to the anesthesiologist, concerned the effects of artificial respiration upon the circulation, particularly cardiac output in response to the so-called "Cournand Curves." The definitive paper was titled, "Physiological Studies of the Effects of Intermittent Positive Pressure Breathing on Cardiac Output in Man," and was published in the *American Journal of Physiology in 1948* (Cournand, A., Motley, H. L., Werko, L. and Richards, D. W.: *Am. J. Physiol.*, *152*: 162 to 174, 1948), and is reprinted below with the kind permission of the authors and the publisher.

PHYSIOLOGICAL STUDIES OF THE EFFECTS OF INTERMITTENT POSITIVE PRESSURE BREATHING ON CARDIAC OUTPUT IN MAN

Andre Cournand, Hurley L. Motley, Lars Werko and Dickinson W. Richards, Jr.

Department of Medicine,
Columbia University,
and the
Chest and Medical Services
of the
Columbia University Division,
Bellevue Hospital, New York,
New York

Am. J. Physiol., 152: 162–174, 1948

The effects of three types of intermittent positive pressure breathing, as differentiated by the shape of the mask pressure curve, were correlated with the changes in cardiac output observed in 33 experiments on 29 human subjects.

The three types of mask pressure curves were as follows: type I, symmetrical with gradually increasing and decreasing slope, expiratory time approximately the same as inspiratory and the end expiratory pressure above atmospheric; type II, asymmetrical with rapidly increasing pressure during inspiration and rapidly dropping during expiration, long inspiratory and short expiratory time intervals and the end expiratory pressure above atmospheric; and type III, asymmetrical with gradually increasing pressure during inspiration and suddenly dropping early in expiration to atmospheric and expiratory time equal to or exceeding inspiratory.

Cardiac output was decreased more or less in proportion to the increase in mean mask pressure with the first and second type curves (Type I, mean mask pressure 7.0 mm. Hg, cardiac output decrease 14.5 per cent; Type II, mean mask pressure 10.6 mm. Hg, cardiac output decrease 16.5 per cent). There was no decrease in cardiac output with the Type III curve (mean mask pressure 5.7 mm. Hg, cardiac output increase 6.0 per cent).

The blood pressure changes produced by the three types of IPPB were small. The arterial pressure, both systolic and diastolic, was increased slightly with Types I and III and decreased by 3 mm. Hg with Type II.

Interpreted in terms of variation in stroke volume, these changes suggest that the deficit in cardiac output incurred during the inspiratory phase is compensated for during the expiratory phase. When the pressure drop is rapid in expiration with the resulting intrapleural pressure low and the right ventricular net filling pressure high, compensation is complete provided expiratory time is of sufficient duration. Expiratory time must equal or exceed inspiratory in order that the number of heart beats during expiration may equal or exceed the number present during inspiration. The time and pressure relationships with the third type of curve permitted compensation to be complete, as the mean right ventricular net filling pressure was not decreased. Compensation was incomplete with the first and second types, because the mask pressure did not drop rapidly after cycling with the first curve, and because expiratory time was too short and the end expiratory pressure still above atmospheric with the second type curve.

A desirable type of IPPB should provide a mask pressure curve that shows: *a*) a gradual increase in pressure during inspiration, *b*) a rapid drop in pressure after cycling occurs, c) a mean mask pressure during the expiratory period as near atmospheric as possible, and d) an expiratory time equal to or exceeding the inspiratory time. Adequate ventilation can be provided with the above type of pressure breathing in man with a minimal disturbance to the circulation.

Published February, 1980

"This Yankee dodge, gentlemen, beats mesmerism hollow."

These were the words purported to have been uttered by Robert Liston to the audience assembled in the operating arena of the University College Hospital of London on the morning of December 21, 1846, after the brilliant surgeon had amputated the leg of one Frederick Churchill.

There were 4 fascinating circumstances in connection with this operation.

The first was that Liston himself had made the operation necessary, a situation still not entirely unknown in the field of surgery today. Churchill, a butler by trade, had fallen and injured his tibia, and a discharging sinus had formed for which he had consulted the great surgeon. Liston had made an incision, probed the sinus with his finger until he felt bone, and then had "plugged" the wound. Quite predictably, Churchill's bodily systems did not appreciate the germs on Liston's finger and responded with fever, sweating, rapid and feeble pulse, headache, nausea, twitching, and exhaustion. In short, septicemia, requiring (Liston's opinion, at least) amputation.

The second interesting feature of the operation was that one of the audience in the crowded surgical amphitheater that day was a handsome Quaker youth by the name of Joseph Lister, who would one day abolish infections such as that which necessitated the operation in the first place.

The third significant point was that the operation is said to have been the first surgery performed outside the United States under the newly discovered ether anesthesia. (It was not, but that is a whole different story in itself. The history books still credit Liston's operation.) The operation on Churchill's festering extremity occurred just 9 weeks and 2 days after Morton's classic public demonstration of the efficacy of ether anesthesia in Boston on October 16, 1846. This may not appear very soon in an age when we can watch a Pope being buried in Rome, or a World Cup soccer match being played in South America, even as the event is happening; but in 1846 that was lightning-fast communications. Jungle drums could have done it faster, or perhaps even the Pony Express, but neither of these could be adapted for Trans-Atlantic transmission.

The final—and most important—aspect were the prophetic words by Liston when he had completed the operation upon the poor butler ("This Yankee dodge, gentlement, beats mesmerism hollow"), for his catchy phrase indeed signaled the beginning of worldwide acceptance of chemical anesthesia and sounded the deathknell for anesthesia produced by the techniques of Franz Anton Mesmer, based on his discovery of animal magnetism.

Certainly one of the strangest chapters in all of the history of anesthesia was that concerning mesmerism and surgery.

The first recorded use of mesmerism for surgical anesthesia occurred on April 12, 1829, when the French surgeon, Jules Cloquet, performed a mastectomy on a patient in mesmeric sleep. The first major surgical operation across the channel in England on a patient in a mesmeric state was an amputation of the leg at the thigh by a British surgeon named Ward, and it was performed at Nottinghamshire in 1842. The first case in the United States was recorded in the August 19, 1843, issue of the *Illinois Telegraph and Review* under the title of, "Case of Excision of a Wen, without pain, in the Mesmeric State," and on February 21 of the same year the *Missouri Republican* reported the removal of a tumor of the shoulder during mesmeric sleep.

There were other cases from America which were reported and published in *The*

Zoist: A Journal of Cerebral Physiology and Mesmerism, and their Application to Human Welfare, during the years 1845–1846: (1) the "Removal of a tumor from the Neck in the Mesmeric State—performed in New York—reported by A. Sydney Doane, M.D. Witnessed among others by Drs. Valentine Mott, J. Kearney Rodgers, Delafield, John W. Francis;" (2) "Removal of another Tumor from the neck of an elderly Medical Man Related in the *Cleveland Plain Dealer*, Performed at Cleveland Medical College by Professor Ackley, assisted by Professors Delamater, Kirkland, and others;" (3) "The removal of a polyp from the nose;" and (4) the removal of a breast by Dr. L. A. Dugas, professor of physiology in the Medical College of Georgia.

These American accounts are of particular interest in that Crawford Long referred to them in his belated paper, "An account of the first use of sulphuric ether by inhalation as an anesthetic in surgical operations," published long after the fact, in 1848:

"At the time I was experimenting with ether there were physicians in high authority, and of justly distinguished character, who were advocates of mesmerism, and recommended the induction of the mesmeric state as adequate to prevent pain in surgical operations. Notwithstanding thus sanctioned, I was an unbeliever in the science, and of the opinion, that if the mesermic state could be produced at all, it was only on 'those of strong imagination and weak minds,' and was to be ascribed solely to the workings of the patient's imaginations. Entertaining this opinion, I was more particular in my experiments in etherization."

It was not, however, the reports in America, or England, or France, or any other European countries, from which the best documented support for mesermism in surgery came—it was from the subcontinent of India.

James Esdaile, son of the Rev. Dr. Esdaile of Perth, was born on February 6, 1808. After graduating from Edinburgh in 1830, he entered the service of the East India Company. In 1845, Esdaile was in charge of the Native Hospital at Hooghly, India.

Having read reports of mesmerism, he was inspired to try it in a surgical case. On April 14, 1845, he performed his first operation on a mesmerized patient. Encouraged by his success in this patient, Esdaile continued his experiments, and by January 22, 1846, he had reported 73 cases of painless operations performed at Hooghly in the 8 month period:

Arm amputated	1
Breast ditto	1
Tumor extracted from the upper jaw	1
Scirrhus testium extirpated	2
Colis amputated	2
Contracted knee straightened	3
Ditto arms	3
Operations for cataract	3
Large tumor of the inguen cut off	1
Operations for Hydrocele	7
Ditto Dropsy	2
Actual cautery applied to a sore	1
Muriatic acid ditto	2
Unhealthy sores pared down	7
Abscesses opened	5
Sinus, 6 inches, laid opened	1
Heel flayed	1
End of thumb cut off	1
Teeth extracted	3
Gum cut away	1
Praeputium cut off	3
Piles ditto	1
Great toe nails cut out by the roots	5
Large tumor on leg removed	1
Seton introduced from ankle to knee	1
Scrotal tumours, weighing from 8 to 80 lbs.	14
removed 17, painless	73

The timing of the advent of mesmerism in surgery was unfortunate, at least from the point of view of its advocates (who were avid and zealous), since it occurred *pari-passu* with the great events of the 1840's, which culminated in the discovery of first nitrous oxide, then ether, and finally chloroform anesthesias. However, certainly from the patient's disadvantage point, it was several steps ahead of being held down by several strong men; and on August 8, 1853, Esdaile, who had returned to Scotland, rushed to mesmerism's defense in a Memorial addressed to Congress in which he indignantly denied that painless surgery had first become possible as a result of the discovery of ether anesthesia. In his deposition to the United States Congress, he drew attention to "the simple and notorious fact . . . that painless surgery by means of mesmerism, years before ether was heard of, was as common in my hospitals, as it has since become in Europe under the influence of chloroform, and nearly three hundred capital mesmeric operations had been performed by me before leaving India, two years ago."

But even the dedicated Esdaile was seduced into a trial of ether as a surgical anesthetic, and he concluded that:

"By cautious and graduated doses, and with a knowledge of the best antidotes, I think it extremely probable that this power will soon become a safe means of procuring insensibility, for the most formidable operations even.

"All mesmerists, who are lovers of truth, and not mere traders, will rejoice at having been the means of bringing to light one truth more, especially as it will free them from the drudgery required to induce mesmeric insensibility to pain, which, although the most striking, is the least important branch of the subject.

"It is only of late years that the application of mesmerism to surgery has been prominently brought forward, principally with the view of affording an ocular demonstration of this great vital agent.

"But the great field for a display of its usefulness is in the treatment of medical diseases, where it often comes to our aid when all other resources have failed."

This passage by Esdaile was revealing and significant, and emphasized that mesmerism failed to survive as an anesthetic method, not only because of the opposition to it (which was loud and clear, particularly by Thomas Wakley, the crusading editor of the *Lancet*, who regarded it as quackery), but more importantly because it was less efficient than ether or chloroform, and the margin of its uncertainty was so much greater. Furthermore, the process of mesmerizing was laborious and time consuming (up to 8 hours, in some cases), and was scarcely suited for emergencies or the parturient. Finally, the advocates of mesmerism were interested in its surgical application chiefly for propaganda purposes, as

demonstrating the existence of mesmeric force. With the appearance of the superior agents, ether and chloroform, interest in the surgical use of mesmerism declined rapidly, although its medical use persisted.

In 1948, Gilbert Frankau published a treatise on Mesmer and Mesmerism (Frankau, G.: *Mesmerism.* London: MacDonald, 1948), which consisted of an introductory monograph by Frankau himself, and then a translation (the first in English) of Mesmer's own *Mémoire sur la découverte du Magnétisme Animal*, which had first been printed at Geneva in 1799. Mesmer's dissertation will be the text of the April issue of "Classical File," and Frankau's introductory monograph is reprinted below.

MESMERISM

G. FRANKAU

MacDonald, London, 1948

INTRODUCTORY MONOGRAPH

In this foreword to Mesmer's treatise, "Dissertation on the Discovery of Animal Magnetism," published in 1799, Frankau reviews in a biographical style the checkered and peripatetic career of Franz Anton Mesmer. That he possessed the personal charm and magnetism of a present-day John Wayne or Billy Graham there seems little doubt. That his influence in Europe in his generation, at least in the "jet set", created much food for conversation appears evident. Frankau would have him be "regarded as the father of modern psychotherapy", and "present-day spiritualism, also, owes some debt—in so far as it is based on the evidence of mediums—to Mesmer: and so does the Church of Christ Scientists, which was founded by Mary Baker Eddy."

However, the academicians of his day believed otherwise in the feats promoted by Mesmer. In 1784, Louis XVI convened a body of 13 commissioners under the presidency of none other than Benjamin Franklin, the newly accredited ambassador of the United States of America, to consider the feasibility of his doctrines. With only one dissenting vote, the verdict was, "the imagination does everything, the magnetism nothing."

Charlatan, honest believer in his doctrines, a Barnum of his generation, who can say? The controversy is still not laid to rest.

Published April, 1980

The story of the use of mesmerism for surgery was surely one of the strangest chapters in the history of anesthesia. That it was also a short chapter was due, of course, to the almost simultaneous introduction, and worldwide acceptance, of N₂O, ether, and chloroform as chemical methods of producing general anesthesia. Elliotson, one of England's foremost advocates of mesmerism and the mesmeric state, wrote of the discovery of ether anesthesia: "If this plan produces insensibility to pain in more instances than mesmerism, and quite as innocently and easily as when mesmerism succeeds, it will indeed be a blessing, and none will hail it more joyously than we mesmerists, who have no other object than the good of mankind. . . ."

The zeal of the mesmerists, as exemplified in Elliotson's writings, led them to claim their fair share of credit for the discovery of anesthesia: "To mesmerism and mesmerists all this is really owing. The idea of proving insensibility for operations had through mesmerism laid such a hold on men that the trial of inhaling ether was made and the success of mesmerism will drive the profession headlong to try the new method and too generally, as in the case of Mr. Liston, out of desire to 'supercede' mesmerism . . . the truth unsuspected by Mssrs. Liston, Wakley, Boott, and the rest of the eager antimesmerists is, that the state induced by ether is somnambulism—*the very same state as the mesmeric*—which varies from deep coma to more or less partial activity of the brain."

Thus, the attitude of even the most ardent mesmerists shifted from advocacy of mesmerism as the method of choice for the achievement of painless surgery to one which claimed, in effect, we-led-you-to-chemical-anesthesia. They readily conceded the much greater reliability of ether anesthesia, and the greater ease with which

it could be produced. The latter point was well documented in the 1846 report of a committee appointed by the Governor General of Bengal "to observe and report upon Surgical Operations by Dr. J. Esdaile, upon patients under the influence of alleged mesmeric agency." The report presented an interesting picture of the manner in which mesmerism was practiced in Esdaile's Hooghly Hospital:

"The patients treated were all native males, from 18 to 40 years old, Hindus and Mohamedans, in all conditions of general health from extreme emaciation to ordinary strength . . . the mesmerists employed by Dr. Esdaile were young men, Hindus and Mohamedans, from 14 to 30 years of age, most of them compounders and dressers from the Hooghly Hospital.

"To each patient a separate mesmeriser was assigned. The room in which they operated was darkened, but from time to time the Committee were enabled to witness, through small apertures made in the door panels, the manner in which the processes were carried on. The patient lay on his back, the body naked from the waist upwards, and the thighs and legs bare: the mesmeriser seated behind him at the head of the bed, leaning over him, the faces of both nearly in contact, the right hand being generally placed on the pit of the stomach and passes made with one or both hands along the face, chiefly over the eyes. The mesmeriser breathed frequently and gently over the patient's lips, eyes and nostrils. Profound silence was observed. These processes were continued for about two hours each day in ten cases, for eight hours in one case in one day, and for six hours in another case, without interruption. Three cases of the ten . . . were dismissed without satisfactory effect."

The Committee's report thus certainly confirmed both the unreliability and the time-consuming nature of mesmerism; but note, additionally, that the induction of the trance, or hypnosis, was accomplished in large part by the "laying on of hands". This has, down through the ages, been an integral part of man's consistent attempt to cure diseases without drugs by some unseen power outside of his own body; in other words, by suggestion. The Greeks appreciated that, to influence the patient's "soul," which in turn would affect an improvement of his physical condition, the physician, or the lay healer, must win the complete confidence, as well as the undivided attention, of the sick person—and that this personal relationship between the patient and physician was brought about by a physical contact. (Plutarch, for instance, records that Pyrrhus of Epirus cured cases of colic by touching the sufferer with his big toe!). Jesus of Nazareth, intuitively one of the greatest of psychologists, firmly believed in the method of laying on of hands. His remarkable cures are still attributed to Divine intervention by vast numbers of people; but at the same time it must be recognized that His own conviction that He would cure the sick was so unshakable and so compelling that His very presence must have had an hypnotic effect on the patient. And He awakened in His disciples, who were to act as healers after him, that perfect confidence, needed by all mental healers, that they would indeed cure the sick; and their conviction, in turn, was transferred to the sick who came to them. Jesus said to them, in the Gospel according to St. Mark, "Go ye into all the world, and preach the gospel to the whole creation; . . . in my name shall they cast out devils; they shall speak with new tongues; . . . and if they drink any deadly things, it shall in no wise hurt them; they shall lay hands on the sick, and they shall recover."

Jesus' cures were in some ways more remarkable than any cures by suggestion of modern psychologists or lay healers. The sufferer's faith in Him, His own conviction that He would cure them, made the establishment of a suggestive atmosphere unnecessary. Mesmer, on the other hand, treated his patients in a darkened room and used complicated "magnetic" equipment. In-

deed, the setting of Mesmer's seances were magnificent and impressive: darkened rooms, soft music, hushed voices, an atmosphere of unreality, heightened his patient's expectancy, their confidence that they would be cured. Mesmer and his assistant wore silk purple coats and carried long wands of beautifully wrought iron, with which they lightly touched the diseased portions of the sufferer's body. The patients sat breathless around a tub filled with perfumed water that also contained magnetic filings so that the patients would be ready to receive the magnetism from the planets. It was the setting of quackery, the acts of the charlatan—yet, it was the origins of modern hypnosis as we know it today, the shadowy no-man's-land which still exists between the charlatan and the conventional therapist. Mesmer's Magnetic Institute in Paris attracted hundreds of the idle rich and was castigated as a hotbed of immorality, and he was eventually banished from the French capital to Switzerland. Yet, there can be no question that in those darkened rooms Mesmer achieved success in relieving the hysterical symptoms of susceptible young females, nor that Mesmer's inadvertent use of hypnotic suggestion led the way to Bernheim and Freud.

In fact, Mesmer's interpretation of "animal magnetism" marked the beginning of mental therapy as we understand it today. Margaret Goldsmith has written, in her book, *Franz Anton Mesmer: The History of an Idea*, "He himself was not a man of sufficient vision to bring his ideas to their scientific conclusion, but he was a great man, for, as an English scientist has pointed out, 'it requires genius to create a subject as a distinct topic of thought.' He deserves all the more credit, because, during the eighteenth century, the belief that the mind can influence the body was being vigorously suppressed. With the growing understanding of drugs, any methods reminiscent of medieval superstition were considered unscientific, and medical men as a whole were intellectual parvenus who clung tenaciously to their knowledge of chemistry. . . . It was chiefly due to Mesmer and his disciples that the power of the mind over the body was slowly emancipating itself from a belief in cures by magic or religion to a more scientific outlook. His theories bridged the gap between ancient superstitions and modern psychotherapy."

The February, 1980, issue of *Survey of Anesthesiology* republished the introductory monograph from Gilbert Frankau's treatise on Mesmer and Mesmerism (Frankau, G.: *Mesmerism.* London: MacDonald, 1948); reprinted below is the second half of Frankau's volume, the translation (the first in English) of Mesmer's own dissertation, *Mémoire sur la découverte du Magnétisme Animal*, which had first been printed at Geneva in 1779.

MESMERISM

G. FRANKAU

MacDonald, London, 1948

DISSERTATION ON THE DISCOVERY OF ANIMAL MAGNETISM

On reading this dissertation, it is apparent that Dr. Mesmer had great difficulty in convincing his peers of the validity of his concepts of curing diseases of the nervous system. The bulk of it is concerned with the trials and tribulations he encountered in trying to refute the pronouncements made against him.

And yet he persisted in his endeavors and continued to treat patients with diverse signs and symptoms, some with apparent success. It is a good question, though, as to whether he created more controversies than cures. Of his sincerity and personal beliefs there seems little doubt.

Published June, 1981

The first recorded pediatric anesthesia was administered on July 3rd, 1842, when Crawford W. Long etherized a young boy with a disease of the toe which necessitated its amputation. The operation was performed without the boy evincing the least evidence of response, and he subsequently stated to Sabrey Hemphill that Dr. Long had cut off his toe without his suffering any pain in the operation.

Five years later, the first textbook of anesthesia, John Snow's "On the Inhalation of the Vapour of Ether," documented Snow's own initial administration of a pediatric anesthesia. This occurred at St. George's Hospital in London on January 28, 1847, when Mr. Caesar Hawkins removed dead bone from the interior of the tibia of William Daphne, aged 6. Young William made a satisfactory recovery and was discharged from the hospital on March 10, 1847.

Pediatric anesthesia as a discipline, however, did not begin to emerge for another hundred years. Prior to World War II, there was not a single pediatric anesthesiologist in this country, and there were only 2 in Canada. Indeed, at the time when Dr. Robert Gross performed his pioneering surgery for ligation of a patent ductus ar-

teriosus at Boston Children's Hospital in 1938 (which was the first successful operation for a congenital heart defect), it was sometimes necessary to call in a resident from the ENT Department to insert the endotracheal tube.

The phenomenal growth of anesthesiology following World War II also included the appearance of the pediatric anesthesiologist. Pediatric surgery was in full flower as a distinct field of endeavor, and these surgeons were technically able to perform more extensive and more difficult operations on ever sicker and smaller patients. The anesthesia requirements for these procedures soon surpassed the skills and experience of the anesthesiologist who administered only occasional pediatric anesthesia, and this inevitably led to the development of Departments of Anesthesiology at various children's hospitals about the country, and the formation of divisions, or sections, of pediatric anesthesia at a number of university medical centers. Knowledge of the often vast differences in the anatomy, physiology, metabolism, and psychology of these little patients, as compared with adults, became recognized, and new techniques and approaches were developed that were based on this knowledge.

Training programs were established and residents were recruited into the blossoming subspecialty; increasing numbers of papers dealing with pediatric anesthesia began to appear in anesthesia, surgical, and pediatric journals. A Section on Anesthesia was formed within the American Academy of Pediatrics and became the first formal subspecialty group within organized anesthesiology. And not least importantly, 3 textbooks devoted entirely to pediatric anesthesia were published: "Pediatric Anesthesia" (Leigh and Belton) in 1948; "Elements of Pediatric Anesthesia" (Stephen) in 1954; and "Anesthesia for Infants and Children" (Smith) in 1959.

The authors of 2 of these textbooks, Dr. C. Ronald Stephen and Dr. Robert M. Smith, 2 of the premier pioneers in the field of pediatric anesthesia, retired during the past year. Between them, they have made some 1134 presentations to medical audiences on the subject of—and in behalf of—pediatric anesthesia; they have published (in addition to their 2 textbooks, one of which is in its second edition and the other in its fourth edition) a total of 352 papers, comments, abstracts, book reviews, editorials, pamphlets and the like; they have taught uncounted numbers of students, interns, fellows, residents, and peers about pediatric anesthesia; and they have probably, through those teachings, made the ordeals of anesthesia and operation less terrifying, less painful, safer, and more bearable for literally millions of young patients. They exemplify the best that the pediatric anesthesiologist can provide. It has been said that, "In spite of new concepts, the day-to-day conduct of pediatric anesthesia is still as much of an artistic endeavor as it is a scientific and technical exercise"; and, indeed, to watch either of these 2 masters give anesthesia is to watch a work of art unfolding.

Pediatric anesthesia, circa 1946, was induced with an ether cone, a few layers of gauze, a can of ether, and then became a matter of devil-take-the-hindmost, as anyone who has conducted anesthesia for T & A with an ether hook can vouch. It was not a pretty sight—esthetically, psychologically, physiologically, or biochemically.

Today, concerns in pediatric anesthesia encompass such important matters as cardiovascular physiology, fluid balance, metabolism, endocrine responses, sophisticated monitoring, and genetic influences. It is simply assumed that airway and respiratory integrity are assured, and that assumption is usually well grounded. There can be no acceptable pediatric anesthesia without complete control of airway and total reliance on the adequacy of both O_2 delivery and CO_2 removal. It was not always thus.

Stephen and Smith both appreciated the fact that the security of the airway and the integrity of respiratory exchange were often lacking during pediatric anesthesia in the early days, and both men played significant roles in ameliorating the situation. In 1948, Stephen (with his colleague Slater) published a landmark article (it was really just a short piece in the "Current Comment and Case Reports" section of *Anesthesiology*), which was a crucial step in the development of the concept of inhalation systems for neonates, infants, and small children assuring the complete removal of CO_2 and at the same time not adding to the work of breathing (Stephen, C. R., and Slater, H. M.: A nonresisting, nonrebreathing valve. *Anesthesiology, 9:* 550, 1948). There was also at this time much opposition to tracheal intubation, and Smith made a significant contribution when he published an unanswerable paper stressing the importance of careful technique and sterile apparatus in the prevention of postintubation sequelae (Smith, R. M.: The prevention of tracheitis in children following endotracheal anesthesia. *Anesth. Analg., 32:* 102, 1953). Both papers contributed handsomely to the homeostasis of the anesthesized pediatric patient and are reprinted below, in chronologic order, with the kind permissions of the authors and the publishers.

A NONRESISTING, NONREBREATHING VALVE

C. R. STEPHEN

AND

H. M. SLATER

Department of Anaesthesia,
Children's Memorial Hospital,
Montreal, Quebec

Anesthesiology, 9: 550, 1948

and

THE PREVENTION OF TRACHEITIS IN CHILDREN FOLLOWING ENDOTRACHEAL ANESTHESIA

ROBERT M. SMITH

The Children's Medical Center,
Boston, Massachusetts

Anesth. Analg., 32: 102, 1953

The mistakes which must be avoided to reduce the incidence of tracheitis include:

1) Mechanical trauma;
   a) use of large, heavy laryngoscopes,
   b) use of larger than necessary endotracheal tubes,
   c) unnecessary roughness
   d) intubation while the child is inadequately relaxed,
   e) faulty positioning of the head,
   f) difficult intubation due to anatomic abnormalities,
   g) continued motion of the tube during anesthesia, and
   g) drying of the mucosa as in nonrebreathing or insufflation techniques.

2) Chemical trauma; avoid use of lubricants on tubes,

3) Contamination:
   a) inadequate cleansing of tubes and laryngoscopes,
   b) improper storage after cleansing,
   c) contamination of tubes immediately prior to use,
   d) use of contaminated lubricants, and
   e) intubation in the presence of upper respiratory infection.

1949

Published June, 1977

There are those who claim—and not without a certain amount of justification—that the origins of regional anesthesia can be traced back to about 3000 B.C., when the use of acupuncture for the treatment of various diseases began to be practised in China. Purists, however, will argue the matter and will pinpoint the date as 1853 A.D., which was the year in which Alexander Wood invented the modern metallic hollow needle in Scotland, and Charles Gabriel Pravaz invented the hypodermic syringe in France. There were intermediary steps along the way between 3000 B.C. and 1853 A.D., of course, such as Sigmund Elsholm in the 17th century and others who attempted to inject opiate in the vicinity of nerves and painful areas in order to relieve pain; but for all practical purposes, the introduction of the syringe and needle must be considered *the* early milestone in the development of conduction anesthesia.

Even in 1853, though, there still was no true local anesthetic drug for the production of regional anesthesia; and the efforts to treat disorders were made by injecting solutions of opiates, of chloroform, of bromides, of tannin, and of other compounds near nerve trunks, with variable degrees of success. In point of fact, it was more than 4 decades after the inventions of the hollow needle and the syringe that a *bona fide* local anesthetic agent was discovered—and then it was discovered by the unlikely collaboration of the man who was to become the Father of Psychoanalysis with another man who was to become one of the leading ophthalmologists in New York City.

Sigmund Freud was primarily interested in the general physiologic effects of cocaine; and more particularly he had employed it, with marked lack of success, in an attempt to cure the morphine addiction of a brilliant young physiologist who had resorted to the poppy to relieve the agony of the neuromata in the stump of his amputated thumb. Carl Koller, a friend of Freud's who was a recent graduate of the medical school of the University of Vienna, and an intern and House Surgeon at the Allgemeines Krankenhaus, was on the other hand interested in finding a substance which would render the cornea of the eye insensitive. Together they carried out numerous experiments with cocaine, identifying the numbing effects when crystals of the substance were placed on the tip of the tongue, and confirming by measurements with a dynamometer that the drug increased physical tolerance to muscular work—a fact which had, of course, been appreciated by the Indians of the Andes mountains in Peru for centuries.

Although Freud's earliest contributions to the medical literature were on the subject of cocaine, and although he recognized the local anesthetizing power of cocaine and its salts, he remained primarily concerned with the general actions of the drug. Nevertheless, Freud might still have been credited with the introduction of cocaine as a local anesthetic drug if the gonadotropic fantasies of his deep subconscious id had not led him off on a long walking tour with his fiancee, the clinical details of which are not available in English translation.

Koller, on the other hand, remained at home in Vienna and continued his experiments in the laboratory on the anesthetic effects of cocaine. He applied a few drops of cocaine solution to an animal's eye, and

stimulated the cornea with the head of a pin: there was no reflex closing of the eyelids, there was no movement of the eyeball, and the animal's head was not jerked backwards. Next he pricked and scratched the cornea with a needle, and there still was no response. He irritated the cornea with a powerful electric current, and the animal continued to be unconcerned. He cauterized the cornea with a silver nitrate pencil until it became milky white, but the animal did not betray any distress. It was time to make the crucial experiment on the eye of a man—naturally, Koller's own eye. (The Walter Reed Society is mis-named: it should be the Carl Koller Society.)

Koller was not present at the Congress of Ophthalmology which was convened in Heidelberg on September 15, 1884, but his friend Josef Brettauer of Trieste carried in his pocket to Heidelberg a brief communication and a vial of cocaine solution forwarded by Koller. The demonstration which Brettauer conducted on a patient from the Heidelberg Clinic was the sensation of the Congress. He instilled a few drops of the cocaine solution into the eye, pressed a probe into the cornea until its surface was indented, seized the conjunctiva with fixation forceps, and moved the globe in all directions. The experiment was repeated the following day, and the second patient also declared that he felt nothing. A thrill was felt by every ophthalmologist in attendance at the Congress, for this gift was the most significant that the specialty had received since Helmholtz presented them with the ophthalmoscope. The era of local anesthesia had arrived, and there would no longer be any operating on the eye of a writhing, screaming patient.

The news from the Heidelberg Congress spread like wildfire throughout the surgical world, and within a matter of weeks (9, to be precise) Dr. William C. Burke, Jr., of South Norwalk, Connecticut, had described the injection of cocaine solution under the skin for the performance of minor surgery; and 4 days later Dr. Richard John Hall of New York City published a report of the experiments which he and the great surgical giant, Dr. William Stewart Halsted, had conducted to produce direct nerve block by the use of the injection of cocaine into their own tissues.

There is absolutely no question that Halsted became a cocaine addict as the result of his self-experimentation. That is about the only dogmatic statement which can be made authoritatively about Halsted's addiction—after that it becomes a question of which book do you read, and which one do you believe? It says right here in this biographical account, for instance, that Halsted was the only man to ever overcome his cocaine addiction. It also says right here, in this other biographical sketch, that Halsted only conquered his cocaine addiction by becoming a morphine addict. An there is even the story—possibly apochryphal—that Halsted's morphine addiction set American Surgery back 50 years by slowing his performance of surgery down so much that The Halsted Technique of dissecting every fiber and tying every capillary (which was mimicked in every medical school in the country) added hours and even days to the surgical schedule.

The only indisputable fact is that cocaine addictions, cocaine toxicity, and cocaine reactions led to feverish attempts to discover newer local anesthetic drugs with no addictive properties, lesser toxicities, and fewer reactions. An unholy number of "caines" were synthesized, tested, and marketed in the next 60 years, but the really important one was procaine (Novocaine), which was synthesized by Einhorn in 1904 and introduced clinically by Braun the following year. There were other drugs, of course, which made their mark; but procaine remained the standard by which all others were compared for a long period of time. Its position as The Leader was not really challenged until the appearance of Xylocaine (lidocaine), which was synthesized by Lofgren and Lundqvist at Stockholm University in 1943, and introduced clinically by Dr. Torsten Gordh in a paper titled, "Xylocain—A New Local Analgesic," which was published in the January, 1949, issue of *Anaesthesia* (*4:* 4–9, 21, 1949), and is republished below with the kind permissions of the author and the publishers.

XYLOCAIN—A NEW LOCAL ANALGESIC

T. Gordh

Department of Anaesthesia, Karolinska Hospital Stockholm, Sweden

Anaesthesia, 4: 4–9, 21, 1949

Xylocaine (lidocaine), a new local anesthetic, w-diethylamino-2.6-dimethylacetanilide, has been subject to trials since 1944.

Clinical investigation began with wheal tests. The different lidocaine solutions (0.5, 1.0 and 2.0 per cent) were tested parallel with procaine and tetracaine. A subcutaneous injection of 1.0 ml. was given. No local reaction was observed. Whereas a 1.0 per cent procaine solution with epinephrine had a duration of action of 60 to 90 minutes, the analgesia produced by 1.0 per cent lidocaine with epinephrine lasted 4 to 5 hours.

For infiltration anesthesia in the emergency department in 400 patients, the amount injected varied from two to 50 ml. of 1.0 per cent solution. The full effect was usually attained within two minutes. No toxic reactions were observed.

For surgery, the drug with epinephrine 1:100,000 was used in goitre operations (80 patients), hernia operations (95), and for infiltration anesthesia along the incision line. Analgesia developed within two minutes and lasted for three to eight hours.

Conduction analgesia was evaluated with mandibular, brachial plexus, sacral and paravertebral blocks. The average dose was 10 to 15 ml. of 2.0 per cent solution with or without epinephrine. Analgesia set in within five to ten minutes and usually lasted 2.5 to 8 hours.

For spinal block, lidocaine 2.0 per cent with 10 per cent glucose produced rapid and satisfactory analgesia for perineal operations.

For surface analgesia, lidocaine is much less toxic than tetracaine and is free from irritation.

With respect to toxicity, the safety coefficient for lidocaine is two to four times higher than for procaine, and five to 10 times higher than for tetracaine.

The recommended dose of lidocaine is a maximum of 0.5 to 1.0 gram. For infiltration analgesia, 0.5 per cent solution is suitable, while for conduction analgesia 1.0 to 2.0 per cent solutions are sufficient. When amounts used were less than 1.0 gram, no toxic reactions were observed.

1950

Published October and December, 1968

Man's utilization of the numbing effects of cold upon physiologic processes is scarcely new. Hippocrates (of Cos) advocated the use of snow and ice to stem hemorrhage, and was well aware of the analgesic nature of cold. The use of cold for refrigeration anesthesia was also employed sporadically both during the Renaissance and subsequently, the most celebrated instance being by Napoleon's Surgeon-General, Baron Larrey, who had noticed that there was no pain during amputations performed on soldiers who had lain on the battlefield at low environmental temperatures.

The concept of total body hypothermia, as contrasted to refrigeration anesthesia, dates back to the time of the illustrious John Hunter, who attempted to freeze carp to a state of suspended animation. Hunter was not successful, and about all that he garnered for his troubles was a witty and satirical piece on the subject in the *Publick Advertiser* of 1770 by James Boswell, Samuel Johnson's famous biographer, entitled, "On The New Freezing Discovery."

Suspended animation has long held man's imagination, however, and total body hypothermia has always appeared to be a reasonable approach to the concept. It was, therefore, not to be unexpected, perhaps, that the technique would be applied to man—at least if one can believe the Bellows Falls, Vermont, *Argus and Patriot,* which published "A Strange Tale" in 1887:

"I am an old man now, and have seen some strange sights in the course of a roving life, but none so strange as one I found recorded in an old diary, kept by my Uncle William that came into my possession at his decease. The events described took place in a mountain town some twenty miles from Montpelier, the Capital of Vermont. I have been to the place on the mountain, and seen the old loghouse where the events I found recorded took place, and seen and talked with an old man who vouched for the truth of the story, and that his father was one of the parties operated on. The account ran in this wise:

"'January 7.—I went on the mountain today, and witnessed what to me was a horrible sight. It seems that the dwellers there, who are unable, either from age or other reasons, to contribute to the support of their families, are disposed of in the winter months in a manner that will shock the one who reads this, unless that person lives in that vicinity. I will describe what I saw. Six persons, four men and two women, one of the men a cripple about 30 years old, the other five past the age of usefulness, lay on the earthy floor of the cabin drugged into insensibility, while members of their families were gathered about them in apparent indifference. In a short time the bodies were inspected by several old people, who said, "They are ready."

"'It was night when the bodies were carried out, and the full moon shone on their ghastly faces, and a horrible fascination kept me by the bodies as long as I could endure the severe cold. Soon the noses, ears and fingers began to turn white, then the limbs and face assumed a tallowy look.

I could stand the cold no longer, and went inside, where I found the friends in cheerful conversation. . . .

"'January 8—Day came at length, but did not dissipate the terror that filled me. . . . After breakfast the men lighted their pipes, and some of them took a yoke of oxen and went off toward the forest, while others proceeded to nail together boards, making a box about ten feet long and half as high and wide. When this was completed they placed about two feet of straw in the bottom; then they laid three of the frozen bodies on the straw. Then the bodies were covered with a cloth, then more straw was put in the box, and the other three bodies placed on top and covered the same as the first ones. Boards were then firmly nailed on the top, to protect the bodies from being injured by carnivorous animals that make their home on these mountains.

"'By this time the men who went off with the ox-team returned with a huge load of spruce and hemlock boughs, which they unloaded at the foot of a steep ledge; came to the house and loaded the box containing the bodies on the sled, and drew it to the foot of the ledge, near the load of boughs. These were soon piled on and around the box, and it was left to be covered up with snow, which I was told would lay in drafts twenty feet deep over this rude tomb. "We shall want our men to plant our corn next spring", said a youngish looking woman, the wife of one of the frozen men, "and if you want to see them resuscitated you come here about the 10th of next May". . . .

"'May 10.—I arrived here at 10 A.M. after riding about four hours over muddy, unsettled roads. . . . We repaired at once to the well remembered spot, at the ledge. The snow had melted from the top of the brush but still lay deep around the bottom of the pile. The men commenced work at once, some shoveling away the snow, and others carrying away the brush. Soon the box was visible. The cover was taken off, the layers of straw removed, and the bodies, frozen and apparently lifeless, lifted out and laid on the snow. Large troughs made out of hemlock logs were placed near by, filled with tepid water, into which the bodies were separately placed, with the head

slightly raised. Boiling water was then poured into the troughs from kettles hung on poles near by . . . a slight twitching of the muscles of the face and limbs, followed by audible gasps, showed that life was not quenched, and that vitality was returning. Spirits were then given in small quantities, and allowed to trickle down their throats. Soon they could swallow, and more was given them, when their eyes opened, and they began to talk, and finally sat up. They were then taken out and assisted to the house, where after a hearty dinner they seemed as well as ever, and in nowise injured, but rather refreshed, by their long sleep.'"

By the time that this apocryphal yarn had been reprinted in *New England Journeys* by the Ford Motor Company in 1953, two authoritative papers had been published which established the rational medical use of cold. The first of these, a masterpiece of clinical logic, introduced the use of hypothermia in cardiac surgery; while the second provided the laboratory documentation which proved the clinical logic. It would be inappropriate to publish the one without the other. In this issue of *Survey*, therefore, is reprinted "Anesthetic Problems in Cardiac Surgery in Children" by William O. McQuiston, M.D. (*Anesthesiology, 10:* 590–600, 1949); while the December 1968 issue will reprint "Oxygen Transport and Utilization in Dogs At Low Body Temperatures" by W. G. Bigelow, M.D., W. K. Lindsay, M.D., R. C. Harrison, M.D., R. A. Gordon, M.D. and W. F. Greenwood, M.D. (*Am. J. Physiol., 160:* 125–137, 1950). Both are republished with the kind permissions of the authors and the publishers.

ANESTHETIC PROBLEMS IN CARDIAC SURGERY IN CHILDREN

McQuiston, W. O.

Anesthesiology 10:590–600, 1949

A report of the first 142 Potts operations on 140 infants with cyanotic congenital heart disease performed by two highly skilled surgeons and one clinically astute anesthesiologist. In addition to the use of topical hypothermia, the author recommended heavy morphine premedication, controlled respiration with cyclopropane, and atropine for bradycardia—all radical departures from the conventions of the time.

OXYGEN TRANSPORT AND UTILIZATION IN DOGS AT

LOW BODY TEMPERATURE

BIGELOW, W. G., ET AL

Am. J. Physiol. 160:125–137, 1950

Anesthetized dogs were placed in a refrigerated room and their rectal temperatures reduced to 18°C. The correlation between decreased oxygen consumption and decreased rectal temperature in the absence of shivering was nicely demonstrated.

Published August, 1965

The road leading to an understanding of the pathways of barbiturate metabolism has been long, circuitous, and, at times, difficult to see clearly. It now appears that there are at least several chemical reactions, rather than a single common one, involved in the detoxification of these drugs.

The first of these is oxidation of substituents in position 5 of the barbiturate ring, which may result in a ketone, an alcohol, or an acid. The brominated barbiturate propallynol (Nostal) is oxidized to ketopropallynol, and butallylonal (Pernoston) to ketobutallylonal. Ketone-like oxidation of a sulfur atom on the side chain can also occur, as in the metabolism of methitural (Neraval) to methitural sulfoxide. Metabolic oxidation to a ketone can be demonstrated, too, in barbiturates possessing a ring structure (rather than a straight chain) as a substituent in position 5: cyclobarbital (Phanodorn) is oxidized to ketocyclobarbtal, heptabarbital (Medomin) is oxidized to ketoheptabarbital, hexobarbital (Evipal) is oxidized to ketohexobarbital, and thialbarbitone (Kemithal) is oxidized to ketothialbarbitone. Side chain oxidation to form an alcohol occurs in the metabolism of pentobarbital (Nembutal) to pentobarbital alcohol, secobarbital (Seconal) to secobarbital alcohol, methohexital (Brevital) to methohexital alcohol (at least in animals), phenobarbital (Luminal) to p-hydroxyphenobarbital, and the antiepilepsy agent primidone (Mysoline) to phenobarbital. Side chain oxidation to form a carboxylic acid occurs in the metabolism of the thiobarbiturates

(such as Pentothal) and pentobarbital (Nembutal).

A second type of chemical reaction that occurs in the detoxification of barbiturates is N-demethylation of one or both of the nitrogen atoms in positions 1 and 3, such as the demethylation of mephobarbital (Mebaral) to phenobarbital and the demethylation of hexobarbital to norhexobarbital. However, these demethylated metabolites retain considerable pharmacologic activity.

A third type of chemical reaction, which resembles N-demethylation of an N-methylbarbiturate (in that the resultant metabolite retains pharmacologic activity) is the conversion of a thiobarbiturate to form the corresponding oxybarbiturate. Thus thiopental is desulfurated to form pentobarbital, thiobutabarbital to form butabarbital (Butisol), and thiobarbital to form barbital.

A fourth type of chemical reaction is hydrolytic cleavage of the barbituric acid ring. Ring cleavage, or hydrolytic opening of the barbiturate ring, has been demonstrated with pentobarbital, amobarbital, cyclobarbital, thiopental, thialbarbitone, and hexobarbital.

A fifth type of chemical reaction is 5-dealkylation, on removal of either of the two substituents from postion 5 of the barbiturate nucleus, which results in a pharmacologically inactive metabolite. This occurs with barbital, cyclobarbital, and seconal.

A final postulated chemical reaction in the detoxification of barbiturates is Nmethylation, or the attachment of a methyl group to one of the nitrogen atoms in position 1 or 3. There is as yet no clear-cut evidence that this occurs in the detoxification of barbiturates in man, and there is only a possibility that, if it does occur, it is an important part of the detoxification process.

This considerable body of knowledge concerning the metabolism of the barbiturates has been built up painstakingly over the course of a number of years. At the time that the thiobarbiturates were introduced into clinical anesthetic practice in the 1930's, a good deal less was known about the fate of the barbiturates, and it was considered that they were ultra short acting because they were detoxified by the body with extreme rapidity. There were, however, certain clinical facts that did not conform to this theory. It was true that thiopental would produce anesthesia of only short duration following the administration of a small dose, and in that respect the drug appeared to be short acting. How-

ever, if the patient was maintained under prolonged anesthesia by successive injections of thiopental, the duration of the subsequent continuing narcosis was also prolonged; in other words, thiopental no longer behaved as an ultra short acting drug. This unpleasant fact, which did not fit in with the concept of rapid detoxification, was conveniently explained away by ascribing such unusual activity to the production and accumulation in the body of less active metabolic transformation products of thiopental which had a very long duration of anesthetic action and a slow rate of detoxification. These myths persisted until the publication of the studies of Brodie and his collegues, "The Fate of Thiopental in Man And A Method For Its Estimation in Biological Materials" (Brodie, B. B., Mark, L. C., Papper, E. M., Lief, P. A., Bernstein, E. and Rovenstine, E. A.: *J. Pharmacol. & Exper. Therap., 98:* 85, 1950), which is reprinted below with the kind permission of the authors and publishers.

THE FATE OF THIOPENTAL IN MAN AND A METHOD FOR ITS ESTIMATION IN BIOLOGICAL MATERIALS*

BERNARD B. BRODIE, LESTER C. MARK,
E. M. PAPPER, PHILIP A. LIEF,
ELEONORE BERNSTEIN AND
E. A. ROVENSTINE

Research Service, Third
(New York University) Medical
Division, Goldwater Memorial
Hospital, Department of Anesthesiology,
New York University-Bellevue
Medical Center and Department of
Biochemistry, New York University
College of Medicine,
New York, N.Y.

J. Pharmacol. & Therap., 98: 85–96, 1950

*   *   *   *

SUMMARY

"1. Methods are described for the estimation of Pentothal and a metabolite of Pentothal in biological fluids and tissues. The method for Pentothal is specific in that metabolic products of the drug are not included in the measurement.

"2. A major step in the metabolism of Pentothal after its intravenous administration to man is oxidation on one of its alkyl side chains to yield a carboxylic acid. This compound, which has been isolated in pure form, has identical ultraviolet properties with that of the parent drug. It has little if any anesthetic activity.

"3. Although Pentothal is transformed almost completely in the body, the rate of this transformation is slow in man, about 15 percent per hour, and even slower in dogs. The rapid decline in plasma levels and quick recovery following a single intravenous dose is probably due to the drug leaving the body fluids and being deposited in the fat.

"4. There is a marked decrease in plasma levels of Pentothal in dogs as the pH is lowered by carbon dioxide inhalation."

Published August, 1959

Almost simultaneously with Morton's classic public demonstration of the clinical efficacy of ether anesthesia on October 16th, 1846, anesthetists became cognizant of the fact that there were varying degrees, or stages, of anesthesia, and that these could be correlated with the amount of ether that had been inhaled. *The Lancet*, on Saturday, January 16, 1847, editorialized: "The insensibility produced by etherization appears to be of a peculiar kind, and to vary considerably in different individuals. In some cases, there is perfect insensibility to pain, and entire loss of consciousness; in others, the operation is felt, and the patient is aware of the different steps of the proceeding, but the pain is extremely slight, merely a sensation of scratching; while some describe the etherized condition as one of partial consciousness of the most exhilarating and agreeable kind; and a few describe their sensations as almost similar to those produced by the inhalation of the nitrous oxide gas; and there are cases in which it appears to act as a violent stimulant, or else it does not act at all. The form of insensibility will have to be examined hereafter by therapeutists, and the etherous inhalation will take its proper place amongst anodyne or narcotic remedies. Probably, the variations observed in different persons may depend, in some measure, on the amount of etherous vapor inhaled, rather than on differences in constitution. . . ."

Two weeks later, in the January 30, 1847, issue of *The Lancet*, Francis Plomley described one of the earliest classifications of depth of anesthesia, which was based in large measure on subjective mental sensations: "I have breathed the ether on several occasions and think its effects may be divided into three stages or degrees. The first is merely a pleasurable feeling of half intoxication; the second is one of extreme pleasure, being similar to the sensations produced by breathing nitrous oxide, or laughing gas; there exists in this stage a perfect consciousness of everything said or done, but generally an incapability of motion; in this stage, also, there is not exactly an insensibility to pain, but rather an indifference, 'a care for nothing sort of feeling;' and if surgical operations are done in this stage the patients almost always recover before the operations are completed, and the results are unsatisfactory. There can be no doubt that most of the failures may be attributed to this cause. . . .

"The third stage, the only one, I think, for performing operations in, is one of profound intoxication and insensibility. The individual is completely lost to pain, and to external impression; the muscles become prostrate, the circulation lessens, and the temperature falls, but the mind is often reveling in the most pleasurable regions, as in a dream, this, no doubt, depending much upon the temperament of the individual, and probably, also, on the physical effects of the operation on the nerves, as very often there is a considerable moaning, and an attempt to move, when under the influence of the knife."

Plomley's classification, dependent as it was mainly on subjective mental sensations, was not of great value in the clinical estimation of depth of anesthesia. The ever-astute John Snow recognized this fact and turned to objective observations of the anesthetized patient, since "the point requiring most skill and care in the administration of the vapour of ether, is undoubtedly, to determine when it has been carried far enough." Snow's classification divided the course of etherization into five degrees and was based upon the anesthetist's use of his own five senses and powers of observation to appraise the depth of anesthesia. The first degree was characterized by retention of consciousness, orientation, and ability to perform voluntary movements, and was not considered by Snow to be practicable for surgery. (However, it is worth noting that Snow observed that once patients had been anesthetized in deeper degrees and subsequently lightened to the first degree, "they are not infrequently free of the pain of an operation which is still

going on, at a time when the mental facilities have returned, together with the special senses of sight and hearing.") The second degree was recognized by the exercise of mental function and voluntary actions performed in a disordered manner and guided by instinct rather than reason. In the third degree, "there is no evidence of any mental function being exercised and consequently no voluntary motions occur." The breathing was deep and regular, and the pupils either stationary or exhibited voluntary motions, but an active lid reflex was retained. The fourth degree was characterized by an absence of all movements except those of respiration, and "an appearance is met with that would be truely alarming if we did not know that it was only due to an agent which is flying away every moment in the breath to leave the patient in a few minutes, without any permanent trace of its having been there." The fifth degree was associated with difficult, feeble, or irregular breathing, followed by paralysis of respiratory movements. Snow did not believe that this last degree was observed in the human.

Snow's classification of the depth of anesthesia, which relied upon the anesthetist's objective observations of physical signs in his patient, has been improved upon, but never fully replaced, during the course of the last hundred years. Many anesthetists have contributed to the development of this classification of depth of anesthesia during the past hundred years, but it was Guedel who finally achieved the ultimate classification of this type, and set down his now world-famous "guide posts" of the depth of anesthesia, which divided anesthesia into four stages, further divided the third stage into four planes, and provided a list of the physical signs characteristic of each stage or plane.

An entirely new approach to the problem of depth of anesthesia was developed by the introduction of electroencephalography as a tool for the anesthetist. Neurologists, laboratory workers and electroencephalographers themselves had, of course, made several studies of the effects of the various anesthetic agents upon electroencephalographic patterns; but it was the group at the Mayo Clinic, which included Raymond F. Courtin, Reginald G. Bickford, and Albert Faulconer, Jr., which made the first serious classification of the depth of anesthesia based upon electroencephalographic patterns, published in the *Proceedings of the Staff Meetings of the Mayo Clinic, 25:* 197–206, April 12, 1950, under the title, "The Classification and Significance of Electro-encephalographic Patterns Produced by Nitrous Oxide-Ether Anesthesia During Surgical Operations."

THE CLASSIFICATION AND SIGNIFICANCE OF ELECTRO-ENCEPHALOGRAPHIC PATTERNS PRODUCED BY NITROUS OXIDE-ETHER

Published April, 1964

The coincidence of identical results produced from simultaneous, but totally independent, investigations by different groups of workers has been remarked upon before in these columns. In point of fact, the coincidence is often more apparent than real, and is usually due to an almost inexorable train of events that leads the same idea, or hypothesis, or imaginative step of deductive reasoning, to occur in two minds at almost the same moment in time. Several examples of this process in action have been seen within recent years in the work and studies that have led to shared Nobel Prizes by scientists from far-separated areas of the world: the emergence of specific facts, data, or knowledge has led them, inevitably but quite separately, to investigations culminating in the same or related conclusions. The discovery of anesthesia was another clear example of this process.

The time was ripe in the eighteen-forties for the development of anesthesia, and it was more than coincidence that Crawford Long in Georgia, in 1842, and Horace Wells in Connecticut, in 1844, had independently, but through making similar chance observations, hit upon the idea of inhaling, in the one instance a vapor, in the

ANESTHESIA DURING SURGICAL OPERATIONS

COURTIN, R. F., BICKFORD, R. G.
AND
FAULCONER, A.

Proc. Staff, Mayo Clinic, 25: 197–206, 1950

Patients were studied during nitrous oxide-ether anesthesia. A consistent pattern of change was observed in the electroencephalogram. Seven levels were described, with the lowest one being complete suppression of any measurable brain-wave activity. These changes were a direct response to the depth of anesthesia and were compared to the peripheral signs of anesthesia generally in use at that time.

other instance a gas, to obtund surgical pain.

Long, the town physician of Jefferson, Georgia, was young enough to enter into the sport of the young men of the vicinity, and he participated in the "ether frolics" of the day in which an evening party was enlivened by the exhilarating effects of the inhalation of ether. He had noted bruises and other painful spots on his body subsequent to such ether inhalations, but had no recollection of having acquired such wounds. Further, he had observed that his friends, while etherized, received falls and blows which should have been sufficient to produce pain; yet on his careful questioning they assured him that they had not experienced the least discomfort from these accidents. Could not the same unawareness to pain as during an "ether frolic" also mitigate the pain of surgery? It could, and it did, during Long's removal of a tumor from the neck of James M. Venable on March 30, 1842.

Wells, a dentist in Hartford, Connecticut, had never heard of Crawford Long or his use of ether, but he came to the use of nitrous oxide for anesthesia in a remarkably similar fashion. He attended an exhibition in Hartford's Union Hall on December 10, 1844, which was put on by an itinerant showman, "Professor" Colton, to demonstrate the chemical wonders and marvels of the day. The high point of the show was a demonstration of the exhilarating effects of "laughing gas" when inhaled by several volunteers from the audience. One of these, a pharmacist's assistant by the name of Cooley, banged his leg badly while under the influence of the gas, yet expressed amazement when Wells pointed out the bloody bruise to him at the end of the exhibition. Wells in turn was amazed that the lad had not felt such an injury; and then he immediately perceived the application to dentistry—why couldn't a man have a tooth extracted under the gas and not feel it? He could, and the very next day Wells himself had his molar tooth removed while he slept tranquilly under the influence of Colton's nitrous oxide.

Thus, the very development of anesthesia itself represents an illustration of the coincidence of identical results produced from simultaneous, but totally independent, investigations by different groups of workers. A more recent example of this process in action in the field of anesthesia is provided by succinylcholine.

Succinylcholine, or diacetylcholine, was described by Hunt and Taveau back in 1911; but they were concerned chiefly with the toxicity and the effect upon blood pressure of the derivatives of choline and its analogues, and it was almost 40 years before the effect of succinylcholine at the myoneural junction was described—simultaneously, but totally independently, by two separate groups of workers thousands of miles apart. Bovet and his colleagues, working at the Instituto Superiore di Sanita in Rome, had noted, as had others, that the presence of two quaternary ammonium groups on a molecule was related to the substance's curarizing activity. They studied a number of aliphatic derivatives possessing two quaternary ammonium groups, among them succinylcholine, and in 1949 they reported the latter drug's paralyzing activity. At the same time, but again stimulated by the knowledge that the presence

of two quaternary nitrogens an optimal distance apart could confer powerful curare-like activity, another group of workers at the Wellcome Research Laboratories in Tuckahoe, New York, undertook to investigate the possibility of producing synthetic curare substitutes from aliphatic dicarboxylic acid aminoethyl esters. They were completely ignorant of Bovet's work when they began their studies; yet their first report, which was also published in 1949, by the chemist, Philipps, indicated that the bis-dimethyl-aminoethyl succinate bis-methiodide (succinylcholine) was the best of the compounds that they had synthesized and possessed potent neuromuscular blocking properties. The more complete report of their studies appeared after the publication of Bovet's original article, which they cited without making any reference to the simultaneous but independent nature of their own work. It was published under the title, "The Neuromuscular Blocking Action of Succinylcholine (Diacetylcholine)," in the *Journal of Pharmacology and Experimental Therapeutics* (Castillo, J. C., and de Beer, E. J.: *J. Pharmacol. & Exper. Therap.*, 99: 458–464, 1950), and is reprinted below.

THE NEUROMUSCULAR BLOCKING ACTION OF SUCCINYLCHOLINE (DIACETYLCHOLINE)

Julio C. Castillo
AND
Edwin J. de Beer

The Wellcome Research Laboratories, Tuckahoe, New York

J. Pharmacol. Exper. Therap., 99: 458–464, 1950

*   *   *   *

SUMMARY

"Succinylcholine (diacetylcholine) has been found to exhibit strong neuromuscular blocking action in the cat, rabbit and mouse but the paralysis is of relatively short duration. This action can be greatly prolonged by eserine and evidence is presented which suggests that the prolongation of

action is due, at least in part, to the inhibition by eserine of certain agents responsible for the inactivation of diacetylcholine."

Published June, 1964

Within the past few decades, a whole new school of medical writers, whose prototypes were Paul de Kruif, Logan Clendening and Howard Haggard, has appeared to explain Medicine to the public and dispel its mysteries. Lay magazines such as *Reader's Digest, Good Housekeeping, Life, McCall's, The Ladies' Home Journal,* and even *The New Yorker,* expound regularly on disease processes, describe the details of the most intricate surgical procedures, explain the advantages and disadvantages of the newest drugs, and advise the readers on the preferred mode of treatment for a specific pathologic condition, often before the reader's own physician has had access to the facts concerning the therapy in his medical journals. And there is nothing, absolutely nothing, that such writers enjoy more than a sensational bit of yellow journalism at Medicine's expense.

Anesthesia and Anesthesiology have come in for their share of such journalism.

For a little more than a year now the controversy over the alleged hepatotoxicity of halothane has raged in the pages of the lay press. Starting innocently as a few dormant sparks that were sporadic case reports in medical journals, it was fanned into a mild flame by two articles and an editorial in the March 7, 1963, issue of the *New England Journal of Medicine,* and then burst forth as an uncontrollable conflagration in *Time, Newsweek,* and newspapers throughout the country. Headlines in *The Wall Street Journal* screamed, "Doctors Debate Use Of Anesthetic Linked To Liver Disorders," and the text of the story continued:

"A 16-year-old girl, operated on in Sacramento, California, recently for a deep wrist cut, was recovering routinely six days later. Suddenly, however, she developed fever and other complications that resulted in her death 13 days after the surgery.

"An autopsy found four-fifths of the

girl's liver destroyed. To doctors at Sutter Community Hospitals in Sacramento the finding had grim overtones. In her operation the girl had been given Halothane, a potent new anesthetic; hers became the tenth reported case in which fatal liver damage had occurred in a surgical patient who had received halothane. In at least as many other instances, liver damage occurred but was not fatal."

Nowhere in the article, of course, did it point out that a direct cause and effect relationship had not been established. Nowhere did it mention that massive liver necrosis can follow surgery performed under any of the known anesthetic drugs. Nowhere did it indicate that a dozen other factors can be as important as, or even more important than, the anesthetic drug itself in the production of postoperative liver dysfunction. It pointed the finger directly at halothane, and left a Thalidomide-inflamed public to berate the anesthetic, whatever the truth may turn out to be in fact.

This is not the first time, of course, that anesthesia has supplied the yellow journalists with their copy. Ten years ago, *Time* blared the bold-print title, "Pain & Patient Killer," and then went on:

"Anesthesia has advanced far beyond the ether mask and morphine stage of 20 years ago. Today, during critical operations. *e.g.,* inside the heart, as many as eight different painkillers may be administered to ease the patient's lot and the surgeon's task. Even in minor surgery, drugs are used lavishly to prevent discomfort. But even the best of the new techniques carry their own hazards. Last week two top Boston anesthesia experts, Henry K. Beecher and Donald Todd, laid down evidence that modern anesthesia is killing not only pain but is still killing a shockingly high percentage of patients.

"Their findings, reported in the monthly

Annals of Surgery:

"Of 599,548 surgical patients studied in ten university hospitals over a five-year period (1948–1952), 384 died of anesthesia, a ratio of one death to 1,560 patients. Nearly one-fourth of all surgical deaths attributed to causes other than patients' own ailments were from anesthesia.

"The anesthesia mortality rate was higher among men than among women. Reason: men, the wage earners, tended to put off hospitalization until disease was advanced, were generally more susceptible to anesthesia's toxic effects because of heart and circulatory ailments.

"Most dangerous of the drugs is curare, a muscle relaxant better known as the poison with which South American Indians tip their arrows. It accounts for one-third of the deaths caused by anesthesia: one death per 370 patients. When used in combination with ether, curare becomes more hazardous, causing one death per 250 patients. Administered during major surgery, the curare death rate soared to one death out of 192 patients."

While the controversy over halothane may still be unresolved, the truth about curare is known: even *Time's* title was wrong, for curare is scarcely a "Pain Killer".

But over the years, one of the best anesthetic sources for lurid newspaper sensationalism has been the after-effects of spinal anesthesia. The famous "Wooley and Roe" case in England, which was tried in the High Courts of Justice in October 1953 provided endless copy, not only for the 11 days that the trial lasted, but also for long periods both before and thereafter. Even the straight-forward statement in the sedate *London Times* (October 20, 1953), "they became partially paralyzed for life following the administration of spinal anaesthetics at the Chesterfield Royal Hospital on October 13th, 1947," incensed the public; and the notorious British tabloids had a field day merely by quoting the plaintiff's testimonies verbatim:

"From the time of the operation I have had no control at all over my bowel functions. I am unconscious of any desire to evacuate, and the motion flows from me without my knowledge . . . my sensation ceases at the level of the lower chest, but during my treatment at the Wharncliffe Hospital at one stage I had spastic tremors in both legs which were so violent that I threw myself out of the chair and out of bed. The result was that I had to be tied down, and in order to obtain relief an operation was performed. When I am in bed in a lying position, I cannot sit up without assistance. When in a sitting position in bed, I do not lie down, I simply fall backwards. I cannot turn over. It is quite impossible for me to dress myself, I can only just manage to wash and shave myself, and of course, feed myself . . . ."

"Prior to the operation I led a very active existence, apart from my job. I have a big garden and spent a great deal of time in it where I grew my own vegetables and flowers. In addition I was a keen pigeon racer. I had about 24 pigeons and have won prizes over 50 and 600 mile distances. I won prizes and raced my pigeons right up to the time of my accident. It was my major hobby. I cannot continue because I cannot get in the cote to handle the birds or get about."

No one can fail to feel whole-hearted sympathy for the pitiful plight of these two helpless victims of a mishap, yet the Court's decision refused the yellow journalists' hue and cry for a blanket condemnation of spinal anesthesia as a technique. The concluding paragraph of Lord Justice Denning's judgment stated:

"These two men have suffered such terrible consequences that there is a natural feeling that they should be compensated. But we should be doing a disservice to the community at large if we were to impose liability on hospitals and doctors for everything that happens to go wrong. Doctors would be led to think more of their own safety than of the good of their patients. Initiative would be stifled and confidence shaken. A proper sense of proportion requires us to have regard to the condition in which hospitals and doctors have to work. We must insist on due care for the patient at every point, but we must not condemn as negligence that which is only misadventure."

This is not the attitude of the courts in the United States, unfortunately, for here the plaintiff is awarded the verdict on the basis of "res ipsa loquitur" (the condition speaks for itself) and not on the fact that the physician has been negligent. The effect of yellow journalism can be devastating in this country, therefore, and can play a major role in governing the choice of anesthesia in a given locality. When such a distinguished neurologist as Foster Kennedy published an article roundly condemning the use of spinal anesthesia in the October, 1950, issue of so respected a journal as *Surgery, Gynecology and Obstetrics*, it was a source of great concern and anguish to the anesthetic community. The lay press went wild. It assailed the use of spinal anesthesia with headlines the likes of, "Will You Be Paralyzed For Life?," and cowed anesthesiologists the country around. The neurologist's view of spinal anesthesia, of course, is beclouded by the fact that he sees those patients who have suffered unfortunate after-effects. The anesthesiologist, on the other hand, also sees the immense number of quite uneventful and successful spinal anesthesias, and he makes a mental comparison of the incidence of those few unfortunate mishaps with the possible morbidities and mortalities that can be expected following other types of anesthesia. Beecher came forward to make this very point in a carefully-worded reply to Kennedy's article:

"The authors certainly succeeded in reminding us that 'spinal anesthesia has many dangers, far too little appreciated by surgeons and anesthetists' (I would have been happier if the word 'some' had preceded 'surgeons and anesthetists.') There are numerous dangers associated with spinal anesthesia. I had supposed everybody was aware of them, but if not, a reminder is a good thing.

"There is, however, a fundamental difficulty here, it seems to me. To say that bad things can follow spinal anesthesia is to state the truth. What we all want to know is how often accidents occur. The article does make some attempt to describe the frequency of occurrence as reported by others, but we are left in the dark as to how many spinal anesthesias were in the pool from which these 12 serious complications drained.

"I could assemble 12 cases of serious central nervous damage following open drop ether, or following any commonly used anesthetic. The point is, how does the frequency of accident compare under the various agents. We don't really know . . ."

The article that stirred up this major controversy was entitled, "The Grave Spinal Cord Paralyses Caused by Spinal Anesthesia" (Kennedy, F., Effron, A. S., and Perry, G.: *Surg. Gynec. & Obst.*, 91: 385–398, 1950). It is reprinted below with the kind permission of the publishers.

THE GRAVE SPINAL CORD PARALYSES CAUSED BY SPINAL ANESTHESIA

Foster Kennedy, M.D., D.Sc., F.R.S. (Edin.),
Abraham S. Effron, M.D.,
and
Gerald Perry, M.D.

The Neurological Service,
Bellevue Hospital,
Cornell University,
New York, New York

Surg. Gynec. & Obst., 91: 385–398, October, 1950

*　　*　　*　　*

SUMMARY

"In summary, we have attempted to review the literature of this subject. We have reported 12 cases of grave paralyses following the use of spinal anesthesia; these in addition to 3 other cases published by one of us in 1945 (44). It is to be noticed that throughout the literature there is a huge variation in the figures given of complicating nervous system symptoms. An explanation for such lack of uniformity in figures may very well be found in the fact that often and in the majority of our cases spinal cord symptoms appeared some considerable time after the patient had been discharged from surgical care, so that the surgeon and anesthetist and, indeed, occasionally the patient were unaware of the relationship of the progressive paralysis of the legs to the previous spinal anesthetic.

"So, spinal anesthesia is accompanied by many definite and terrible dangers which are far too little appreciated by surgeons and anesthetists.

"From a neurological point of view, we give the opinion that spinal anesthesia should be rigidly reserved for those pa-tients unable to accept a local or general anesthetic.

"Paralysis below the waist is too large a price for a patient to pay in order that the surgeon should have a fine relaxed field of operation."

1952

Published April, 1971

Narcotic is a dirty word today. To an extent, this has always been true, for by far the most important and unwanted side effect of the narcotic drugs is addiction. They remain, however, unsurpassed in the alleviation of severe pain; and since the alleviation of pain is fundamentally what anesthesia is all about (the intensivists to the contrary notwithstanding), the narcotic analgesics are extremely important drugs to the anesthesiologist.

The use of naturally occurring narcotics—as compared to the thousands of synthetic narcotic analgesics which have been prepared—goes back many centuries. The Greeks, well before the advent of Christianity, used opium as a narcotic and hypnotic; and Dioscorides (A.D. 60) is said to have recognized the superior quality of the juice extruded from the poppy head as compared to that extracted from a mixture of crushed heads and leaves of the poppy plant.

The "spongia somniferum," dating back to the 12th century, was one of the first applications of narcotics to the surgical patient. It was a sponge soaked with the juices of opium, hyoscyamus, mulberry, mandragora, and other drugs. Not surprisingly there was tremendous variation in the potency of these sponges, which led to complications when the concentrations were on the heavy side, and their use was occasionally associated with asphyxia, "congestion," and even death. In fact, Swerdlow states that, "By the 17th century the use of nar-cotics had become so discredited that when Nicholas Bailly, a surgeon of Troyes, administered a narcotic potion to a patient before operation he was arrested and fined for practicing witchcraft."

The use of narcotics to relieve the pain of surgery was a subject of repeated controversy from the 12th to the 19th century, but from the early decades of the latter century onward there are numerous records of the preoperative administration of opium for this specific purpose. Some of these attempts were apparently quite successful, but the great variability of the opium content and rate of absorption could produce inadequate analgesia on the one hand and coma and death on the other.

Three events of the 1800's changed the picture completely. The first of these was the isolation by the chemist, Sertürner, of the active principle of opium, morphine. This provided a drug the effects of which were predictable and placed the use of opiates on a scientific basis for the first time. The second was the invention of the modern metallic hollow needle in 1853 by Alexander Wood in Scotland, which provided a means by which the opiate could be introduced into a vein, a muscle, or subcutaneously. The third event was the invention of the hypodermic syringe, also in the year 1853, by Charles Gabriel Pravaz, who attached an improved hollow needle to his syringe.

There soon followed an increasing use of morphine during surgery, and as premedication prior to surgery. The latter use is generally attributed to the great Claude Bernard, but according to Archer, W. W. Green of the Maine Medical School should receive the credit for advocating the hypodermic use of morphine before inhalation anesthesia. The addition of scopolamine to the morphine premedication was thought to counteract the ill effects of the morphine, and allowed sufficiently large doses so that surgery could be performed under this combination alone.

The early part of the present century saw an increasing use of morphine as part of the actual anesthetic procedure, both to supplement waning regional anesthesia and as the anesthetic procedure itself for minor surgical manipulations. The introduction of the intravenous barbiturates and the less frequent use of the potent inhalation agents heralded the use of narcotics as an inherent part of general anesthesia, as did also the introduction of the muscle relaxant drugs. These two milestones permitted the development of the thiopental-nitrous oxide-narcotic-muscle relaxant combination, which has developed into one of the most important anesthetic techniques in use today.

The icing on the cake was the development of the narcotic antagonists, which provided the anesthesiologist with a safe, reliable means of preventing or correcting some of the ill effects of large doses of opiates. The clinical introduction of Nalline was reported by Eckenhoff, Elder, and King at the May 15, 1951, session of the Physiological Society of Philadelphia, but the definitive paper was published under the title of "N-Allyl Normorphine: An Antagonist to the Opiates" (*Anesthesiology, 13*: 242–251, 1952) by Eckenhoff, Hoffman, and Dripps, and is reprinted below with the kind permission of the authors and the publisher.

N-ALLYL NORMORPHINE: AN ANTAGONIST TO THE OPIATES

ECKENHOFF, J.E., HOFFMAN, G.L.
AND
DRIPPS, R.D.

Anesthesiology, 13:242–251, 1952

By measurement of tidal volume and respiratory rate, the authors showed that nalorphine given after operation stimulated respiration in seven patients depressed by large doses of several narcotics given during operation. They also administered nalorphine 10 mg. intravenously to a large number of patients in labor and shortened the time required for first respiration of infants of those mothers who were moderately depressed by narcotics.

Published April, 1967

One of the major accomplishments of modern anesthesia has been civilizing the South American Indian arrow poison, curare, by using it to help in saving human lives rather than as a deadly weapon. Curare was the first of the muscle relaxants to be employed in anesthesia, and it has proved to be an excellent drug. In the first place, curare does its job, when it is employed intelligently and in proper dosage, admirably well: that is to say, it produces profound muscular relaxation with great consistency. In the second place, curare is quite specific in its action: no drug is entirely specific under all circumstances, of course, but the purity of the curare which is available today is such that the major action of the drug is at the target organ, the myoneural junction, and permits predictable and quantitatively controllable poisoning of that organ. Finally, curare has the great advantage, which is always desirable when a toxic substance is to be administered to man, of having an effective antidote in the form of neostigmine and other anticurare drugs.

Nevertheless, curare is not the ideal muscle relaxant drug on several counts. There is, as an example, the matter of its duration of action. When curare is administered intravenously in a dosage of 0.15 to 0.20 mg. per kg., its action may be expected to last for 25 to 30 minutes, with some variation in either direction, depending upon the individual patient as well as a number of other factors which may influence the magnitude and duration of the myoneural blockade produced by the drug. This length of action can be disadvantageous under certain circumstances, and particularly when only brief and fleeting muscle relaxation is necessary: if a muscle relaxant drug is being employed to facilitate endotracheal intubation, or to provide momentary relaxation for the reduction of a fracture, or to soften the convulsions associated with electroshock therapy, 25 to 30 minutes of relaxation is scarcely necessary and can be a distinct nuisance.

There is also the matter of the time of onset of drug action. Full neuromuscular block is not effected until about 2 to 3 minutes after the injection of curare, although again this will vary somewhat, depending upon the individual patient and certain other factors, such as circulation time, the state of hydration, blood volume, and the like. Furthermore, since the administration of curare should always include a test dose and a period of observation of that dose, the onset of full muscular relaxation is necessarily longer than 2 to 3 minutes by a factor of, at the very least, 2. This delay means that anticipatory administration is necessary if relaxation is to be provided at the precise moment that it is needed during surgery; and while this aim is generally possible, circumstances do arise in which operation must be delayed to await the onset of the action.

Not only is the time of onset of action a problem on occasions, but also the manner in which that action is dissipated may be a disadvantage. For the myoneural block produced by curare is not terminated crisply, but tends to wane slowly over a period of time. As a result, the anesthesiologist is often confronted with the decision whether to administer a further incremental dosage for peritoneal closure, which will produce relaxation that will outlast the end of the surgery, or attempt to squeeze by with a weakening relaxation that can be insufficient for the requirements of operation at that juncture.

There are other liabilities of curare in addition to these inherent characteristics of the drug. Myasthenia gravis, for instance, although a rare disease with an incidence that is less than 1 per 15,000 population, is characterized by a defect of neuromuscular transmission which renders the victim exquisitely sensitive to curare and other nondepolarizing drugs. When the disease is unsuspected and latent, the administration of curare will produce extremely long—and at times even irreversible—degrees of muscle paralysis which may lead to tragedy. This sequence can occur, furthermore, not only in patients with latent myasthenia, but also in some patients with neoplasm (and particularly oat-cell carcinoma of the lung) who react to curare as do patients with frank myasthenia gravis.

Curare is also allegedly capable of inducing the release of histamine in patients with bronchial asthma or other manifestations of allergic diathesis. Under such circumstances, histamine will produce both intense bronchospasm and severe hypotension; and in addition there have been reports of swelling of the eyelids, edema of the face and neck, giant hives over most of the body, and pharyngeal and epiglottic edema. There can be little doubt, however, that, although histamine *can* be the basis of these complications, most instances of bronchospasm which occur during clinical anesthesia associated with the administration of curare are due to an inadequate depth of anesthesia, insufficient analgesia, or a failure to obtund noxious reflex activity.

Ganglionic blockade is also a by-product of curare administration, and produces peripheral vasodilation and hypotension—at least in the experimental animal. It must be added, however, that, although ganglionic blocking action can occur after large doses of d-tubocurare in the laboratory, normal clinical doses produce little or no significant blockade in man. This finding is in contrast to the prevalent belief some 20 years ago, when a great deal was made of curare's anti-shock properties, presumed to be due to its ability to produce ganglionic blockade (perhaps a prophetic forerunner of today's belief that Dibenzyline is useful in the therapy of shock because it interrupts the flow of sympathetic vasoconstrictor impulses).

For all of these various reasons, real or imaginary, the medical profession and the pharmaceutical industry have been constantly on the prowl looking for a new and better muscle relaxant. Most authorities today are agreed that the ideal solution to the problem would be the synthesis of a short-acting, nondepolarizing relaxant, which would require no antagonist. No such drug is at present available, or even dimly visible on the horizon, although diallylnortoxiferine dichloride (Alloferin), which is not as yet commercially available in this country, could represent a right step in that direction. An earlier step in that direction was the demonstration that diacetylcholine (succinylcholine) exhibited neuromuscular blocking action of extremely short duration. This fact was elucidated by the simultaneous, but totally independent, work of Bovet and his colleagues in Rome, and Castillo and de Beer at the Wellcome Research Laboratories in Tuckahoe, New York. The clinical applications of this muscle relaxant drug were soon under study on both sides of the Atlantic; and one of the first clinical reports was by von Dardel and Thesleff, which was entitled, "Succinylcholine Iodide as a Muscular Relaxant. A report of 500 Surgical Cases" (*Acta chir. Scandinav.*, *103:* 321–336, 1952). It is republished below with the kind permission of the authors and the publishers.

SUCCINYLCHOLINE IODIDE AS A MUSCULAR RELAXANT A REPORT OF 500 SURGICAL CASES

O. Von Dardel

AND

S. Thesleff

Department of Anaesthesiology,
Karolinska Sjukhuset, and the
Department of Pharmacology,
Karolinska Institutet,
Stockholm, Sweden

Acta chir. Scandinav., 103: 321–336, 1952

*   *   *   *

SUMMARY

"A report is given of the use of succinyl-choline iodide as a muscular relaxant in surgical operations. The series comprises 500 patients (224 men and 276 women) belonging to all age groups and risk groups. Succinylcholine iodide was given as an intravenous drip infusion to 55 of these patients.

"One of the characteristics of the preparation is its short-term action. It was therefore found suitable for use on occasions when relaxation of short duration only was required. It was also found to be eminently suitable for lengthier operations, when easily regulated muscular relaxation was desired.

"Muscular relaxation was found to be satisfactory in every case. No cumulative effect or tachyphylaxis was observed.

"No complications or toxic actions were encountered, either during anaesthesia or post-operatively, that could be ascribed to the use of succinylcholine iodide as a muscular relaxant."

Published December, 1975

The physician anesthetist has been a gadgeteer from the very beginnings of anesthesia for the simple reason that he had nobody to turn to for equipment and, of necessity, had to develop his own. Probably because of the almost century-long dominance of the volatile inhalation agents after the discovery of anesthesia, vaporizers have always received an inordinate amount of attention by those designing anesthesia apparatus.

The first was Morton's inhaler, which was used in the classic public demonstration of ether anesthesia at the Massachusetts General Hospital on October 16, 1846. It consisted of a two-necked glass globe in which there was a sea sponge which held the ether and served to enlarge the evaporating surface. One aperture admitted the air to the interior of the globe, and the vapor-charged air was then drawn through the second into the lungs. The subject held the mouthpiece, which was shaped for the purpose, in his lips. The brass cylinder which connected the globe with the mouthpiece contained a leather flap hung in such a way as to open during inspiration and close during expiration. The expiratory breath passed forth through the protrusion at the side of the cylinder. This side port, which was approximately square and had a sloped cover of appropriate shape, was fitted with a leather flap hung so as to open during expiration and close at the beginning of inspiration. Thus a unidirectional flow was obtained through the ether chamber to the patient and out at the side. The first nonrebreathing valve!

When Professor Jacob Bigelow wrote his famous "My Dear Boott" letter from Boston on November 28th, 1846, to his friend in London, describing the success of the October 16th etherization at the Massachusetts General Hospital, Boott immediately recognized the enormity of the accomplishment—and within a matter of days a second ether inhaler had been designed. This British inhaler, made by "Hooper of Pall Mall" from specifications supplied by Boott and Mr. Robinson, looked for all the world like a Turkish hookah, with a glass vessel shaped like a sea captain's decanter and a long elastic breathing tube. It, too, like Morton's inhaler, featured sponges to increase the evaporating surface and a valve system to make it, in essence, a nonrebreathing circuit. This apparatus was used on Saturday, December 19th, 1846, in Boott's own home to extract a "firmly fixed molar tooth" from the jaw of a Miss Lonsdale "without the least sense of pain, or the movement of a muscle."

Two days later, at the University College Hospital in London, Robert Liston undertook the first surgical operation performed in England under ether anesthesia, amputating the leg of a butler by the name of Frederick Churchill. The ether vapor was administered "by means of an ingenious apparatus extemporaniously contrived by Mr. Squire of Oxford Street." Squire's inhaler was strikingly similar to Hooper's in looks and design; and for the very good reason that both shared the common heritage of being descendants of Nooth's apparatus. Dr. Nooth was a contemporary of Joseph Priestley, and he designed an apparatus for impregnating water with carbon dioxide, the bottom part of the apparatus being a glass vessel similar in size and shape to those used by Hooper and Squire in making their inhalers.

By the spring of the next year, 1847, the pages of the medical journals all across the continent were full of descriptions and illustrations of inhalers. The incomparable John Snow (who added a couple of inhalers of his own to the scene) commented in his book, *On The Inhalation of Ether In Surgical Operations*, of the inadequacies inherent in these inhalers:

"Many of the apparatuses first invented did not allow of easy respiration, but offered obstructions to it—by sponges, by the ether itself, by valves of insufficient size, but more particularly by tubes of too narrow calibre: and there is reason to believe that in many instances, this was the cause of failure, and that the insensibility, when produced, was partly due to asphyxia."

Ten years later, in 1858, Snow again wrote on the subject in his second book, *On Chloroform And Other Anaesthetics:*

"When the inhalation of ether was first commenced, the inhalers employed consisted generally of glass vases containing sponge, to afford a surface for the evaporation of the ether. Both glass and sponge being very indifferent conductors of ca-

loric, the interior of the inhalers became much reduced in temperature, the evaporation of ether was very much checked, and the patient breathed air much colder than the freezing point of water, and containing very little of the vapour of ether. On this account, and through other defects in the inhalers, the patient was often very long in becoming insensible, and, in not a few cases, he did not become affected beyond a degree of excitement and inebriety."

All of this indicates that within the first few years of the introduction of inhalation anesthesia, the basic principles of vaporization—particularly the need for a large evaporating surface and the effect of temperature—were understood and appreciated. However, during the next century, despite the fact that literally hundreds of vaporizers and inhalers were designed and built, none provided constant vernier control of the vapor concentration until Morris designed the "copper kettle." This he reported in the November, 1952 issue of *Anesthesiology* in an article entitled, "A New Vaporizer for Liquid Anesthetic Agents" (Morris, L. E.: *Anesthesiology, 13:* 587, 1952), which is reprinted below with the kind permission of the author and the publisher.

A NEW VAPORIZER FOR LIQUID ANESTHETIC AGENTS

Lucien E. Morris, M.D.

Madison, Wisconsin

Received for publication
June 12, 1952

Anesthesiology, 13: 587, 1952

* * * *

"The distinguishing feature of the circuit is the additional and completely separate flow of oxygen which is bubbled through the liquid anesthetic agent. This oxygen is metered through a rotameter provided with a by-pass so that the entire required range of both fine and coarse flow may be read on the same tube. This separate stream of oxygen containing anesthetic vapor is then joined with the main stream of gases from all the other meters in a special small mixing chamber situated just before the point of delivery of the gases from the machine. The value of such a circuit lies in the fact that the increase in vapor concentration delivered to the patient may be gradual and steadily progressive in proportion to the amount of oxygen metered through the liquid and in inverse relationship to the total flow of other gases.

* * * *

"Copper, because of its high specific heat, is the material from which the container is made. It is well known that heat is required to vaporize any liquid. If vaporization takes place without addition of heat from an outside source, then the heat necessary to vaporize the liquid is taken from the liquid itself. As the temperature of the liquid goes down, the efficiency of vaporization is reduced because of the fall in partial pressure of the vapor above the liquid. The copper container, therefore, plays an important role as a source of heat and in the transfer of heat from the room air and all the metal parts of the machine to the liquid to be vaporized. The temperature of the liquid anesthetic agent in this vaporizer has been observed during use with ether to be never lower than 15 C. less than the room temperature.

THE VAPORIZING SURFACE

"The gas flowing through the liquid anesthetic is finely dispersed by passing through a sintered bronze disk (porex). The multitude of tiny bubbles leads to maximal vaporization efficiency by providing a greatly increased surface for the liquid-gas interface. In addition, this disk conducts directly to the liquid the heat required for vaporization."

1953

Published August, 1975

The specialty of anesthesiology lost one of its most distinguished ladies last year when Ginny Apgar died on August 9. She was a physician in every sense of the word, a true scientist, everybody's friend—but above all, a lady.

Dr. Virginia Apgar was born in Westfield, New Jersey, on June 7, 1909, and 20 years later she graduated with the degree of Bachelor of Arts from Mount Holyoke College in Massachusetts. Four more years, and she received the degree of Doctor of Medicine from Columbia University's College of Physicians and Surgeons. She stayed on at Presbyterian Hospital as a surgical intern from 1933 to 1936, and then as a fellow in anesthesiology at the same institution for 6 months. She then served as a resident in anesthesia at Wisconsin General Hospital in Madison, Wisconsin, under Dr. Ralph Waters, and finished her residency training at Bellevue under Dr. Rovenstine in 1938. She was certified by the American Board of Anesthesiology in 1939, the second woman to achieve the Board's Diploma.

She returned to Presbyterian Hospital as an Attending Anesthesiologist and as an Assistant Professor of Anesthesiology at Columbia University in 1938, the first woman physician to work in the specialty there; and 11 years later, in 1949, she became the first woman to receive a full professorship at Columbia. She remained at Presbyterian Hospital as Attending Anesthesiologist until 1959 when, at the age of 50, she earned the degree of Master of Public Health from Johns Hopkins. She then became Vice-President and director of basic research for the National Foundation-March of Dimes, going on to become Senior Vice-President of the Foundation in charge of medical affairs.

Dr. Apgar was the recipient of the 1961 Distinguished Service Award of the American Society of Anesthesiologists, and in 1973 she received the P & S Alumni Association Gold Medal for distinguished service. That same year she was presented on national television as Woman of the Year. She was an Honorary Associate Fellow of the American Academy of Pediatrics, and also an Associate Fellow of the American College of Obstetricians and Gynecologists.

But, as Dr. Leonard Brand wrote in the *P & S Quarterly*, Winter 1975, Volume XX, No. 1, "these credentials don't tell the true story of the 'Ginny' we knew." Dr. Brand's obituary does, however, and it is quoted extensively in the following, with his kind permission and that of the *P & S Quarterly*:

"Anyone who met her had a 'Ginny' story to tell, whether it had to do with her interest in music, playing the violin and cello, or building her own string instruments. She was an accomplished musician and was a member of the Teaneck Symphony of New Jersey, the Amateur Music Players and the Catgut Acoustical Society. Or whether it had to do with her love of fishing, having fished most of the famous fishing grounds of the world, be it the Great Barrier Reef off Australia or the streams of Scotland. There were stories about her stamp collecting and her love of baseball and golf. There were stories of her driving her automobile as if it were an airplane. There were scores of stories about the little human things she did, visiting the relative of a friend in a small town in New Zealand or in a village in Norway or doing some small thoughtful favor for one of her friends or acquaintances. The tales of her adventures in traveling over the face of the earth were legion. She always had just arrived from somewhere or was on her way to catch the next plane.

"All of these stories tell a great deal about Ginny. Most of them are true and if they're not, they could have been. The important thing was that in spite of her travels and constant movement, when Ginny stopped for a moment she accomplished more than the dozens of people who were watching her fly by. She delivered her lectures with such a rapid flow of words that you had to sit on the edge of your chair and listen intently or you'd miss several paragraphs. Time was precious to her and her mind and hands were never still. I remember once watching a World Series baseball game on television with my children when the game was interrupted by rain and simultaneously our phone rang. My daughter said, 'That must be Ginny. She only calls during rain delays.'

"Let's turn our attention to Ginny's career here at the Medical Center. Her four years at P & S from 1929 to 1933 were very impressive and she came on the staff as a Junior Fellow in Surgery. In 1936 Dr. Hugh Auchincloss, Sr., suggested to Ginny that the Medical Center was in dire need of a strong Department of Anesthesiology and that this new developing specialty required skills which she had in abundance. She accepted his advice and spent six months learning rudimentary clinical anesthesia from Miss Anne Penland, an experienced nurse-anesthetist who was with the Presbyterian Hospital Unit in France during World War I. In 1937 Ginny spent seven months in Dr. Ralph Waters' department at the University of Wisconsin and returned to New York to complete her training with Dr. Emory A. Rovenstine at NYU. In 1938 she was appointed Director of the Division of Anesthesiology at the Medical Center here, starting a residency program and slowly building a full time staff of physician-anesthesiologists. At that time there were no accommodations for her two new residents and she personally bore the cost of their accommodations at $100 a month. In 1938 she also instituted the first formal undergraduate training in anesthesia for the third and fourth year medical students and in 1943 offered an elective course for medical students.

"Several generations of medical students will always remember Ginny's machine-gun style lectures and her very practical and unembarrassed teaching of anatomy. Ginny had an outstanding caudal hiatus and hundreds of medical students learned to do caudal blocks by palpating her caudal hiatus. She appreciated the bright ones and had infinite patience with the slow ones. No one could ever lie to her successfully because she could see right through you and she herself was so trusting that the most flagrant liars didn't have courage to betray her trust. She had little tolerance for sham or pompousness and everyone was treated equally with genuine interest and friendliness. She took a sincere personal interest in every one of her students so that they almost always did well because they didn't have the heart to disappoint her.

"Her first published paper from the *Anesthesiology Service* was 'Experience with Pontocaine Spinal Anesthesia' in 1939. In the next decade her published papers and the quality of the residents she trained had made her a national figure. In 1949 it was apparent that continued progress toward a truly academic department demanded strengthening in the areas of basic and applied research and with Dr. Apgar's support her good friend Dr. Emmanual M. Papper was appointed Executive Officer and Professor of Anesthesiology. Dr. Apgar applied her talents from 1949 until she left the Medical Center in 1958 primarily to the Sloane Hospital for Women, where she developed the Apgar Score used throughout the world to evaluate newborn infants. She wrote many scientific papers concerning the anesthetic management of obstetrical labor and delivery and participated in the delivery of almost 20,000 babies.

"It was interesting to see the variety of distinguished people who came to pay their respects at her memorial service. But I also saw the check-out lady from the local supermarket and the traffic policeman from her home town who did so much business with her."

As Dr. Brand's obituary implies, Ginny Apgar left a great many heritages, but her name will always be associated with the method of evaluating the newborn infant which she devised. While more sophisticated methods of psychophysiologic testing of the effects of analgesic drugs and anesthesia on the fetus have been introduced in a research setting—tests such as the habituation of the auditory orienting reflex and the Neonatal Behavioural Assessment Scale—the Apgar Score remains the method by which the practicing clinical anesthesiologist evaluates the condition of the newborn infant. The concept was presented first before the Twenty-Seventh Annual Conference of Anesthetists—a joint meeting of the International Anesthesia Research Society and the International College of Anesthetists which was held at Virginia Beach, Virginia, September 22–25, 1952—in a paper entitled, "A Proposal for a New Method of Evaluation of the Newborn Infant." This was subsequently published in *Current Researches in Anesthesia and Analgesia* (Apgar, V.: Anesth. Analg., *32:* 260–267, July–August, 1953), and is reprinted below with the kind permission of the Publisher.

A PROPOSAL FOR A NEW METHOD OF EVALUATION OF THE NEWBORN INFANT

Department of Anesthesiology,
Columbia University, College of
Physicians and Surgeons and
the Anesthesia Service,
The Presbyterian Hospital

Anesth. Analg., 32: 260–267, 1953

*   *   *   *

"The purpose of this paper is the reestablishment of simple, clear classification or "grading" of newborn infants which can be used as a basis for discussion and comparison of the results of obstetric practices, types of maternal pain relief and the effects of resuscitation.

*   *   *   *

"The signs used are as follows:
(1) Heart Rate.—This was found to be the most important diagnostic and prognostic of the five signs. A heart rate of 100–140 was considered good and given a

score of two, a rate of under 100 received a score of one, and if no heart beat could be seen, felt or heard the score was zero.

*　　*　　*　　*

"(2) Respiratory Effort.—An infant who was apneic at 60 seconds after birth received a score of zero, while one who breathed and cried lustily received a two rating. All other types of respiratory effort, such as irregular, shallow ventilation were scored one. An infant who had gasped once at thirty or forty-five seconds after birth, and who then became apneic, received a zero score, since he was apneic at the time decided upon for evaluation.

"(3) Reflex Irritability.—This term refers to response to some form of stimulation. The usual testing method was suctioning the oropharynx and nares with a soft rubber catheter which called forth a response of facial grimaces, sneezing or coughing. Although spontaneous micturition and defecation are not a response to an applied stimulus, they were considered to be favorable signs if they occurred.

"(4) Muscle Tone.—This was an easy sign to judge, for a completely flaccid infant received a zero score, and one with good tone, and spontaneously flexed arms and legs which resisted extension were rated two points. We are unable to agree with Flagg's description of spasticity as a sign of asphyxiation of the infant. The use of analeptics in the baby did not influence this score because of the standardized early time of observation and rating.

"(5) Color.—This is by far the most unsatisfactory sign and caused the most discussion among the observers. All infants are obviously cyanotic at birth because of their high capacity for carrying oxygen and their relatively low oxygen content and saturation. The disappearance of cyanosis depends directly on two signs previously considered—respiratory effort and heart rate. Comparatively few infants were given a full score of two for this sign, and many received zero in spite of their excellent score for other signs."

*　　*　　*　　*

Published February, 1962

Today the Classical File is 5 years old— as is *Survey of Anesthesiology* itself—and a fifth anniversary is always a milestone. Indeed, marriage counsellors regard it as a particularly significant milestone, for they believe that the fourth and fifth years of matrimony are amongst the most dangerous to wedded bliss (there's no way of telling how much consideration they've given to the Seven Year Itch). The honeymoon is over by the fifth anniversary, and marriage has settled down to the serious business of day-to-day living. Perhaps the same is somewhat true of journalism: the novelty and first flush of creative pride have waned, and the serious business of meeting the deadline and getting out the journal has become ingrained.

But the fifth anniversary is also a time of pleasant reminiscence and happy planning for the future. The ground rules for the Classical File, as laid down 5 years ago, were—and remain—fairly simple: an arti-

cle pertaining to any phase of anesthesia, published at least 5 years previously and considered of "classical stature," would be republished in each bimonthly issue of *Survey*. It is, of course, the term "classical stature" that has been the guiding factor. A paper might be of purely historical, purely scientific, purely clinical, or even of merely anecdotal, interest: if it possessed "classical stature," it warranted inclusion in Classical File. A chronologic approach to the literature pertaining to anesthesia was thus totally unfeasible: the early years of Classical File would contain only history, subsequent years would become almost wholly clinical, and future years would become increasingly (stated hopefully) scientific. It was deemed more advisable to make the Classical File a *pot pourri*, alternating the republication of the old with the new, the clinical with the scientific, and the truly historical with the anecdotal.

The result, no doubt, has often seemed

helter-skelter to the casual reader; yet there has been a carefully detailed plan in back of it. The first issue of each volume has contained a "first" of historical significance: the report of Morton's first public demonstration of ether, Horace Wells' tract on his clinical use of nitrous oxide, the first recorded anesthetic death, Crawford Long's initial use of anesthesia in surgery, and Simpson's introduction of chloroform into anesthetic practice. The second issue of each year has been devoted to a historical "first" of recent vintage: the introduction of curare, of thiopental, of cyclopropane, of ethylene, and of decamethonium. The third issue has been concerned with regional anesthesia: Sise's use of pontocaine-glucose for spinal analgesia, the technique of continuous caudal anesthesia, Halsted's infiltration blocks with cocaine, Corning's initial attempts at spinal injections, and Pages' development of epidural anesthesia. The fourth issue of each volume has contained a concept of important clinical significance: the anatomy of endotracheal intubation, the unreliability of the recognition of cyanosis, the utilization of electroencephalography in anesthesia, and the measurement of blood pressure during anesthesia. The last two issues of each year have emphasized basic laboratory work, preferably an article of monograph-length to run on a "to-be-continued" basis and filling the Classical File space in both issues: Haggard's papers on the absorption and distribution of ether; Courville's monograph on the asphyxial effects of nitrous oxide; Quastel's measurements of cerebral oxygen utilization; Scott Smith's self-experimentation on the lack of cerebral effects of curare; the Hardy-Wolff-Goodell measurement of the intensity of pain; the studies of Pike, Guthrie and Stewart on cardiac resuscitation; and Claude Bernard's century-early experiments on the mechanism of curare's activity.

One important aspect of anesthesia has been neglected to date in Classical File: the socioeconomic advances. There are those who believe that undue emphasis has been placed on these advances during the past two decades; and there are also many who would agree. Yet, there is no gainsaying that the progress in this area has been

tremendous, if not, indeed, revolutionary. And there is also no gainsaying that much of the other progress in anesthesia has been an indirect (if not, indeed, a direct) result of this socioeconomic advance. For this reason, Classical File departs from its usual sequential plan in order to reprint an article of "classical stature" that has been republished many times before in medical journals and all over this country and abroad; republished so often, as a matter of fact, that its presentation here could almost be considered *de trops*—except that Classical File would be derelict in its duty to ignore such a communication any longer. For those who have read this classic before, it is hoped that rereading will only serve to intensify the enjoyment; for those who have never read it, *Survey* is delighted to present Richard Gordon's "Sleeping Partner," published in the October 7th, 1953, issue of *Punch* and reprinted below, with the kind permission of the author and publisher.

SLEEPING PARTNER

Richard Gordon

Punch, Oct. 7, 1953

Surgeons are traditionally accused by the medical profession of introducing two necessary evils—wound infection and anaesthetists. In the past hundred years both of these have fortunately become less dangerous to human life.

When chloroform was still a novelty and gas a luxury, the anaesthetist was a seedy practitioner, a Coroner's familiar, creeping round hospitals and nursing homes with a rag of lint in one pocket of his coat tail and a bottle of ether in the other. With this equipment he could perform his shaky tricks instantly and anywhere, like a strolling conjurer. The surgeon took the limelight and ninety per cent of the fee: the anaesthetist at his best was only a Jeeves, ready to smooth the surgical progress of his master, to encourage him in clinical distress, and to temper discreetly his operative enthusiasms. He was a butt for all the hearty surgical fun that battens on blood and sterile towels—how relieved the nurses were when Sir Lancelot's wrath at a moving target was canalized into: "If the patient can keep awake, Mr. Anaesthetist, so can you!" From his perch at the head of the table he yawned beneath his mask at weary accounts of forgotten anatomical battles, and he left the hopsital by bicycle in the dust of the surgical limousine.

As operations became longer and anaesthetists had more hours of comparative inactivity to mediate over their humility, they invented a scheme to assert their personalities in the operating theatre. The trick was simple: they repudiated the rag-and-bottle, and invented a machine a-glitter with chromium plate and taps to administer the anaesthetic for them. At first the surgeons pretended amusement, and made jokes about "The Gas, Fight, and Choke Company." But they were mystified and intimidated particularly when the anaesthetist strolled away for a cup of coffee and left his patient tranquilly freewheeling. It has previously been plain to everyone in the theatre that any damn fool with a bottle and a roll of lint could give an anaesthetic, but even the dullest junior probationer could now see that the manipulation of this secret machine needed the fused skills of an engineer, pilot, and safebreaker.

The anaesthetists cooly pressed their advantage. The machines became bigger and more aggressive, forcing the surgeon to operate uncomfortably in the remaining corner of the theatre. Anaesthetists boldly told their own stories across the towel clips, and the daily operating list ended politely with "General Anaesthetic, Dr. Tompkins, please." Surgeons who once began an operation by plunging knife into abdomen with a roar of "Is he asleep, Bill?" waited patiently for permission, with sterile gloves meekly clasped. Afterwards they bowed over the swab bucket, as the anaesthetist neutralized his apparatus with a pair of spanners, and said "Thank you, Dr. Tompkins—a very beautiful anaesthetic. We shall have the pleasure of working together next week, I presume?" Two limousines now left the hospital courtyard together.

When surgeons and anaesthetists reunited after the war they were faced with problems of readjustment as powerful as those of any other long separated couple. The surgeons had seen Army doctors at work with squares of flannel and ether cans, and had learnt so much about lorries, guns, tanks, and radio sets from enthusiastic brother officers that they were no longer frightened of an anaesthetist's civilian equipment. But they were infuriated to find that anaesthetists had assumed the grand simplicity; heavy apparatus was pushed into theatre sister's store room, and modern anaesthesia conducted with a single syringe.

This consecration in the anaesthetist's armament was permitted by purification of the curare arrow-poison from South America: the Brazilian pigmy blows a curare-tipped dart into his victim before eating him, and the British anaesthetist sticks a curare-filled syringe into his patient before dishing him up to the surgeon. But as more and more unwanted side-effects of the arrow-poison were discovered, and more and more drugs were invented to counteract them, the anaesthetist's syringe grew into a battery of violent poisons and antidotes.

Today he arrives at the hospital in a van, which contains his assistants and a number of expensive electronic machines to let him know the pulse rate and blood pressure without having to count them. The surgeon is allowed to operate as long as his manipulations do not disturb the anaesthesia: to complain that narcosis is not sufficiently profound is as unthinkable as sending back the speciality at a famous restaurant. Anaesthetists are friendly men, and have no malignancy in their new mastery: every one of them thoughtfully thanks the surgeon at the end of the operation for making, with his skill, their superb anaesthetic necessary.

Published October, 1962

The condition of the heart and circulation during anesthesia is of interest to all those concerned with the operative care of the surgical patient, but it is of fundamental concern to the anesthetist. As the primary function of the heart is mechanical, in that it serves as a pump to distribute blood to the entire body, the main interest centers in its ability to continue to supply a sufficiently large amount of blood to meet the body's needs. Until comparatively recently, this ability was evaluated by simple palpation of the peripheral pulse, or by the measurement of blood pressure with a sphygmomanometer. John Snow, the first professional anesthetist, noted that, during the "fourth degree of etherization" (or surgical anesthesia by his classification), "The integrity of the functions of respiration and of circulation is not impaired . . . the pulse is distinct and of good volume."

With the passage of time, however, and the accumulation of a considerable experience in the administration of anesthesia to patients, clinicians came to realize that anesthesia was not always quite so innocuous to the action of the heart and the integrity of the circulation as John Snow and some of his early colleagues had imagined. Deaths occurred during anesthesia that seemed to be associated with—if not, indeed, caused by—failure of the heart and deterioration of the circulation. Some attributed these tragedies to "surgical shock" and the inability of the patient to "stand the anesthesia," a rather nebulously defined lack of physiologic reserve that quickly became one of the most ample and frequently filled wastebaskets in medicine. The suspicion persisted in many quarters, nonetheless, that anesthesia exerted a direct, and a deleterious, effect upon cardiac function. It was not until the introduction of precise physiologic measurements of cardiac output that there appeared to be any hope of bringing scientific fact out of this chaos of differing opinion.

Alas! The introduction of precise measurements of cardiac action during anesthesia served only to compound the chaos and differing opinions. There was almost universal agreement that severe hypotension occurred rather commonly, and cardiac arrest occasionally, during clinical ether anesthesia; but there was no unanimity of opinion as to the mechanisms of these occurrences. In fact, there was, at times, bitter disagreement. On the one hand, physiologists and pharmacologists, working with heart-lung preparations of experimental animals in their laboratories, regularly and emphatically reported a direct myocardial depression and decrease in cardiac output during the ether anesthesia. On the other hand, those who investigated the cardiac output in the intact organisms frequently reported either no change or even an increase in the cardiac output. Blalock, for instance, who studied the cardiac output of the dog during ether anesthesia by means of the Fick principle, demonstrated that the cardiac output was increased in all but three of his 19 experiments. The studies of Johnson on the hemodynamic effects in man confused the issue still further: five of his 13 patients showed an early increase in cardiac output and then a fall later, while the other eight patients all showed early and sustained decreases in cardiac output.

It is now recognized that it is rarely possible to draw conclusions about the mechanisms of circulatory effects of any drug from the changes it may cause in a single dependent variable such as the cardiac output. It is further recognized that this is true because the normal circulation always initiates circulatory reflexes which may act on various aspects of circulatory dynamics to prevent overall change in a single parameter, or to accentuate change in that parameter in one direction or another. One of the most important of these circulatory reflexes is the release of endogenous substances which exert powerful effects on circulatory dynamics. This fact explains the variance in the effects of ether on cardiac output that were revealed by the use of the heart-lung preparation, in contrast to those that were revealed in the intact organism. It was beautifully demonstrated by William R. Brewster, Jr., James P. Isaacs, and Thorkild Wainø-Andersen in the report of their studies entitled, "Depressant Effect of Ether on Myocardium of the Dog and Its Modification by Reflex Release of Epinephrine and Nor-epinephrine," which was published in *The American Journal of Physiology*, *175:* 399–413, December, 1953, and is reprinted below, with the kind permission of the authors and the publisher.

DEPRESSANT EFFECT OF ETHER ON MYOCARDIUM OF THE DOG AND ITS MODIFICATION BY REFLEX RELEASE OF EPINEPHRINE AND NOR-EPINEPHRINE

WILLIAM R. BREWSTER, JR.,
JAMES P. ISAACS
AND
THORKILD WAINØ-ANDERSEN

From the Anesthesia Laboratory
of the Harvard Medical School
at the Massachusetts General Hospital,
Boston, Massachusetts

Am. J. Physiol., 175: 399–413, 1953

*   *   *   *

SUMMARY

"Evidence has been presented to show that diethyl ether exerts a direct depressant (negative inotropic) effect upon the myocardium of the dog which is quantitatively sufficient, in the absence of circulating epinephrine and nor-epinephrine, to produce either a substantial decrease in cardiac output or cardiac arrest at blood ether concentrations required for surgical anesthesia.

"A major factor in the safety of ether anesthesia, insofar as the effect of diethyl ether upon the myocardium is concerned, is the quantitative reflex release from the adrenal medullae and sympathetic nerve endings of epinephrine and nor-epinephrine which, by virtue of their positive inotropic effect upon the myocardium, antagonize the myocardial depression of diethyl ether."

1954

Published June, 1970

The fascinating thing about the history of anesthesia is that we are all living it. Most of us in the specialty, who are now middle aged (*i.e.*, over 30) and grandparents, see changes in our practices in the space of but 2 or 3 years, the likes of which the pediatricians have not seen in 10 years and the obstetricians will not see in 50. A few of these changes have been evanescent and fleeting, but the vast majority have been of a more permanent nature—cyclopropane, controlled respirations, thiopental, *d*-tubocurare and the other muscle relaxants, induced hypotension, recovery rooms, ventilators, hypothermia, monitoring equipment, drug antagonists, new local anesthetic drugs which can outperform procaine, intensive care units, halothane, respiratory wards—the list goes on and on.

One of the fortunately evanescent and fleeting changes was the near loss of spinal anesthesia from our armamentarium.

The history of spinal anesthesia from the very beginning has been one of waves of wild enthusiasm followed by periods of condemnation and rejection, and the 1930's and 1940's belonged to the former. Babcock, as the period commenced, wrote "Spinal anesthesia has emerged from the dangerous period in which it was considered necessary merely to inject a solution of local anesthetic within the spinal dura and then to operate with little further attention to the patient. The need for a very precise technique and for the constant supervision of the anesthetized patient is now recognized. The physiologic changes due to the blocking of the spinal rami are now evident. Methods for localizing the block to designated segments of the spine have been developed. The control of the duration and intensity of the analgesic is possible within limits. The pain of operation may be abolished with or without complete loss of tactile sense and of muscular contraction."

This happy period came to a close in October, 1950, when the subscribers to *Surgery, Gynecology and Obstetrics* received their monthly copy of that journal and in it the article by Foster Kennedy on "The Grave Spinal Cord Paralyses Caused by Spinal Anesthesia."

Kennedy was born in Belfast, Ireland, on February 7, 1884, the son of William Archer Kennedy and Hessie Foster (Dill) Kennedy. He was educated at Queen's College in Belfast, and then received the M.D. degree from the Royal University of Ireland in 1906. He became Resident Medical Officer at the National Hospital in London, and by 1910 was chief of the clinic at the New York Neurological Institute. World War I took him back to Europe, where he served with distinction in the Medical Corps of the British Army in France. He was promoted to captain, and then to major, and "was mentioned in dispatches." After the war, he returned to New York and became a distinguished and world famous neurologist, serving as President of both the Neurological Society of New York and the American Neurological Association, and receiving honorary memberships in the Neurological Societies of Paris, Hungary, Cuba, Mexico and Sweden. He was Professor of Neurology at Cornell University Medical School, and Attending Physician in Charge of the Neurological Service at Bellevue Hospital. He was a prolific writer and the author of numerous articles on neurologic and psychiatric subjects. Unquestionably, the best known of these was, "The Grave Spinal Cord Paralyses Caused by Spinal Anesthesia."

"Unfortunately," wrote Kennedy, "it is not generally known, and still less widely accepted, that spinal anesthesia may result in temporary or permanent neurological complications: paralyses or continuing root pain."

He then described in detail some 12 instances of spinal cord paralyses which had appeared in patients following spinal anesthesia—and sometimes following spinal anesthesia "by some considerable time after the patient had been discharged from surgical care, so that the surgeon and anesthetist and, indeed, occasionally the patient were unaware of the relationship of the progressive paralysis of the legs to the previous spinal anesthesia." He concluded:

"We do not question the advantages of the excellent and admirable relaxation of the abdominal musculature produced by spinal anesthesia. On the other hand, one cannot underestimate the gravity of the many possible complications nor the probability of their permanence . . . spinal anesthesia is accompanied by many definite and terrible dangers which are far too little appreciated by surgeons and anesthetists . . . from a neurological point of view, we give the opinion that spinal anesthesia should be rigidly reserved for those patients unable to accept local or general anesthetic . . . paralysis below the waist is too large a price for a patient to pay in order that the surgeon should have a fine relaxed field of operation."

The impact of Kennedy's words on the medical profession was immense; and when Time, Good Housekeeping, and similar important journals had picked up and broadcast the story, the future of spinal anesthesia in this country looked not just grim, but nonexistent. It was saved by the brilliant, timely, and important series of articles by Dripps and Vandam, the first of which, "Long-Term Follow-up Of Patients Who Received 10,098 Spinal Anesthetics; Failure To Discover Major Neurological Sequelae," was published in the December 18, 1954 issue of the *Journal of the American Medical Association* (*156:* 1486–1491, 1954). It is reprinted below with the kind permission of the authors and the publisher.

LONG-TERM FOLLOW-UP OF PATIENTS WHO RECEIVED 10,098 SPINAL ANESTHETICS; FAILURE TO DISCOVER MAJOR NEUROLOGIC SEQUELAE

Dripps, R.D.

AND

Vandam, L.D.

J.A.M.A., 156:1486–1491, 1954

During 1948 to 1951, patients of the Hospital of the University of Pennsylvania who received spinal anesthesia by a rigidly standardized technique were carefully examined at frequent intervals postoperatively for sequelae and were contacted by mail or phone 6 months later. They obtained six month follow up reports for 86% of the anesthetics and were able to describe with precision the early and late neurologic sequelae of spinal anesthesia. They reported separately sequelae of lumbar puncture alone (*J.A.M.A. 147*:1118–1121, 1951) and in this paper, sequelae attributable to the injection of the anesthetic solution alone.

Published August, 1971

Probably the first written description of the effects—and alleged side effects—of curare was contained in the book on the New World, *De Orbe Novo*, published by the Italian monk, Peter Martyr d'Anghera, in 1516: "They like to use bows and poisoned arrows . . . . Whoever is wounded by one of these poisoned arrows dies, but not instantly, and no Spaniard has yet found a remedy for such wounds. The natives know some, but the remainder of one's life, after being cured, is sufficiently disagreeable; for it is necessary to abstain from many things one likes. First of all from sexual pleasure for two years, and afterwards, during a lifetime, from liquors, excessive pleasures of the table, and all exertion. Otherwise death quickly follows. Our monks have seen many wounded Indians, for they live in a state of perpetual war, but they assisted at the death of only one woman, who was unwilling to undergo the cure; the women fight by their husbands' sides. Nobody has been able to extort from them the secret of this antidote."

During the past 30 years, since the day on which, as T. Cecil Gray has pointed out, curare revolutionized clinical anesthesia for all time by permitting the production of utter muscle flaccidity without the necessity of resort to deep and dangerous levels of general anesthesia, a number of more authentic side effects have been identified. Some of these have been due to interactions with other drugs; some have been due to such characteristics as the effect of temperature on the effects of the drug itself; some have been due to the inherent pharmacologic properties of the drug; some have been due to the patient; and some have been due to the presence of intercurrent disease states.

Cullen, one of the first clinicians to employ curare, came early to the realization that there was an interaction between curare and ether—and a danger from that interaction—when curare was administered during ether anesthesia: "Curare can be used during ether anesthesia, but the dose must be reduced to one-third of that used during cyclopropane anesthesia. Experience gained during the use of curare with ether prompted investigation into the effect of several anesthetic agents on the humoral transmission of nerve impulses. The agents studied were cyclopropane, ethylene, ether, tribromethanol with amylene hydrate (avertin fluid), and sodium ethyl (1 methylbutyl) thiobarbiturate (pentothal sodium). It was found that humoral transmission of nerve impulses was not greatly interfered with by cyclopropane and ethylene. In high concentration, but within the anesthetic range, pentothal sodium and avertin fluid produced a moderate interference. Ether had a marked curariform action which, interestingly enough, had been ascribed to it as early as 1914.

These studies helped to make clear not only the increased depression which occurs with the concomitant use of ether and curare, but also assisted in elaborating the clinical observation of unequal muscular relaxation during equal levels of anesthesia with cyclopropane and ether."

Furthermore, the interaction of curare with other drugs is not necessarily confined to ether or other anesthetic agents that the patient receives during surgery; any of the drugs which are administered to the patient is potentially capable of interacting with curare or other muscle relaxants which the patient receives during operation. A most important case in point is the administration of an antibiotic drug, and there is now considerable experimental evidence to show that some antibiotics have an action at the myoneural junction. Molitor and Graessle were the first to note this effect when, in 1950, they studied the toxicity of streptomycin and observed that the survival rate of their animals was increased if artificial respiration was used. Brazil and Corrado subsequently demonstrated that intravenous doses of streptomycin administered to dogs or pigeons produced hypotonia and respiratory impairment, and that neostigmine reversed this block to an extent, although not as rapidly as calcium chloride. It has since been shown that neomycin, streptomycin, dihydrostreptomycin, polymyxin B, and kanamycin are all capable of producing neuromuscular blockade. The clinical significance of this work, of course, lies in the accidental deaths associated with the combination of anesthetic and antibiotic drugs. A number of these have been reported, so it is wise to ensure that muscle relaxants have worn off if intraperitoneal antibiotics are to be used.

Not only the concomitant administration of a variety of drugs, but also many other factors may alter or affect the pharmacologic response to muscle relaxant drugs. There are, for instance, effects of changes in acid-base balance upon the activity of curare and other muscle relaxants. An increase in pH serves to decrease the activity of d-tubocurarine, while a lowering of pH potentiates the neuromuscular effect of curare. Exercise also increases the intensity of the block produced by d-tubocurarine, while it facilitates recovery of neuromuscular transmission after decamethonium induced depolarization block: the potentiating effect of exercise parallels a concurrent rise in plasma level of lactic acid, suggesting that increased glycolysis and lactic acid production caused by exercise may be involved in the increased sensitivity to d-tubocurarine. Dehydration diminishes both the plasma volume and the volume of extracellular fluid, so that an intravenous dose of a muscle relaxant will result in higher initial concentration of the drug at the endplate, and a slower diffusion from the plasma and the endplate to the extracellular compartment. Both of these factors serve to intensify and prolong the neuromuscular effect of blocking drugs. Disturbances of fluid balance also are generally accompanied by disturbances of electrolyte balance, and the latter can have a profound effect upon both neuromuscular transmission and the action of muscle relaxants. Inorganic ions may influence neuromuscular transmission in several ways, by affecting the nerve fiber, by affecting the nerve terminal, by the release of the neurohumoral transmitter substance, or by changing the sensitivity of the postjunctional membrane and muscle fiber to depolarization. A change in temperature may also influence the effects of the various muscle relaxant drugs. In the experimental animal, for instance, lowered muscle temperature, either of the whole animal or of a single limb alone, reduces both the speed of onset and the intensity of the nondepolarization block produced by d-tubocurarine, effects which are reversed by rewarming. Conversely, the depolarization block produced by decamethonium or succinylcholine is prolonged and intensified by lowered temperature.

Finally, there are a number of disease states and pathologic situations which significantly affect the response to muscle relaxant drugs. Liver disease can increase the patient's sensitivity to both the nondepolarizing and the depolarizing types of relaxants—although for different reasons—so that both types of these drugs must be employed with great caution in patients with liver damage. Another disease state that can affect the sensitivity to the myoneural blocking drugs is carcinomatous neuropathy. There have now been several reports of patients suffering from neurologic and neuromuscular disorders associated with carcinoma (bronchogenic, prostatic or sigmoid, but particularly oat cell carcinoma of the lung), without the presence of any metastases in the central nervous system itself, who have responded to muscle relaxants in an abnormal manner. The mechanism of the increased sensitivity to both the depolarizing and the nondepolarizing drugs in these patients with carcinoma remains obscure, but the necessity of employing a test dose in patients suffering from carcinomatous neuropathy is obvious. By far the most important disease state in relation to the use of the muscle relaxant drugs, however, is myasthemia gravis. The neuromuscular junction of the myasthenic patient exhibits a greatly increased sensitivity to curare and other nondepolarizing drugs, and this effect has been used as the basis for a diagnostic test for latent myasthenia gravis. On the other hand, these patients generally have a decreased sensitivity to decamethonium due to increased resistance of the endplate for depolarizing influences. The mechanisms involved have not been elucidated; but the altered sensitivity of the myasthenic to neuromuscular

blocking agents in general necessitates great care in the administration of these drugs to each such patient.

The blessings of curare, therefore, are not unmixed. At a meeting of the Section on Anaesthetics of the Royal College of Medicine which was held on April 2, 1948, it was pointed out that side reactions and, in some instances, idiosyncrasy could occur and could "place the anaesthetist in an embarrassing and difficult position." There was agreement, however, as to the "comparative nontoxicity" of the drug. On the other side of the Atlantic there was no such agreement. Indeed, quite to the contrary, even as the British anaesthetists were meeting at the Section on Anaesthetics, a major hassle over the dangers of curare in anesthetic practice was taking place in the United States. The report which in large measure precipitated the furor was published in the July, 1954, issue of *Annals of Surgery* under the title, "A Study of the Deaths Associated with Anesthesia and Surgery, Based on a Study of 599,548 Anesthesias in Ten Institutions 1948–1952, Inclusive" (Beecher, H. K. and Todd, D. S.: *Ann. Surg., 140:* 2–34, July, 1954). It is republished below in two parts in this and the subsequent issue of *Survey of Anesthesiology* with the kind permissions of both the authors and the publisher.

Published October, 1971

The so-called "Beecher-Todd Report on Curare Deaths," the republication of which was begun in the last issue of *Survey* and is completed in this issue, was in fact neither the Beecher-Todd report nor a report on curare deaths. It was a survey of the deaths associated with anesthesia and surgery as they occurred in 10 university medical centers in the United States between January 1, 1948, and December 31, 1952 (*i.e.*, a 5 year period). During the course of those 5 years, 21 physicians and 11 secretaries worked continuously on the collection of data on 599,548 anesthesias administered at the university hospitals involved in the study: The Massachusetts General Hospital (Harvard University); The Presbyterian

Hospital of New York (Columbia University College of Physicians and Surgeons); The Hospital of the University of Pennsylvania (The University of Pennsylvania); The George Washington University Hospital and the Gallinger Municipal Hospital (George Washington University); The Duke University Hospital (Duke University); The Vanderbilt University Hospital (Vanderbilt University); The Charity Hospital of Louisiana (Tulane University); The University of Minnesota Hospitals (University of Minnesota); The Salt Lake County Hospital (University of Utah); and the Stanford University Hospitals (Stanford University). The data collected represented 105 man years of professional effort in which the material was painstakingly observed, recorded, gathered, and checked.

This retrospective survey was concerned with the role that anesthesia might have played in the total surgical care of the patients involved, and in particular with the extent to which anesthesia contributed to mortality in the surgical patient. It recognized that death in the surgical patient could be due to: (1) the patient's disease (the unavoidable progression of the patient's primary illness); (2) error in diagnosis (whether or not surgery was performed: *i.e.*, death following generalized peritonitis from a ruptured appendix in a patient being treated conservatively under the erroneous diagnosis of acute pancreatitis or death from a perforated peptic ulcer in a patient in whom a misdiagnosis of acute appendicitis had been made and simple appendectomy performed); (3) error in surgical judgment (failure to digitalize when digitalization was clearly indicated, failure to administer blood in adequate amounts in hemorrhagic shock, or the performance of the wrong operation); (4) error in surgical technique (death due to postoperative hemorrhage because a ligature slipped, infection not present at the time of operation, or leakage of the contents of a hollow viscus at the surgical suture line); or (5) death due to anesthesia ("anesthesia death").

The statistics obtained from this study were impressive. Those included in the part of the report republished in the last issue of *Survey* described the types of anesthetists (and the number of anesthesiologists) administering the anesthetics, the incidence of the varying anesthetics used, and the techniques involved. Those concerned with mortality rates and their causes are contained in the concluding portion of the report (Beecher, H. K., and Todd, D. S.: A study of the deaths associated with anesthesia and surgery: based on a study of 599,548 anesthesias in 10 institutions, 1948–1952, inclusive. *Ann. Surg., 140:* 2–34, 1954), which is reprinted below, again with the kind permissions of the authors and the publisher.

A STUDY OF THE DEATHS ASSOCIATED WITH ANESTHESIA AND SURGERY: BASED ON A STUDY OF 599,548 ANESTHESIAS IN TEN INSTITUTIONS 1948–1952, INCLUSIVE

BEECHER, H.K.
AND
TODD, D.P.

Ann. Surg., 140:2–34, 1954

Quite apart from the controversy surrounding the interpretation of the massive data summarized in this report, this study was a landmark in the evolution of multiclinic trials and of clinical pharmacology. By no means a model study, it did, however, demonstrate the feasibility of investigating rare events by combining the efforts and experience of many institutions to gain sufficient experience for study. This method, in a more refined design, was used subsequently in the National Halothane Study.

1956

Published April, 1966

Without almost any question, the past decade in clinical anesthesia has been dominated by halothane. There have been a number of other developments which have been important, of course—the technique of hypothermia, monitory, the intensive care unit and the respiratory ward, extracorporeal circulation, hyperbaric oxygenation, the refinement of ventilators, instrumentation for blood gas analysis, to name only a few—but by sheer weight of numbers, if nothing else (although there has been a great deal else!), halothane has been *the* milestone in clinical anesthesia during the last 10 years.

The anesthetic drugs employed in the past have often been discovered by happenstance, but halothane represents the result of a determined effort to produce a compound with specific physical and chemical properties. This search was instigated, really, because of the experiences during World War II, when it became apparent that there was an urgent need for a safe, potent, nonexplosive, volatile anesthetic drug. This need was further accentuated after the war because of the increasing use of electrocoagulation and other electrical equipment during surgery, the rising costs of constructing operating rooms which would be safe against fires and explosions, and the imperative requirement for a simple yet safe anesthetic for use in the event of a nuclear holocaust.

One group undertaking such a search was the Research Department of the General Chemical Division of Imperial Chemical Industries, Ltd. (I.C.I.) in England, and Suckling has described the efforts of this team of physicists, chemists, engineers, and pharmacologists in their attempt to develop a compound with all of the necessary properties: *i.e.*, absence of chemical toxicity, absence of inflammability and explosive hazards, and anesthetic potency itself.

The I.C.I. team noted, first, that one way to reduce toxicity was to employ compounds which were chemically inert and therefore unlikely to be involved in metabolic processes within the body; and they further noted that one group of chemicals which possessed a high degree of chemical stability was the fluorinated hydrocarbons. The chemical inertness of these compounds is the result of the strong bond between carbon and fluorine, as a consequence of which the fluorine atom is quite unreactive. It therefore seemed a reasonable hypothesis that chemicals consisting of the groups CF_3- or CF_2- would be highly stable and unlikely to be involved in metabolic processes within the body. By 1951, I.C.I. had, in fact, decided to concentrate their studies on compounds containing these groups in order to obtain a stable molecule and (hopefully) therefore one with low toxicity.

It was also appreciated that nonflammability and nonexplosiveness could be facilitated, if all other things were equal, by keeping the percentage of hydrogen in the molecule at a low level. The substitution of such halogen atoms as fluorine and bromine for hydrogen will reduce flammability and explosiveness, and, indeed, the halogenation of hydrocarbons tends to decrease flammability in proportion to the number of halogen atoms which are substituted. The group of compounds with which the I.C.I. team planned to work—the fluorinated hydrocarbons—could thus be made nonflammable and nonexplosive by the presence of chlorine and bromine atoms in the molecule in place of hydrogen.

And, finally, the problem of anesthetic potency was approached from the point of view of the thermodynamic activity of the substance in question. Ferguson had shown that the saturated vapor pressure was an important factor in explaining the differences in potency between anesthetic compounds, and that the ratio (Pa/Ps) of the partial pressure producing anesthesia (Pa) to the saturated vapor pressure of the compound at a given temperature (Ps) is approximately equal to thermodynamic activity. It was thus possible, from Ferguson's work, to calculate the approximate anesthetic potency of a compound in advance.

On the basis of these precise reasonings, I.C.I. began with a series of fluorinated paraffins which they themselves manufactured under the trade name Arcton and sold for use as refrigerants and aerosols. These Arcton compounds owe their use as refrigerants and in aerosols to their volatility, low toxicity, and nonflammability; and the decision was made to search among these, as well as other fluorinated compounds, for a substance which would be a safe, potent, nonexplosive, volatile anesthetic agent. Arcton 4 (CF_2HCl) and Arcton 7 ($CFHCl_2$) were tested as anesthetics, but both produced convulsions in mice; and it became evident that compounds of the Arcton type which are gases at room temperature frequently do produce convulsions. However, the physical and chemical considerations mentioned above indicated that 2-bromo-2-chloro 1,1,1-trifluoroethane ($CF_3CHBrCl$), which is a liquid at room temperature and also a compound from the Arcton series, might fulfill all of the stated requirements. The substance (which was an unknown compound at the time) was therefore synthesized, screened, and eventually subjected to detailed pharmacologic study. The results of these studies were reported in 1956 in the British Journal of Pharmacology by Raventós (Raventós, J.: The action of Fluothane—a new volatile anaesthetic. *Brit. J. Pharmacol., 11:* 394, 1956) and are reprinted below with the kind permissions of the author and the publisher.

THE ACTION OF FLUOTHANE A NEW VOLATILE ANAESTHETIC

J. Raventós

From the Research Department,
Imperial Chemical
(Pharmaceuticals) Ltd.,
Hexagon House,
Blackley, Manchester, 9

With an Appendix by
R. R. Goodall

(Received May 31, 1956)

Br. J. Pharmacol., 11: 394, 1956

* * * *

SUMMARY

"1. Fluothane ($CF_3CHClBr$) is a volatile liquid with a b.p. of 50.2°C. and an S.G. of 1.86. It is not inflammable when mixed with O_2 in concentrations from 0.5 to 50% (v/v). It is stable over soda lime.

"2. It is an inhalation anaesthetic more potent than ether and chloroform on experimental animals. Its therapeutic ratio is about twice that of ether. Induction of anaesthesia and recovery are both rapid and free from excitement. It produces good muscular relaxation. It does not cause salivation or vomiting.

"3. With the exception of hypotension, it does not produce any serious functional disturbances. It does not produce cardiac irregularities, but increases the sensitivity of the heart to adrenaline. It does not increase capillary bleeding.

"4. The inhalation of high concentration (3.5%) stops the respiration, but this apnoea is easily reversible.

"5. The only pathological lesion found in animals after its use is a mild dilatation of the proximal tubules of the kidney. This lesion is not associated with alteration of the renal function."

Published October, 1977

It is said that fat people are happy people. They are cheery in countenance, they get along well with their fellow humans, they are stoical in disposition, they have a bright outlook on life, and they are complacent. Shakespeare understood this well when he had Caesar say, "Let me have men about me that are fat, Sleek-headed men, and such as sleep o' nights: Yond Cassius has a lean and hungry look; He thinks too much: such men are dangerous." Washington Irving made the same point in *Knickerbocker's History of New York:* "Who ever hears of fat men heading a riot, or herding together in riotous mobs?"

But fat people in operating rooms are anything but jolly sights. The morbidly obese who are to undergo jejunoileal or other gut-bypass procedures are, of course, a legend unto themselves. The just plain obese should also strike terror into the heart of any anesthesiologist: the anesthetic problems of obesity shorten the lives of many surgical patients—and also the lives of some of their anesthetists. Venepuncture is technically difficult, and there is the danger of both extravascular injection and inadvertent intraarterial injection; bony landmarks for conduction anesthesia are hard to palpate; upper airway obstruction is common, with the often inelegant induction sequence of bucking, salivation, breath-holding, and cyanosis; satisfactory laryngoscopy may frequently be impeded by supra- and antesternal pads of fat, and trauma to the mouth and oropharynx is common; and most particularly, there are significant changes from the normal in terms of cardiopulmonary function.

The abnormalities in respiratory function are many—as Gertrude, Queen of Denmark, said of Laertes, "He's fat, and scant of breath." And so he was. In the obese, the total lung capacity is reduced; the inspiratory capacity (IC) is reduced; the expiratory reserve volume (ERV) is reduced; the vital capacity (VC) is reduced; the functional residual capacity (FRC) is reduced; the closing volume (CV) is increased; and the combination of an increased closing volume and decreased expiratory reserve volume leads to underventilation of the dependent portions of the lung, and hence hypoxemia, due either to overperfusion of underventilated areas of the lung or to perfusion of totally unventilated lung tissue.

The cardiovascular problems are also immense (no pun intended). There is a positive correlation between increased weight and increase in arterial blood pressure; and although blood pressure measurement, by the Riva-Rocci armlet sphygmomanometer method, is often inaccurate in the obese (because of the cuff size of the armlet), it is well documented that hypertension and obesity go, if not arm in arm, at least cheek by jowl. Cardiac output is increased, up to 10 liters per minute with a 100 kilogram weight gain. Total blood volume is also increased; and this, combined with the increased stroke volume, forces the increased cardiac output into a relatively unaltered peripheral resistance, leading to the hypertension. There is cardiomegaly by chest x-ray, estimated at 1 millimeter for every 1.32 kilogram increase in weight above normal by the Ponderal or Somatic Index (height in centimeters divided by the cube root of weight in pounds); and there may be electrocardiographic changes in some patients and increased left ventricular end-diastolic pressures. The cardiomegaly is not due to fatty infiltration of the heart, but rather to true left ventricular enlargement (muscle hypertrophy), which may or may not be associated with right ventricular enlargement.

These cardiopulmonary changes are common to almost all obese patients. There is, however, an association of signs and symptoms, occurring in an estimated 10 per cent of these patients, which is unique. These were described by a former Dean of Harvard Medical School and his colleagues in delightful fashion as "The Pickwickian Syndrome." Mr. Pickwick was fat, of course; but the reference is not to him, as

so many people mistakenly believe, but rather to Mr. Wardle's boy, "Fat Joe," in Charles Dickens' "The Pickwick Papers." The original paper (Burwell, C. S., Robin, E. D., Whaley, R. D. and Bickelmann, A. G.: Extreme obesity associated with alveolar hypoventilation: a Pickwickian syndrome. *American Journal of Medicine, 21*: 811, 1956) is reprinted below with the kind permission of the authors and publishers.

EXTREME OBESITY ASSOCIATED WITH ALVEOLAR HYPOVENTILATION—A PICKWICKIAN SYNDROME

C. SIDNEY BURWELL,
EUGENE D. ROBIN,
ROBERT W. WHALEY
AND
ALBERT G. BICKELMANN

Department of Medicine,
Harvard Medical School,
Boston, Massachusetts

Am. J. Med., 21: 811, 1956

This article considers the association of obesity, somnolence, polycythemia and excessive appetite, illustrated by a case history. A classic description of this association of signs and symptoms was written by Charles Dickens in 1837 in his "Pickwick Papers", and for this reason the authors call it the Pickwickian syndrome. Clinical features include marked obesity, somnolence, twitching, cyanosis, periodic respiration, polycythemia, right ventricular hypertrophy, and right ventricular failure.

The authors describe a patient, 5 feet 5 inches tall and weighing 263 pounds, who portrayed most of the above signs and symptoms, all of which disappeared during a weight loss from 121.4 to 103.6 kg.

1957

Published December, 1973

When succinylcholine was introduced into clinical practice in 1952—after having sat on the shelf with its myoneural blocking properties unrecognized for more than 45 years!—it was widely hailed as the ideal muscle relaxant. By one definition, that is "a drug which hits, runs, and leaves no memory," succinylcholine appeared to fill the bill. An early clinical report concluded, "One of the characteristics of the preparation is its short-term action. It was, therefore, found suitable for use on occasions when relaxation of short duration only was required. It was also found to be eminently suitable for lengthier operations, when easily regulated muscular relaxation was desired. Muscular relaxation was found to be satisfactory in every case. No cumulative effect or tachyphylaxis was observed. No complications or toxic actions were encountered, either during anesthesia or post-operatively."

An ideal drug, indeed!

Almost before that ink was dry, however, reports of complications, toxic reactions, undesirable pharmacologic effects, and drug interactions began to appear in the literature.

One of the first of these to be documented was the feeling of muscle stiffness and pain caused by the fasciculations which follow i.v. administration of the drug. Generally this occurs in the neck and shoulders, chest, abdomen, and back, but occasionally in the jaw or limbs. The pain usually appears within 12 to 24 hours (sometimes as soon as 3 hours or as late as 4 days), and lasts 1 or 2 days (but can last for as long as 5 or 6 days). The mechanism involved is not really understood, but presumably is related to depolarization, although there is no correlation between the magnitude of the visible fasciculations and the incidence or severity of the pain. The frequency of this complication is variously reported as 0.7 per cent, 26 per cent, 34 per cent, 36 per cent, 40 per cent, 49 per cent, 59 per cent, 49 per cent again, 72 per cent, 76 per cent, 83 per cent, and 89 per cent! There does appear to be a higher incidence in the middle age groups (20 to 50 years as opposed to children or older adults); in females; and following early ambulation. Its occurrence can be reduced by thiopental, pretreatment with gallamine or d-tubocurarine, and by high doses of i.v. procaine or lidocaine.

Transient increase in intraocular tension was another pharmacologic effect which caused early concern. It was attributed to compression of the globe by the succinylcholine induced contraction of the extraocular muscles, and fear was expressed as to the effect of such increased pressure in acute glaucoma and its occurrence during intraocular surgery with the globe incised. In point of fact, a case of vitreous expulsion was reported under the latter circumstances, and the presence of an eye injury or "open eye" surgery became a firm contraindication to the use of succinylcholine.

There were also reports of a rise in intragastric pressure following the use of succinylcholine, a matter of some moment in relation to the "crash induction" so commonly employed in an effort to prevent regurgitation and aspiration in patients with full stomach. Any sudden increase of intragastric pressure, added to the pressure already exerted by the gastric tone produced by the full stomach, could be sufficient to open the cardia and allow stomach contents to pass upwards. The increase in intragastric pressure was presumed to be related to the occurrence of pronounced fasciculations; and, again, as in the case of the muscle pains, thiopental or pretreatment with a nondepolarizing relaxant were advocated to prevent the fasciculations.

The early pharmacologic experiments in anesthetized cats and dogs had indicated that succinylcholine had no effect on the cardiovascular system, but clinical experience soon proved that this was also not true. The first of the adverse cardiovascular effects reported was that of hypertension, originally believed due to a direct effect upon the myocardium, but now attributed at least in part to the release of catecholamines by a ganglion stimulating action of succinylcholine. More disturbing have been the many reports of bradycardia, sinus arrest,and supraventricular and ventricular arrhythmias following repeated i.v. injection of succinylcholine, particularly in infants and children. Ventricular arrhythmias also occur in digitalized patients following succinylcholine, possibly related to myocardial ionic movements of potassium, and represent a potential hazard, particularly in the fully digitalized patient.

While histamine release associated with the use of muscle relaxants is usually thought of in terms of d-tubocurarine, there have been a number of reports of bronchospasm following the use of succinylcholine, presumably secondary to histamine release. In at least one instance, the situation deteriorated to death. An allergic reaction has also been described, consisting of a rash on the trunk, head and extremities, facial edema, and a fall in blood pressure (from 155/100 to 70/40), which was attributed to histamine release by succinylcholine.

Generalized myotonia has been reported following the use of succinylcholine in patients suffering from myotonia dystrophica or myotonia congenita, and this has also occurred in patients with these diseases after the administration of other depolarizing muscle relaxants. In some patients it became exceedingly difficult to inflate the lungs, and marked cyanosis resulted. These generalized muscle spasms may be associated with myoglobinuria, which is usually an indication of muscle damage and perhaps is related to gross fasciculations. In any event, it would seem prudent to avoid the use of succinylcholine (or other depolarizing drugs) in patients known to have either myotonia dystrophica or myotonia congenita.

The effect of succinylcholine upon muscle tissue may also be involved in the production of the terrifying syndrome of malignant hyperthermia. The precise etiology of this syndrome remains unknown, and certainly it can occur in both susceptible laboratory animals and in patients without exposure of either to succinylcholine. Nevertheless, it is also true that the drug can trigger the syndrome in susceptible animals, and has been a common denominator in a great many of the patients who have been victims of the syndrome. Indeed, an abnormal response to succinylcholine is often the first sign of malignant hyperthermia, and usually consists of exaggerated fasciculations following the initial dose, failure to produce muscle relaxation, or even frank muscle spasm to the point of opisthotonus. It is not clear in such instances whether the succinylcholine actually triggers the syndrome, or whether the abnormal reaction to the drug merely represents part of the picture of a fundamental biochemical defect of the muscle.

Succinylcholine can produce hyperkalemia to dangerous levels (i.e., cardiac arrest) in patients in whom the response to the drug has been altered by severe burns; neurologic damage such as paraplegia, hemiplegia and multiple sclerosis; muscular dystrophy; or massive trauma. The mechanism is probably related to the fact that succinylcholine, by virtue of its depolarizing mode of action, produces an efflux of potassium from the muscle cell and a rise in potassium level, and this response becomes exaggerated in the types of patients just enumerated. The critical period appears to be between 20 to 60 days following burns; and a similar, although less well defined, period following neurologic damage or gross trauma. Cautious observers, however, believe that the vulnerable period should be considered to extend from as early as 24 to 48 hours and to as late as 90 days.

The earlier belief that succinylcholine is freely compatible with all other drugs has also had to be altered, since it is now recognized that prolonged apneas can follow the use of the drug when certain other compounds are being employed simultaneously. The anti-tumor agents, AB-132 and cyclophosphamide, have been reported to produce a prolonged response to succinylcholine, presumably by depression of the plasma cholinesterase level; and echothiophate eye-drops—an opthalmologic favorite for the management of chronic glaucoma and accommodative esotropia—also cause prolonged apnea when the patient is given succinylcholine. In fact, a great many organophosphorous compounds (of which echothiophate is one) have this property; and a case has been reported from Germany in which an agricultural worker who was the victim of organophosphorous poisoning (the organophosphates are the world's most commonly used pesticides, now that DDT has lost its ecologic status) was prepared for craniotomy in the mistaken belief that he had a brain lesion, received succinylcholine for intubation, and as a result remained apneic for hours. In the case of organophosphate poisoning with echothiophate or a pesticide like parathion, it is not a matter of depression of plasma or pseudocholinesterase levels, but rather of phosphorylation of the cholinesterase, which renders the enzyme totally inactive. A number of disease conditions do actually lower pseudocholinesterase levels, however, by interfering with its hepatic production: liver disease itself, of course; carcinomatous neuropathy; pregnancy; and cachexia or malnutrition from whatever cause. The local anesthetic drugs, procaine and lidocaine, compete with succinylcholine for plasma cholinesterase hydrolysis, and can potentiate the muscle relaxant's action clinically on this basis if they are used in large amounts in the treatment of persistent arrhythmias or as part of the anesthetic technique.

Prolonged apnea following the administration of succinylcholine, however, is most often due to frank overdosage, and results from one of two mechanisms. The first of these relates to the metabolism of succinylcholine. The short duration of action of succinylcholine is the result of its extremely rapid hydrolysis by pseudocholinesterase, to succinylmonocholine and choline. Succinylmonocholine is then hydrolyzed at a much slower rate to succinic acid and choline again (presumably) by pseudocholin-

esterase, but perhaps by other cholinesterase or cholinesterase-like enzymes. Succinic acid and choline have no clinically significant actions at the myoneural junction (succinic acid will enhance the activity of succinylcholine if injected intraarterially, but this is a laboratory exercise of no clinical importance), but succinylmonocholine is a depolarizing muscle relaxant, much less potent than succinylcholine ($\frac{1}{20}$th to $\frac{1}{80}$th, depending upon whom you read), but also much more slowly metabolized. When larger doses of succinylcholine are infused, therefore, considerable amounts of succinylmonocholine can accumulate and produce a prolonged apnea.

The second method by which frank overdosage can produce a prolonged apnea relates to the fact that the block produced by succinylcholine may undergo a change to a nondepolarizing type of block, a so-called "phase II" or "desensitization block." The occurrence of this type of block does not necessarily mean that a prolonged apnea will follow, but a prolonged apnea may well be associated with—if not caused by—a phase II block.

The complication following the administration of succinylcholine which has received the most attention, however, is that relating to prolonged apnea due to atypical pseudocholinesterase. It is interesting that this particular complication should receive so much attention because it is really comparatively rare, occurring in perhaps 1 : 2500, depending upon the population under study. The study which led to its discovery was important, though, not because of the atypical cholinesterase itself, but because it focused attention on the role which genetic factors can have in the reactions to anesthetic drugs and other drugs employed in the surgical patient. It was entitled, "A method for the detection of atypical forms of human serum cholinesterase. Determination of dibucaine numbers" (Kalow, W. and Genest, K.: *Can. J. Biochem. Physiol.*, *35:* 339–346, 1957), and is reprinted below with the kind permission of the authors and the National Research Council of Canada.

A METHOD FOR THE DETECTION OF ATYPICAL FORMS OF HUMAN SERUM CHOLINESTERASE. DETERMINATION OF DIBUCAINE NUMBERS

W. KALOW

AND

K. GENEST

Can. J. Biochem. Physiol., 35: 339–346, 1957

ABSTRACT

"Cases with atypical esterase activity were found by determining esterase inhibition in numerous sera. A suitable inhibitor was the local anaesthetic dibucaine (cinchocaine, TN Nupercaine, Perkain) A good discrimination between typical and atypical sera was obtained under the following conditions: The esterase activity of human serum diluted 1 : 100 was measured with a recording spectrophotometer at 240 mμ. The substrate was 5×10^{-5} M benzoylcholine dissolved in $M/15$ phosphate buffer, pH 7.4. The concentration of the inhibitor was 10^{-5} M. With the experimental temperature around 25° C., the average inhibition of the typical enzyme was 78.8 ± 0.3%. The inhibition of the atypical esterases was less; in rare cases the inhibition was only 16%. For each person, the inhibition characteristics were constant over a period of several months, and independent of the esterase level. The degree of inhibition measured under these conditions and expressed in per cent has been termed "Dibucaine Number"."

Published June, 1979

In a letter to the Editor of the British Medical Journal on January 28, 1950, Dr. F. H. Winterbottom described an incident involving his administration of anesthesia to a woman who was undergoing subtotal pancreatectomy for a carcinoma of the head of the pancreas:

"I saw the patient on the third day after operation and during conversation casually inquired about when she came around. Her reply was somewhat shattering—'As a matter of fact, Doctor, I woke up in the theatre! I remember going to sleep after your injection in my arm, and some time later I was awakened by the most excruciating pain in my tummy. It felt as if my whole inside were being pulled out: I wanted to cry out or otherwise indicate my suffering, but I couldn't move any part of me. I heard the doctors talking about the gall-bladder and about doing something with it to the small intestine. Then I went to sleep again and later woke up back here in bed.'"

Dr. Winterbottom had performed the anesthetic with "thiopentone, nitrous oxide, and tubarine," and his query to the readers of the British Medical Journal was whether any other anesthetist had had the misfortune of having a curarized patient very definitely conscious at some stage of an operative procedure. His letter was entitled "Insufficient Anaesthesia," and he commented that, if faced with a similar type of case again, he would perhaps be a little more generous with the thiopentone.

Awareness during anesthesia is scarcely a new phenomenon: it has been a potential hazard from the very beginning. In fact, probably the first documented instance of awareness during anesthesia occurred on the occasion of the classic public demonstration of the efficacy of ether anesthesia by William Thomas Green Morton on October 16, 1846. Dr. John Collins Warren, the Senior Surgeon at the Massachusetts General Hospital, who performed the operation for the removal of a tumor from the neck of Gilbert Abbott, has left us perhaps the best description of that operation:

"The patient was arranged for the operation in a sitting posture and everything made ready . . . the patient was then made to inhale . . . from a tube connected with a glass globe. After four or five minutes he appeared to be asleep and was thought by Dr. Morton to be in a condition for the operation. I made an incision between two and three inches long in the direction of the tumor and to my great surprise without any starting, crying, or other indication of pain. The fascia was divided, the patient still appearing wholly insensible ... I was not satisfied myself until I had, soon after operation and on various other occasions, asked the questions whether he had suffered pain. To this he always replied in the negative, adding, however, that he knew of the operation, and comparing the stroke of the knife to that of a blunt instrument passed roughly across the neck."

Note Warren's careful language: "To this he always replied in the negative, adding, however, *that he knew of the operation*, and comparing the stroke of the knife to that of a blunt instrument passed roughly across the neck." This is awareness without pain, comparable, but not identical, to the ether analgesia during recovery from ether anesthesia described by John Snow a year later: "Commonly, the patient would feel pain if any part of an operation were performed in this stage, but not always; for, in some instances, the special senses of sight and hearing, and complete consciousness and volition, return before common sensibility, and the operation may be going on, for a short time, without his feeling it, and perhaps, whilst he, thinking that it is concluded, is remarking that he did not feel it."

Indeed, many of the anesthetics of the first decades, following Morton's successful use of ether, were performed at such light levels of anesthesia that accounts at the time indicate that it was customary to inquire, immediately after commencement of surgery, whether the patient was feeling any pain—conversation among surgeon, anesthetist, *and patient* was the rule, just as it still is today when conduction anesthesia is used. As surgical horizons expanded to intra-abdominal operations, the demand for muscular relaxation and even utter flaccidity led to much deeper levels of anesthesia, and little was heard of awareness during anesthesia with such potent inhalation anesthetics as ether and chloroform.

With the introduction of curare, however, the problem of awareness began to re-emerge. The instance described in the letter from Winterbottom, quoted above, was followed by a spate of Letters to the Editor in the British Medical Journal, but 9 years were to elapse before the next published report appeared in the literature. This described a 40 year old woman undergoing vaginal hysterectomy under thiopental, N_2O, succinylcholine infusion, with assisted respirations. It was noted that there were occasional episodes of resistance to inspiratory assistance, and at one point during the operation the patient (in the lithotomy position) suddenly moved her right leg. Graff and Phillips reported: "Despite this apparently uneventful anesthetic course the patient had a most unpleasant experience to relate to the surgeon and anesthetist .... She had been intermittently conscious and unconscious during the three-hour anesthetic period .... She volunteered the information that an airway had been inserted in her mouth and removed at some time later .... She reconstructed details pertaining to the discussion of the blood loss and the decision to start administration of the second unit of blood .... She also experienced dull, unbearable pelvic, lower back, and perineal pain during much of the operation."

There was little doubt in the minds of the attending physicians that the patient was conscious during phases of this procedure and suffered considerable discomfort.

Graff and Phillips documented this case in 1969, and during the intervening 20 years, which have witnessed a widespread use of so-called balanced techniques of anesthesia, the anesthesiologist has become very concerned over the problem of awareness during anesthesia. A number of investigations have been undertaken and have clearly identified the problem of awareness, with or without pain, as being related to the use of muscle relaxants. Henderson, in one of the first retrospective studies, could identify no instances of awareness during 181 anesthetic administrations which did not include the use of a muscle relaxant; only 2 instances of awareness in 201 patients to whom a short-acting muscle relaxant was administered to facilitate endotracheal intubation (and these could undoubtedly be accepted as instances of redistribution of thiopental before the inhalation agent could take hold of the situation); but 6 instances of awareness in 216 patients to whom a long-acting muscle relaxant was administered, combined with the use of controlled respirations. She found, in short, a 2.8 per cent incidence of awareness when a long-acting muscle relaxant was employed to produce total paralysis, with ventilation then being maintained by artificial means.

The problem, of course, is the difficulty of judging the "depth" (and that is a most inappropriate word for it) of hypnotic-nitrous oxide-relaxant-narcotic anesthesia. There is no precise classification of the stages and signs of anesthesia such as Guedel developed for the administration of ether anesthesia. It has been said that, with this mode of "balanced anesthesia," there is a floor under the anesthesia, in the sense that the patient is unlikely to become too "deep" (in the classical sense), but that there is no ceiling over it, and it is all too possible for the patient to become too "light" and enter a stage of awareness. Indeed, one wag has classified the stages of "balanced anesthesia" as too light, too deep, and just right. Every anesthesiologist develops his or her own criteria indicative of insufficient doses of the individual drugs employed in "balanced anesthesia", and these do not always coincide with the criteria which would be employed by another observer. The blood pressure, the pulse rate, sweating, grimacing, movement, tearing, straining, sternocleidomastoid tension, and the like mean different things to different people, and even many of these disappear as useful signs in the fully paralyzed, ventilated patient.

Gordon Wyant described the problem eloquently in a sensitive and thought-provoking Letter to the Editor of the Canadian Anaesthetist's Society Journal:

"Dear Sir:

General anaesthesia, by definition, involves total loss of consciousness and the patient who is told that a general anaesthetic will be administered is entitled to expect not only freedom from pain during the surgical procedure but also total oblivion. That patients much too frequently become aware of their surroundings in the course of their operation and moreover, although happily more rarely, that pain sensation is not totally abolished must in the vast majority of instances and in the absence of equipment failure be a reflection upon the anaesthetist's competence and choice of technique.

"Awareness in the course of a general anaesthetic used to be a rarity when reliance for the maintenance of the anaesthetic state was placed upon potent but easily adjustable inhalation agents and relaxants were used only to the extent that relaxation of skeletal muscles was required. The introduction of techniques which combine light sleep and analgesia with large doses of relaxants has changed all that. Even experienced anaesthetists do not always find it easy to determine when unconsciousness is on the wane or when further doses of analgesics are required since the classical signs of tachycardia and tearing are by no means constant and in retrospect have not occurred in some patients who, by their own account, have been awake during all, most, or part of the operation. Hence errors of judgment as to the need for deeper anaesthesia and further analgesics do occur and they happen more frequently the less experienced the anaesthetist."

Many people have pondered these problems at considerable lengths, but the first to attempt to unravel the conflicting signs and devise a rational scheme of things was Philip D. Woodbridge, in a paper which he wrote on the need to develop a new classification to describe the levels of nervous depression during anesthetic polypharmacy or "balanced anesthesia."

Woodbridge was way ahead of his time, of course; but in addition he made a fatal mistake. He had a friend who was a Professor of Classics, and together they plotted to outdo Oliver Wendell Holmes and come up with an even worse word than anesthesia to describe the state that Woodbridge was so brilliantly documenting. They did. They came up with the term *nothria*, which, translated from the Greek, means torpor. Then they compounded the error by coining the following words derived from *nothria; nothrogen*, noun, a drug which produces nothria; *nothretic,* adjective, insensible, inactive, stuporous; *nothretize,* verb, to produce nothria; *nothreusis,* noun, the process of producing nothria; *nothretist,* noun, one who produces nothria; *nothrology,* noun, knowledge or study of nothria; and *nothrologist,* noun, one who makes a study of nothria. No one ever really took the paper seriously after that, which was too bad, because it was precisely the type of concept that was needed to classify and evaluate the various levels of the hypnotic-nitrous oxide-narcotic-relaxant sequence. It was a landmark paper on a matter of great concern to the anesthesiologist, and it deserved to be taken seriously.

Woodbridge's paper, "Changing Concepts Concerning Depth of Anesthesia," was published in the July-August, 1957, issue of *Anesthesiology* (*18*: 536, 1957) and is reprinted below with the kind permission of the publisher.

CHANGING CONCEPTS CONCERNING DEPTH OF ANESTHESIA

Philip D. Woodbridge

Anesthesiology, 18: 536, 1957

"Before each operation and before each phase of each operation the *nothrologist* needs to ask himself: how much *sensory* blocking is needed? how much *relaxation* is needed? how much blocking of *reflexes* is needed? how much *mental* blocking is needed? and with what drug will I produce each of these actions? He may decide on a single drug which, combined with suitable preliminary medication, will cover the needs of the operation, with a wide margin; or, on the other hand, he may fit the effect more closely to the need in each component by using drugs having more specific actions. The currently discussed question of the use of a single agent as contrasted to "polypharmacy" seems to resolve itself mainly into the questions of how closely the proposed drug or combination of drugs fits the anticipated pattern of needs for a given operation, and what undesirable side effects it may produce.

* * * *

"The pattern of signs of depth of "general anesthesia" formulated by Guedel and others was designed primarily for ether and similar drugs. We are now using drugs having more limited or specific action, and a new pattern of signs is needed to use with them. Such a pattern is offered, for further elaboration by others, in which the process until now known as "general anesthesia" is divided into the four components of sensory block, motor block, block of reflexes, and mental block. Since the word anesthesia properly refers to sensory block only, the word *Nothria* is introduced, to refer to combinations of these components."

1959

Published February, 1967

Today, Classical File is ten years old—as is *Survey of Anesthesiology* itself—and a tenth birthday party is always a wonderfully exciting event. There are presents to open, games to play, and ice cream and cake galore. At least, so it is with ten year old boys and girls.

With ten year old Classical Files it is a little different. There is no ice cream and cake, and the name of the game has just recently become Find-Something-Good-That-Faulconer-And-Keys-Haven't-Already-Republished. But there are lots of presents—and have been for ten whole years. Perhaps the biggest and best has been from The Editor of *Survey of Anesthesiology*, who has scrupulously refrained from changing so much as a comma (although he thinks that there are too many of, them) in the Introductory Comments to Classical File. A second wonderful present has been from the publishers, who have cooperated completely and uncomplainingly to fulfill requests for translations, reproductions of illustrations, and myriad other outlandish demands. And, finally, there have been all those presents from other journals, books, authors, and publishers which have made Classical File possible and for which public acknowledgment of thanks are due:

*   *   *   *

All of these goodies are bound to put one into a gay, holiday mood; and faithful readers of these columns may recall that on the occasion of a similar joyous anniversary 5 years ago, Classical File indulged in a bit of whimsey concerning the socio-economic status of anesthesia by republishing Richard Gordon's "Sleeping Partner." This light-hearted approach failed to precipitate irate letters either from or to the Editor of *Survey of Anesthesiology*, a fact which has been interpreted as license for Classical File to shed its strict concern with science and musty archives once every 5 years in favor of some consideration of the more mundane aspects of the practice of anesthesia.

For this reason, Classical File departs from its usual sequential plan to present an article that has been republished many times in medical journals all over this country and abroad; republished so often, as a matter of fact, that its presentation here could almost be considered *de trops*—except that Classical File would be derelict in its duty to ignore such a communication any longer. For those who have read this classic before, it is hoped that rereading will only serve to intensify the enjoyment; for those who have never read it, *Survey* is delighted to present the editorial, "A Fable of Anesthesia For Our Times," which was published in the September, 1959, issue of the *Journal of Community and Social Medicine* (*J. Comm. & Soc. Med., 3:* 47–53, 1959)

and is reprinted below with the kind permissions of the editor and the publishers.

A FABLE OF ANESTHESIA FOR OUR TIMES

J. Comm. Soc. Med., 3: 47–53, 1959

Once upon a time there was a mouse who was an anesthesiologist.

He was a very well-trained mouse, and he held a number of degrees to prove this fact, including an A.B., a C.D., and E.F., and an F.F.R.R.S.T.U.V.A.

He was active in a number of scientific societies, among which were the International Rodent Anesthesia Research Society, the Amalgamated Association of Mice Anesthesiologists, and the United Society for the Prevention of Laryngospasm.

He also held a faculty appointment at The Medical School and of this he was exceedingly proud; whenever he gave anesthesia for the Chief of Surgery—who naturally was a bear—he made a special effort to have things go well, for he knew that it was the Bear who dispensed faculty appointments.

One day the Bear was in an especially bad humor.

In the first place, there had been that ridiculous incident of the porridge bowls the night before, and it had been well after midnight before they had gotten the little girl back to her family.

And then, when he finally had gone to bed, he hadn't been able to sleep. He was still seething over the letter of rejection from *The Leading Surgical Journal*. Having the article rejected was bad enough in itself, for Lord knows he had published very little that year, and one didn't stay Chief of Surgery just by doing good surgery. As a matter-of-fact, doing good surgery didn't have anything to do with being Chief of Surgery: a lot of the other bears didn't realize this, but a couple of the residents were beginning to suspect it. But the thing about the letter that he really resented was the insinuation by The Editor that the work had been plagiarized from some research of one of The Editor's own junior colleagues. Why, he remembered the very night at last year's Grand Surgical Meeting when he had told The Editor, at dinner, of his idea that the serum rhubarb level was drastically reduced after operation, and might account for some of the cardiovascular complications encountered in the postoperative period. (He had forgotten the name of the interne who had first suggested this at rounds one day; but in any case, the boy had been very indefinite and hadn't expressed it at all well.)

The Bear finally had drifted off to a fitful sleep, only to get up in the morning to that hideous family argument at breakfast over where to go to hibernate the next winter. The argument had been dominated by the unpleasant, but inescapable, fact that Junior Bear was doing so poorly at school that he would have to be tutored again, and they wouldn't be able to afford a hibernation in any event.

The crowning blow, though, was to arrive at The Hospital and find that two operating rooms were closed again for lack of anesthesia. Now this didn't affect the Bear's own operating schedule, of course, for as Chief of Surgery he had a goldplated priority (he had objected to this priority system when it had first been set up some years before he was made Chief of Surgery, but he was beginning to see the wisdom of it now). But besides, that little pipsqueak, the Mouse, wouldn't dare give anesthesia for anyone else if he were operating. No, his own cases would get done, all right; that wasn't the problem. The problem was that some of the other bears would be raising cane about two operating rooms being closed again because there were not enough anesthesiologists—and particularly those bears who had been bumped off the schedule would be raising cane. And this *did* affect the Bear, because you didn't stay Chief of Surgery just by doing good surgery.

The Mouse had been intuitively aware of the Bear's foul mood the minute the Bear had come into the operating room. Perhaps it was the Mouse's keen perception of people—his mother, who used to do interpretations of the dreams of each member of the family at breakfast, had always said that he was so sensitive to people that he should become a psychiatrist—but it also might have been the fact that the Bear started off by glaring at him so viciously that he felt like climbing right inside the reservoir bag of his anesthesia machine.

"Well, what the blankety-blank-blank are you going to do about those two rooms being closed again, huh?"

The Bear's roar almost blew the mouse right off his stool.

"S-S-ir?"

"I said, what the blankety-blank-blank are you going to do about those two rooms being closed again?"

"Well, its . . . it's awfully hard to get anesthesiologists, you know."

"Why? Why is it so blankety-blank hard to get them?"

"Well, there's . . . there's a very real shortage . . . all over the country . . . a real shortage."

The Mouse paused. He wanted to go on, but then he thought that discretion was the better part of valor. On the other hand, it was wise to strike while the iron was hot. He went on.

"Besides, it's not easy to get them to come here. The working conditions aren't the best, you know." He hurried on, lest he lose his nerve. "And with all those ward cases, the income isn't very good for all the work we do, you know. And the cheese isn't terribly good."

"Cheese, schmeese," roared the Bear. "Who gives a blankety-blank about cheese. We've got to get this surgery done, and that's all there is to it. Now over at Elsewhere Hospital they don't have any trouble running *all* of their operating rooms *all* the time. My friend Grizzly is Chief of Surgery over there, and he says that they have a troupe of trained canaries to give anesthesia and they're never short of anesthetists. They don't have to cancel half a dozen cases every day: they get *all* of their cases done every day."

The Mouse had known this was coming and he had been dreading it.

"But wouldn't you rather have a trained mouse anesthesiologist than a registered canary given anesthesia for you?"

"I don't give a blankety-blank who gives my anesthesia so long as I can cut," roared the Bear. That's beside the point, anyway," he added as an afterthought, "You'll give my anesthesia for me if you want to stay here. But we've got to get those other two rooms opened. *And that's final.*"

That afternoon the Mouse and the Bear went downstairs to the office to see the Fox—who naturally was the Hospital Superintendent.

The Fox was a very pleasant fox, always cordial and smiling—and very clever. The Mouse had never trusted the Fox. In the first place, he didn't trust people who were always smiling. And in the second place, he'd been around long enough to know that the Fox was an Empire Builder—and he didn't trust Empire Builders, either.

That afternoon the Fox was all smiles, and all cordiality, and all pleasantness. He agreed with the Bear that something must be done about the situation in the operating room. The Hospital was losing a great deal of money with those two operating rooms closed; it was running a deficit for that fiscal moon which was just too large to ignore any longer. But quite aside from the deficit, the Board of Directors—who naturally were all Eagles—was getting very upset. After all, the Board of Directors had a responsibility to the Community, and that responsibility was to see that The Sick in the Community were cared for in the best possible manner. Surely, the Mouse could see that responsibility—and as a physician he must share that responsibility. The Community had a right to expect The Hospital and its physicians to care for The Sick. Surely, the Mouse could appreciate that right—after all, that's why he had gone into Medicine, wasn't it, to care for The Sick? Of course it was. Well, now, there was the problem: how were they going to solve it. What was needed was more anesthesiologists. The Mouse sighed wanly, and explained again that there was a big shortage, all over the country. The Fox just smiled and listened. Besides, the Mouse went on, even more wanly, the working conditions weren't the best, the income wasn't too good in view of the arduous call schedule and all the work that they had to

cover, and the cheese wasn't terribly good. The Fox just smiled some more, ignored the remark about the cheese (although it burned him up inwardly—that little pipsqueak), and directed himself to the Bear.

"Well, if we can't get anesthesiologists, we'll have to find some other solution, I guess. Perhaps we should consider what you phoned me about this noon."

"You mean a troupe of trained canaries?", asked the Bear.

"Yes, I don't like it as a solution; in some ways it's a backward step," went on the Fox smoothly, "but there just doesn't seem to be any alternative. We have a responsibility to The Community, and that responsibility is to see that The Sick are cared for in the best possible manner."

"But they won't be cared for in the best manner," cried the Mouse.

"The best *possible* manner," went on the Fox, even more smoothly, "The best *possible* manner. And I don't think that canaries who have been well trained and are registered with the Association of Canary Anesthetists would be all that bad. There are lots of simple anesthesias that they can do very adequately; and you and the other mice could supervise them and take over the more difficult cases yourselves. After all, you've said many times that an anesthesiologist is really working to save the difficult 10 per cent from trouble, that the rest of the anesthesias are fairly routine. Like obstetrics, where the obstetrician is really working to keep the few problem cases out of trouble."

The Mouse blushed right down to the tip of his tail. He had said that, of course, and in some ways it *was* partly true. But the trouble was, you could never tell who the 10 per cent were going to be, in most instances. He tried to explain this to the Fox, but the Fox just smiled and said, well, in any event, there didn't seem to be any other alternative. They had a responsibility to The Community to care for The Sick, and he was going to have to recommend a troupe of trained canaries to the Board of Directors as the best possible solution to the problem.

The next few months were a nightmare for the Mouse. One of the younger mice on the Staff got called into Service, and they had to close a third operating room. The neurosurgeon—who naturally was a Wildcat—told the Mouse that if something wasn't done, and done soon, he was going to the Board of Directors himself, for some of them were very close personal friends of his and they would listen to him, you better believe it. The Mouse tried desperately to find replacements. He wrote or called all of his friends to see if they knew of someone who could fill in; he advertised in all of the journals; he even wrote to some of the Placement Bureaus, although he knew that they couldn't usually get anybody very good that way. The bears were roaring all the time now, and the Fox kept calling him downstairs for more and more conferences about getting a troupe of trained canaries and even starting a school to train canaries, for the Mouse had pointed out that even a troupe of trained canaries wasn't going to be easy to hire—there was a shortage of them, too.

It all came to a head one day when the Fox put out a letter to the entire staff outlining the situation and stating that, as of the next full moon, the Hospital would hire a troupe of trained canaries as anesthetists. The mice would supervise the canaries, and the Hospital hoped that the mice would become fulltime employees of the Hospital, as that would make things much easier administratively. The salary policy would be very liberal: each mouse would be paid just as much as he had earned as income from private practice the previous fiscal moon; and, of course, the Hospital was in a position to add all kinds of fringe benefits—pension, life insurance, health insurance, cheese insurance, and the like. Naturally, all the mice refused to become salaried employees of the Hospital; they told the Fox to go to, and stayed in private practice.

On a Tuesday afternoon soon thereafter—the Weasel—who naturally was the Assistant Superintendent of the Hospital—telephoned the Mouse.

"The Fox is away," the Weasel explained, "a National Symposium for Foxes on Cost-accounting, but he wanted me to call you to let you know that we have hired a troupe

of trained canaries and the first of them will be arriving to start work next week. He wants you to set up their work schedule and a schedule for their supervision by the other Mice."

"Now wait a minute," cried the Mouse, "This is a big step backwards—things aren't all that bad."

"Well," said the Weasel smoothly (he wasn't as smooth as the Fox, but he was smooth enough), "we now have three operating rooms closed because we don't have enough anesthesiologists. That's 12 sick people in this Community who can't be operated on each day. That's 72 sick people in this Community who are being neglected each week. That's 3,744 sick people in this Community who are not receiving the proper Medical Care, which is their birth-right, each year. We have a responsibility to this Community—you, and I, and the whole Hospital Family—we have a big and sacred responsibility to this Community."

"But they aren't being neglected," wailed the Mouse, "lots of those operations aren't necessary. Doing or not doing a rhinoplasty on a Pelican has nothing to do with proper Medical Care."

"That's beside the point," went on the Weasel. "And furthermore we can't run the Hospital with all those empty beds," he added as an afterthought. "Anyway, the Board of Directors has ordered it, and it's been done. You can expect the first canary to arrive next Monday."

The next few months were even more of a nightmare for the Mouse. Some of the canaries weren't really trained at all, even if they were registered with the Association of Canary Anesthetists, and he had to train them himself. And then he'd just get a canary to the point where she was moderately safe when she'd leave to join another troupe of trained canaries. He never could rely on the canaries all being there when they were supposed to be, either: they were always calling in and saying that they were nesting or laying an egg or something.

But the worst problem was the bears. They were roaring continuously now, complaining that this was a really bad risk patient, and demanding that one of the mice give the anesthesia. "Canaries are all right,

Mouse, but this D. & C. is a real bad risk. Let the canary do Joe Bear's case—he's just doing a portacaval shunt."

The Mouse was close to tears with distraction. Here they had said that they just wanted to be able to cut, but now they all wanted mice anesthesiologists for all of their cases, and there were no more mice to go around than there had been before. In fact, there were less, for two others had resigned rather than supervise canaries and run a school to train canaries.

Then one day the Fox called the Mouse down to his office again.

The Fox was very pleasant, and very cordial, and all smiles, as usual. He'd had a phone call from another Fox, he said, a friend of his who was Medical Superintendent at the Mecca Hospital. They had a young Rat who was just finishing his training in anesthesiology who would like to work at The Hospital. He apparently was a very good anesthesiologist, although young, and very well thought of at the Mecca Hospital. He had a young and growing family, though, and he couldn't afford to take chances financially. He had to be able to count on enough income to feed the young and growing family. What the Fox proposed to do was put the Rat on a salary: this would guarantee his income, and he could take over some of the supervising and training of the canaries. This would give the mice more time to do their own private cases, and still keep an eye on the canaries. That was one of the things that the mice had been complaining about, the Fox went on smoothly, and this would be a good solution.

Now the Mouse didn't like this idea at all, for he knew where this would lead. But the Fox kept answering all of his objections and emphasizing that it would give them another trained anesthesiologist and so improve patient care—which after all was their aim, and their responsibility to the Board of Directors and the Community. The Mouse couldn't very well say that he just didn't trust the Fox, which is really what it came down to; but short of saying that, there wasn't any valid argument that the Fox couldn't answer. The Mouse spent three hours that afternoon arguing with

the Fox, and when he left the fox's office he felt as though he'd been locked in a closed barn for a month with a Cheshire cat.

The Rat arrived a month later. He was a very arrogant rat, and he had a great deal to say about the way anesthesia was being given in The Hospital. He thought that the equipment was terrible and immediately put in an order for six Cyclone anesthesia machines and four Tornado ventilators. The Mouse was very disturbed about this, for the budget for equipment for the year wouldn't possibly cover that amount of new purchases; and besides, the order should have gone over his signature. He told the Rat this, but the Rat just laughed and said that there would have to be some changes made. The Rat refused to be on call at night or on the weekend to supervise the canaries. He said that his salary wasn't *that* big: if the mice wanted to be on call, that was their business, but he wasn't going to be. What should be done, he said, was to make one of the canaries a Head Canary, and let her worry about supervision at night and on the weekends. That's the way it had been done at the Mecca Hospital.

It was almost a year after the Rat had come when the Fox called the Mouse down to his office one day.

He was all smiles, and pleasantness, and cordiality. How were things going? The Mouse didn't think that things were going at all well, but he didn't say so. He said all right, he guessed. Yes, well, said the Fox, there was a knotty problem from the administrative point-of-view, and he'd been talking to the Board of Directors about it. The fact of the matter was that the Hospital was losing a great deal of money on the Anesthesia Department, what with all the new equipment and all the salaries for the canaries, and the Rat, and all, and something would have to be worked out so that the Hospital didn't run into such a big loss. Now his idea was that if the mice were to go on salary too, guaranteeing them as much income as they had earned from private practice the previous fiscal moon, of course, as well as such fringe benefits that the Hospital could provide as a pension plan, health insurance, life insurance, and even cheese insurance, why then the Hospital could make up the deficit without passing the cost on to the patient, and the mice would be even better off than they were at present.

The Mouse said that he couldn't see how that could be so at all: how could The Hospital pay even more money to run the Department and not have a deficit that would be passed on to the patient?

"Well," said the Fox smoothly, "after all, there would be income from the private cases that is going to the mice as private fees now."

The Mouse thought about this for a while. But how, he asked, would that money, which was going to the mice now, more than just cover what would be paid them under the Fox's plan? Why wouldn't there still be a deficit?

"I was just coming to that," said the Fox; "we won't need as many mice as there are now."

And so the Mouse resigned (if that's what you call it) from the Hospital Staff and the Medical School Faculty. He also dropped his membership in the Amalgamated Association of Mice Anesthesiologists, for he realized now that you didn't have to be a Mouse to be an anesthesiologist—you could be a Rat. Then he went down to the Virgin Islands on the advice of his psychiatrist—who naturally was an Owl. He has stayed on there even after he recovered from his acute melancholia: he does some general practice in St. Thomas and some part time anesthesia at the hospital in Charlotte Amalie.

The Bear retired from private practice and took a full time job as Coordinator of Surgical Research at The Hospital. He was given a gold watch by the troupe of trained canaries at the testimonial dinner marking his retirement as Chief of Surgery. The Bear family hibernates at the same cottage in Palm Springs every winter now.

The Fox built a 250 bed wing on The Hospital, and then hired two more Assistant Superintendents because The Hospital was so much bigger.

And the moral to this story, of course, is that the horns of a Dilemma are equally sharp if you happen to be a mouse.

Published February, 1975

Christopher Wren was undoubtedly the best known of England's architects. He was responsible for the reconstruction of St. Paul's Cathedral following its damage in the The Great Fire of London in 1666. Furthermore, he designed 52 churches and buildings in London, including the additions to both the Kensington and Hampton Court Palaces. As noted previously in these columns, he was a man of many parts and myriad talents. He held the degrees of Bachelor of Arts, Master of Arts, Doctor of Civil Law, and Doctor of Law; and he was at one time Savilian Professor of Astronomy at Oxford. He was an authentic genius, with a wide range of interests. Perhaps not unreasonably, these came to include experimental medicine; and in 1665, some 188 years before the invention of the hollow needle and syringe, he made use of a quill and an animal bladder ("in the manner of clysterpipes") to inject fluids intravenously—a fact recorded in the Monday, December 4, 1665, issue of the *Philosophical Transactions of the Royal Society*, under the title, "An account of the rise and attempts, of a way to conveigh liquors immediately into the mass of blood."

Within a year, the British physician, Richard Lower, made use of the knowledge of Sir Christopher Wren's demonstration that substances could be introduced directly into the blood stream by making a transfusion, which he also reported in the *Philosophical Transactions of the Royal Society* in an article entitled, "The method observed in transfusing the bloud out of one animal into another." It must be deduced from his account that Lower was a remarkable scientist and doctor. His final paragraph read, "The most probable use of his experiment may be conjectured to be, that one animal may live with the bloud of another; and consequently, that those animals, that want bloud, or have corrupt bloud, may be supplyed from others with a sufficient quantity, and of such as is good, provided the transfusion be often repeated, by reason of the quick expense that is made of the bloud."

The technique of transfusion had been born—and transfusion reactions were not far behind. Within 7 months, Jean Baptiste Denis reported from Paris on the first:

"December 19 (Sunday—Gregorian Calendar). We used what art we could to dispose the fancy of our patient to suffer the transfusion, which we resolv'd should be tried upon him that night about 6 o'clock. M. Emmerez open'd the Crural Artery of a Calf and did all the necessary preparations . . . and after he had drawn from the patient about ten ounces of blood out of a Vein of the right arm, we could give him no more again than about five or six ounces of that of the calf, by reason that his constrained posture and the crowd of spectators, interrupted very much this operation.

"Meanwhile he found himself, as he said very hot all along his arm, and under the Armpits, and perceived that he was falling into a swoon, we presently stopped the blood running in, and closed the wound; yet he supped two hours after, and notwithstanding some dulness and sleepiness he was now and then, he yet passed that night with singing, whistling and other extravagances usual with him.

"We therefore prepared ourselves to repeat it upon him the next Wednesday at 6 o'clock in the presence of several persons. . .

"We took but two or three ounces of blood from him, and having put him into a convenient posture we made the second transfusion into his left arm more plentiful than the first. For considering the blood remaining in the calf after the operation, the Patient must have received more than one whole pound.

"As this second transfusion was larger, so were the effects of it quicker and more considerable. As soon as the blood began to enter into his veins, he felt the like heat along his arm, and under his armpits, which he had felt before. His pulse rose presently, and soon we observed a plentiful sweat over all his face. His pulse varied extremely at this instant, and he complained of great pain in his kidneys, and that he was not well in his stomach, and that he was ready to choke unless they gave him his liberty. Presently, the Pipe was taken out that conveyed the blood into his veins, and while we were closing the wound, he vomited of Bacon and Fat he had eaten half an hour before. He found himself urged to urine, and asked to go to stool. He was soon made to lie down, and after two good hours straining to void divers liquors, which disturbed his stomach, he fell asleep about 10 o'clock, and slept all that night without awakening till next morning, was Thursday, about 8 o'clock. When he was awakened, he shewed a surprising calmness, and a great presence of mind, in expressing all the pains, and a general lassitude he felt in all his limbs. He made a great glass full of urine, of a colour as black, as if it had been mixed with the soot of chimney. . .

"Friday morning he filled another urinal with his water, almost as black as that of the day before. He bled at the nose very plentifully . . . Saturday morning . . . the same day; his urine cleared up and after that time it resumed little by little its natural color."

The clinical symptoms and signs of a hemolytic transfusion reaction in the conscious patient can include chill (55 per cent), temperature elevation (47 per cent), shock (hypotension—2 per cent), increased pulse rate (28 per cent), tightness in the chest (7 per cent), dyspnea (7 per cent), rales (3 per cent), nausea and vomiting (7 per cent), lumbar pain (5 per cent), urticaria (35 per cent), red urine (5 per cent), jaundice (1 per cent), and such miscellaneous signs and symptoms as singulitis, a feeling of numbness in the face, a throbbing feeling in the arms, difficulty in breathing through the nose, a swollen feeling in the jaw, a burning sensation on voiding, uncoordinated speech, and headache. It is interesting to note that Jean Baptiste Denis also described a number of these in his report more than 300 years ago!

The diagnosis of a transfusion reaction during general anesthesia is dependent upon far less evidence, since of course there are no symptoms whatsoever, and even the signs may be modified by the effects of general anesthesia itself. The anesthetized patient does have one thing going for him, however, in terms of having a correct diagnosis made—the anesthesiologist. The anesthetized patient is watched far more closely in the operating room than any patient is observed at the bedside, so that the meager signs that do accompany a transfusion reaction during anesthesia have far more chance of being observed than the more liberal supply of diagnostic clues in the conscious patient. The problem in the anesthetized patient, however, is formidable, despite the anesthesiologist's close attention to his patient's well-being. The factors of concern have been beautifully documented in the April, 1959, issue of the *British Journal of Anaesthesia* in an article titled, "Incompatible blood transfusions during operation" (Binder, L. S.; Ginsberg, V.; and Harmel, M. H.: *Br. J. Anaesth., 31:* 217–228, 1959), which is reprinted below with the kind permissions of the authors and the publisher.

INCOMPATIBLE BLOOD TRANSFUSIONS DURING OPERATION

LEE S. BINDER,
VICTOR GINSBERG
AND
MEREL H. HARMEL

The Departments of Anesthesiology and Medicine, State University of New York, Downstate Medical Center and the Kings County Hospital Center, Brooklyn, New York

Br. J. Anaesth., 31: 217–228, 1959

*   *   *   *

SUMMARY

"Eleven case reports are presented which illustrate the circumstances surrounding the administration of incompatible blood and the development of incompatible transfusion reactions during anaesthesia. Unlike the clinical picture manifested by conscious patients, the signs of transfusion reaction in this group of patients were generally limited to hypotension, generalized oozing, or both; and incompatible transfusion reactions which develop during operation may be classified on this basis. Because the coagulation defect may be unrecognized, and because both hypotension and increased bleeding are commonly attributed to other causes, the incompatible transfusion reaction is not suspected until late and the patient therefore treated with still more incompatible blood.

"The coagulation defects associated with incompatible transfusion reactions are not clearly defined. The authors suggest that fresh whole blood is the only substance which provides all clotting factors, and should therefore be the initial therapy of any acute coagulation defect.

"Since diagnosis and treatment of incompatible transfusion reactions are uniquely difficult during operation and in the immediate postoperative period, the authors stress that the greater hope for decreasing the incidence of incompatible transfusion reactions in the surgical patient lies in more adequate preparation of the patient with regard to pre-operative blood volume replacement and more judicious use of blood during operation."

1960

Published April, 1968

The Lancet had quite a tale to tell on August 4th, 1934:

"The patient was a middle-aged man, rather thin and pale. He said that for a number of years he had suffered at times from pain in the region of the stomach after food. Recently vomiting had troubled him. This took place at irregular intervals, the amount being copious. On going into details he remembered bringing up matter which he had eaten many hours before. The vomit was offensive as a rule. He also was prone to violent and foul-smelling eructations. But what really distressed him more than anything else was the following startling occurrence.

"One evening he had taken his wife to the cinema. There, in the darkness, feeling inclined to smoke, he had taken out a cigarette, and put it between his lips; he struck a match, bringing it up in his cupped fingers. Just at that minute a violent eructation occurred. To his alarm and astonishment, and of those seated near him, there was a flash and a sharp explosion; the cigarette was blown from his lips away across several rows of seats; his mustache was singed, and his lips and fingers burnt. In pain and confusion he had hurriedly to leave the cinema. The astonishment of the neighbours at this 'fiery exhalation' can well be imagined.

"The diagnosis of pyloric obstruction was fairly clear. Gastric peristalsis was easily seen. The barium meal showed the usual prolonged delay in the stomach. The gastric contents were copious, with yeast cells, sarcinae, and lactic acid. No doubt the gas from the stomach mingled with the air in the mouth and cupped hands in just the right proportions, the cavities forming an explosion chamber, which required only a naked flame to produce this unpleasant occurrence. At laparotomy a cicatrised ulcer was found at the pylorus."

This was certainly a novel story, but hardly a unique one. Back in 1886, *The British Medical Journal* had one of its own to tell, under the heading of "Surgical Memoranda:"

"I have thought it right to put on record the following case, as it seems to me to be one of some rarity, and to have some importance from a medicolegal point of view. I cannot do better than give the facts in the words of the patient himself, who communicated them to me by letter. He writes as follows:

" 'A rather strange thing happened to myself about a week ago. For a month or so I was troubled very much with foul eructations. I had no pain, but the smell of the gas which came from my stomach was disagreeable to myself, and to all who happened to be in the room. About a week ago, as I said, I got up in the morning, and lighted a match to see the time, and when I put the match near my mouth, to blow it out, my breath caught fire, and gave a loud crack like the report of a pistol. It burnt my lips, and they are still a little sore. I got a terrible surprise and so did my wife, for the report awakened her.'

"From the above occurrence it would appear that the condition known as 'halitosis' or diseased breath, is not only a source of misery to the sufferer, and those compelled to associate with him, but may, under certain circumstances become a condition of danger to the unfortunate possessor of it. In the present instance, the gaseous results of the imperfectly digested food had their atoms of carbon and hydrogen so arranged as to give rise to the presence of carburetted hydrogen, the inflammable and explosive qualities of which came into play when mixed with due proportion of atmospheric air in the presence of the unguarded light of the burning match. I may add, that the patient to whom this accident happened, is a most intelligent and observant man, and that the diet I prescribed for the indigestion from which he suffers from time to time has alcohol excluded from it, and I know that my instructions in that respect are acted upon."

Four years later, the same journal had another "fiery exhaler" to report. This was a 24 year old factory worker, whose work required him to rise early, "and on one occasion after striking a match to see the time, and when holding it near his mouth, an eructation of gas from the stomach took place. To his consternation the gas took fire, burned his face and lips considerably, and set fire to his moustache."

The Lancet reported yet another case in 1902:

"An elderly man under my care has been suffering for some weeks from severe atonic dyspepsia. A marked feature of his case is fermentative decomposition of the contents of the dilated stomach with frequent eructations of foul gas which he says 'tastes like rotten eggs.' On Sept. 19th, two hours after a light breakfast, he was obliged to eructate just as he was lighting his pipe with a match; instantly there was a blinding flash and a slight report due to ignition of the gases released from the stomach. The patient's beard and eyebrows were thoroughly singed but happily no further damage was done."

Alexander Pope had foreseen, perhaps not the problem itself, but at least its ingredients, when he wrote:

"Behold the stomach: crammed from every dish,
The tomb of boiled and roast and flesh and fish.
Where bile and wind, and phlegm and acid jar,
And all the man is one intestine War!"

But Pope was writing of visceral "wind" more than a century before the clinical introduction of anesthesia precipitated the problem of explosive anesthetic mixtures retained in the stomach and intestines during the postoperative period. It is a little recognized hazard; yet during the administration of a flammable gaseous or volatile anesthetic *via* a face mask, the anesthetic vapor or gas may be introduced into the stomach, particularly when assisted or controlled respirations are employed, and then remain there as a potential source of fire or explosion well into the recovery stage.

Indeed, deNava and McDermott have reported an ignition of anesthetic vapors emanating from a patient some 2½ hours after the termination of an ethylene and oxygen anesthesia. This led them to investigate the retention of flammable anesthetics in the stomach by instilling various mixtures of anesthetic gases into the stomachs of sleeping dogs by Levine tube and periodically sampling for ignitibility. They found that an ethylene-oxygen mixture retained in the stomach might still be flammable some 4 hours after the anesthesia was over; that mixtures of nitrous oxide, oxygen and ether were flammable for about 50 minutes; of cyclopropane and oxygen for 35 minutes; and of ether and oxygen for 25 minutes. They pointed out that the problem is dealt with only vaguely in the medical literature; that the average clinical anesthesiologist is almost blithely unaware of the danger; and that postanesthesia recovery rooms are seldom considered a hazardous location from the point of view of explosion.

The same can hardly be said of the anesthetic period itself. Untold amounts of ingenuity, effort, time and money have gone into attempts to safeguard the patient and the operating room against the dangers of fire and explosions brought about by the presence of flammable anesthetic drugs. Some of the devices and practices recommended in the literature include safety wiring; mercury switches; elevated electric outlets; grounding; intercoupling; ventilation; humidification; wire screens; banning of wool and silk; sparkproof motors; grounded floor plates; conductive flooring; conductive rubber; dilution of flammable mixtures with inert gases; nonsparking metals; elimination of flame, cautery, smoking, x-ray, etc. in the presence of a combustible gas; rebreathing technique; intercepting valve; continuous contact with hand and mask before beginning and during anesthesia; banning of ordinary rubber soles and metal shoe spikes; ionization of the air; rinsing tubes and mask with water or with calcium chloride solution; washing floors with calcium chloride solutions; eliminating ordinary rubber from the operating room; washing out the anesthetic machine with carbon dioxide at the end of each anesthesia; wet flowmeters; turning on cylinder valves very slowly; blowing off some oxygen when starting a new cylinder; keeping nitrous oxide and ethylene on separate machines; and avoidance of unnecessary movements by the anesthetist and of frequent adjustments of the mask. Undoubtedly, at least some of these measures have been helpful; yet by 1940, when ethylene and cyclopropane had become well established as anesthetic agents, it was estimated that there was a gross incidence of one fire or explosion in from 8000 to 70,000 anesthetics, and that each year several patients' lives were lost, a number of operating room personnel were injured, and much property damage occurred. It became evident that, despite the prodigious efforts aimed toward safety, the only sure way to prevent fires and explosions was to eliminate the use of flammable anesthetic agents.

This need has been compounded in the past couple of decades by the tremendous increase in the use of cautery during surgery, of diagnostic x-ray techniques at the time of operation, and of electronic monitoring devices in the operating room. Accordingly, much effort has been expended in the attempt to develop nonflammable and nonexplosive inhalation anesthetic

agents which would be potent, safe and controllable. One of the most promising of these was reported by Artusio and his colleagues at Cornell Medical College in a paper entitled, "A Clinical Evaluation of Methoxyflurane in Man," in the September-October, 1960, issue of *Anesthesiology* (Artusio, J. F., Jr., Van Poznak, A., Hunt, R. E., Tiers, F. M. and Alexander, M., *Anesthesiology, 21:* 512, 1960), which is reprinted below with the kind permissions of the authors and the publisher.

A CLINICAL EVALUATION OF METHOXYFLURANE IN MAN

ARTUSIO, J.F., JR., VAN POZNAK, A.,
HUNT, R.E., TIERS, F. M.,
AND
ALEXANDER, M.

Anesthesiology 21:512, 1960

This first report of the clinical use of methoxyflurane describes its administration to 100 patients by closed, semiclosed and open drop techniques. Anesthetic signs and stages, effects on circulation, ECG, EEG and muscle relaxation are described.

1961

Published August, 1972

The danger of fire or explosion associated with the use of flammable anesthetic vapors and gases has been of concern almost from the beginning. Indeed, a Dr. J. J. Black wrote a note entitled, "Caution Against the Use of Ether Near Fire or Light," in the *Philadelphia Medical Times* as early as 1874: "Some time since, in removing a tumour from a woman's neck, I had occasion to use the actual cautery, and whilst doing so the ether on the towel took

fire, and disconcerted for a while all present, but did no damage except very slightly burning the patient's face. Fortunately, the bottle did not come in contact with the flame. I remember almost serious trouble to have arisen from this accident in this very way in the clinic of a distinguished surgeon. I mention it in order that it may serve its part in this important matter, and keep all on their guard when using ether near fire or light."

Since that time, almost every textbook on the subject of anesthesia has contained a chapter on fire and explosion hazards, and the anesthesiologist has come to be considered an authority on their prevention. The latter has cost literally millions and millions of dollars, for the construction and maintenance of operation rooms free of these hazards is an expensive game. In fact, in a number of hospitals the use of flammable anesthetic agents such as ether, cyclopropane or ethylene is either restricted or totally banned; and there is no question that the development of nonexplosive techniques and agents such as trichlorethylene, halothane, methoxyflurane, and the newer intravenous agents—Innovar, ketamine, diazepam, and the like—has been much hastened by the fire and explosion hazard.

The textbook chapter on fires and explosions almost always lists the flammable and explosive agents, of course; and it also almost always includes one or more tables showing the lower and upper percentage limits (v/v) of flammability in both oxygen and air. There is then a discussion of the use of inert diluents to render the explosive drug safe, the diluent acting either by absorbing the thermal energy of an incipient explosion or by absorbing free radicals which result from the absorption of thermal energy by a molecule of an explosive gas and which, if not deactivated, will combine with oxygen and initiate a chain reaction producing an explosion. Finally, the chapter will almost certainly detail the various factors necessary for the initiation of a fire or explosion: i.e., (1) combustible material; (2) an oxygen supply; and (3) a source of ignition. Among the sources of ignition, of course, are the open flames and fires referred to by Dr. Black; heated materials such as diathermy or cautery; and sparks from static electricity, electric shorts, electric arcs, motors, induction coils, switches, extension cords, loose light bulb connections, photographic power packs, x-ray and fluoroscope, electric recording devices (EKG, EEG, etc.), and other electronic monitoring devices.

Electricity is more than just a hazard in causing explosions in the hospital environment, however, for modern developments in diagnostic and therapeutic procedures have greatly expanded the ways in which patients, and staff personnel too, are exposed to its dangers. Non-fatal, but frightening and annoying, shocks are of course the most common in human exposure to electricity. These are followed closely in incidence—at least in the operating room, recovery room, intensive care unit, coronary care unit, and cardiac catheterization laboratory—by electrosurgical burn injuries, since improper connection between the unit and the patient ground plate, or between the ground plate and the patient, can result in serious burns to the patient.

The really important, and frequently fatal, danger, however, is that to the heart, and particularly its conduction system. Zoll and Lilienthal noted this danger in an editorial reviewing the utilization of electrical pacemakers for Stokes-Adams disease in 1960. They pointed out that direct electrical stimulation of the heart carries a risk of ventricular fibrillation from technical accidents, and reported knowing of several instances in which transient fibrillation was inadvertently produced. They emphasized the danger of attaching a number of different types of electrical apparatus to the patient when a pacemaker is used unless all such instruments are properly grounded.

Their warning was almost immediately followed by reports of fatalities and injuries from the use of electrical equipment, and today the anesthesiologist is as much concerned with electrical hazards as he was with fire and explosions 20 or 30 years ago. Within the past year, for instance, the National Fire Protection Association has issued a manual on electrical hazards; the American Society of Anesthesiologists has signaled its concern by changing its Committee on Fires and Explosions to a Committee on Flammable Hazards and Electrical Equipment; the National Research Council has believed the matter important enough to hold a 2 day symposium on electric hazards in hospitals; and almost every anesthesia journal has published at least one paper on the subject.

The article which ushered in this era of

intense activity and interest in the dangers to the patient of electrical devices and equipment was a report from Leiden of two electrocutions which occurred in precisely the way which Zoll and Lilienthal had predicted. It was entitled, "Myocardial Electrodes and the Danger of Ventricular Fibrillation," and appeared in the May 6, 1961, issue of *The Lancet* (Noordijk, J. A., Oey, F. T. I. and Tebra, W., *Lancet 1:* 975–977, 1961). It is reprinted below with the kind permissions of the authors and the publishers.

MYOCARDIAL ELECTRODES AND THE DANGER OF VENTRICULAR FIBRILLATION

J. A. NOORDIJK, M.D.,
F. T. I. OEY, M.D.,
W. TEBRA

Published April, 1978

The tenement corridor was dingy, dark and dirty. A trash pile of candy wrappers, soda cans and styrofoam cups filled the corner immediately to the left of the doctor's waiting room. The air was rank with the smell of orange rinds and frying food. The hallway itself was full of addicts on the nod, gaunt-eyed and listless, or nervously birdlike. They sat on the bannister or leaned against the graffiti-covered walls, chain-smoking or murmuring amongst themselves.

The door to the doctor's office opened and an emaciated woman of indeterminate age glided out as if walking on shadows. She rejoined her group on the second floor landing and they came to life and surrounded her to inspect the prescription that she had just obtained, examining it as eagerly as a group of high school students would a newly awarded diploma. Then they whooped down the creaking stairs to the drugstore below, where the innocent little piece of paper was to be exchanged

From the Department of Thoracic Surgery of the University Hospital, Leiden

Lancet, 1: 975, 1961

*   *   *   *

SUMMARY

"On the basis of two case-histories, attention is drawn to the risk of ventricular fibrillation resulting from the use of electrical apparatus (*e.g.*, an electrocardiograph) in patients connected with a mains-powered pacemaker-monitor by means of electrodes embedded in the myocardium.

The fibrillation is caused by the passage of an electric current through the heart. This current may arise from imperfect insulation of the electrocardiograph or from a "standard" leak in it, or from the capacity effect in the instrument. The current passes, via the electrodes in the myocardium, to the earth connection of the pacemaker."

for the highly prized packet of little blue pills.

The little blue pills were Valium (diazepam).

Valium is classified as a minor tranquilizer, but traffic in it—from street to Board Room—is anything but minor: it is probably the most abused drug in this country today. The argument over whether it causes true addiction is academic: two "blue bombers" (10 mg. apiece) are worth a dollar on the street, which indicates something, whether it is true addiction or not. Some 60,000,000 prescriptions for the drug are written each year and sales amount to some $500,000,000, and if this does not constitute misuse, it at least certainly represents overuse. Reliance on antianxiety medications in today's Anxious World is quite understandable, but these figures are overwhelming and astounding.

In point of fact, however, Valium *is* one of the most abused and misused drugs today, as witnessed by the fact that, of the

10,000 poison victims seen at the Rocky Mountain Poison Center in Denver, 1,000 were due to Valium. The most common adverse reactions are fatigue, drowsiness, and ataxia; but abrupt withdrawal can lead to convulsions, tremors, abdominal cramps, vomiting and sweating. There are also "infrequently encountered" bad reactions which include depression, jaundice and vertigo; and "paradoxical reactions" are sometimes seen consisting of hallucinations, rage and—of all things from a so-called tranquilizing drug—anxiety.

The anesthesiologist does not often see these reactions, or at least does not always recognize them as being due to Valium, although surely many of the patients whom the anesthesiologist does see are taking Valium, some on a long-term basis and some only for the time since they entered the hospital for work-up prior to surgery.

This is by no means to say that the anesthesiologist does not see reactions to Valium, but merely that they are more immediate reactions due to the acute method of administration, which is almost always intravenous. These immediate and acute reactions to intravenous Valium can be extremely serious, including as they do cardiac arrest, cardiovascular collapse, respiratory arrest, laryngeal incompetence, asthma, and acute allergic reactions; but with the exception of thrombophlebitis, which can have an incidence as high as 3.5 per cent, these reactions do not occur with great frequency, and certainly not with sufficient frequency to diminish the ever-burgeoning use of the drug in anesthetic practice.

One of the early papers introducing Valium to the clinician was by Randall, Heise, Schalleck, Bagdon, Banziger, Boris, Moe and Abrams, which was titled "Pharmaco-

logical and Clinical Studies on Valium, a New Psychotherapeutic Agent of the Benzodiazepine Class" (*Curr. Ther. Res.*, 3:405–425, 1961), and which is republished below with the kind permission of the authors and the publisher.

PHARMACOLOGICAL AND CLINICAL STUDIES ON VALIUM$^{(T.M.)}$. A NEW PSYCHOTHERAPEUTIC AGENT OF THE BENZODIAZEPINE CLASS.

L. O. RANDALL, G. A. HEISE,
W. SCHALLER, R. E. BAGDON,
R. BANZIGER, A. BORIS,
R. A. MOE AND W. B. ABRAMS

Departments of Pharmacology and Clinical Pharmacology, Hoffman-La Roche Inc., Nutley 10, New Jersey.

Curr. Ther. Res., 3:405–425, 1961

Diazepam was evaluated in nine patients attending a psychiatric clinic for eight to 17 weeks (average 12.5 weeks). The starting dose ranged from 10 to 15 mg. daily and it was increased to a maximum of 75 mg. per day. The patients with anxiety reactions, anxiety with depression and involutional syndrome had an excellent clinical response to diazepam. Minor subjective side effects, such as fatigue, dizziness, drowsiness and incoordination, were seen in seven patients. In some patients, the side effects disappeared with continuation of the medication.

Published April, 1970

Scientists have been trying to come up with an explanation for the mechanism of anesthesia for the last century and a quarter, and enough "Theories of Narcosis" have now been proposed so that one can be fairly sure that there is not yet an

entirely acceptable answer. In view of this long search and the continuing inconclusive status of the subject, it is not surprising that there is scarcely anything in the physical or biologic sciences that can be considered irrelevant to the quest. It is equally unsurprising that each new theory has been a reflection of the advances of science up to the time at which the new theory was propounded. The ultimate and final theory—when it succeeds, in fact, in unraveling the mystery—will undoubtedly come only when there is a sufficient knowledge of molecular biology so that the make-up and functions of the cell itself can be explained on a molecular basis.

One of the earliest theories of the mechanism of action of anesthesia, and one which was put forth soon after Morton's classical demonstration of the efficacy of ether as an anesthetic at the Massachusetts General Hospital on October 16, 1846, explained the phenomenon on the basis of the mechanical changes in the blood supply of the brain. This was in truth a "theory," without data to support it even in the heydays of anatomy and physiology, and it was justifiably shortlived.

Next came the first biochemical theory of narcosis—that of Bibra and Harless in 1847–which was based on a series of experiments on frogs and mammals with ether, acetic ether, and ethyl chloride. Their hypothesis was that these and other anesthetic substances were excellent solvents for fat, and that anesthetic action was based on the fact that anesthetics dissolved fat from the brain cells and redeposited the brain's fatty constituents in the liver. They proceeded to anesthetize one group of animals with ether, while another group of unanesthetized animals of the same age and weight served as controls, and then determined the quantity of fat in the brains and livers of each group. They concluded in favor of their hypothesis, but critical examination of their data did not substantiate these conclusions.

Claude Bernard, the titan among 19th century physiologists, was one of the early proponents of what have come to be called the Precipitation Theories. These theories have been based on changes in the colloid of the cell, during or following anesthesia, by coagulation or flocculation of the protein, or by increase in viscosity of the cytoplasm, or by the combination of the anesthetic with the protein of the cell. Over the years there has been a considerable accumulation of evidence that coagulation or flocculation of protein does cause dehydration and reduction of metabolism, and that the narcotic (anesthetic) may combine with protein and other constituents of protoplasm. There are 2 fundamental problems with the Precipitation Theories, however. The first is that, in all of the evidence produced in regard to the precipitation of proteins by narcotics, the concentrations required seem to be more than those necessary to produce narcosis in animals or depression of the reflex reactions of tissues or cells. The second, and perhaps the more telling, objection is that the precipitations are in most cases irreversible, and therefore cannot account for the reversible protoplasmic poisoning which anesthesia is assumed to be (of course, we could be wrong there, too!).

The Dehydration Theories were closely related to the Precipitation Theories, and were based upon the fact that shrinkage of cells due to loss of fluid was noted following exposure to narcotics (anesthetics) or depressants. This observation suggested to the proponents of these theories that the cause of anesthesia was the loss of water from the anesthetized cell, produced by the action of the anesthetic upon it. There were several roadblocks to the acceptance of these theories. One was the fact that the process was not always proven to be reversible. Another was the very high concentrations of anesthetics employed, which undoubtedly caused death of the cells. By far the greatest objection, however, was the fact that, if the theory were true, then any process of dehydration would lead to narcosis or cessation of function, and clearly narcosis does not always follow dehydration and fluid loss in a cell.

In 1893, Richet called attention to the fact that, in many cases, the lower the solubility of a narcotic in water, the greater its narcotic strength, and the Water Solubility Theory was born. Its problem was one common to many theories of narcosis: by no means all narcotics or anesthetics conformed. Obviously, water solubility is a factor (if the narcotic is to reach the cell), but water insolubility is not necessarily related to narcotic strength: paraffin, for instance, is totally insoluble, and also totally without narcotic action.

In 1902, Winterstein, working in Verworn's laboratory, performed an experiment which formed the basis for the Asphyxial Theory of narcosis. He administered strychnine to a frog, and then stimulated the amphibian until exhaustion set in. He then "perfused the frog with saline free from oxygen and repeatedly stimulated, so that any supposed oxygen stores were exhausted, and the waste products formed were washed away. Then it was perfused with oxygenated blood-saline containing chloroform, thus giving the frog (or its cord) a chance to take up and bind oxygen if it could do so in the presence of the narcotic. Then oxygen-free saline was perfused to wash away the chloroform. No sign of recovery was shown until it was perfused with blood-saline when tetany soon occurred. It was thus proved that a cell under a narcotic could not take up and store oxygen." These, and similar experiments performed by others, were considered by Verworn to show that during anesthesia the oxygen absorbing activities of the cells were lost; and that since oxygen disappeared from the cells during narcosis at the same rate as before narcosis, an asphyxia must occur, which could account for the production of the narcosis. There are two major arguments against the Asphyxial Theory. The first of these is that nonoxidative processes are also depressed by narcotics, and consequently narcosis cannot be due to any form of asphyxia in these cases and hence cannot form the basis of a general theory of narcosis. The second is that diminished oxidation is the result and not the cause of narcosis, and narcotics do not interfere with the accessibility of oxygen to the cell.

It was but a short step from the Asphyxial Theory to the Inhibition of Oxidation Theory, and the latter has been proposed in several guises, one being the inhibition of oxygen consumption of the brain by narcotics, and another being the inhibition of certain enzyme systems. Again, however, the statement that narcotics depress cellular oxidation tells nothing about the mechanism, and it is probable that lowered cellular respiration is a result rather than a cause of anesthesia.

The Absorption Theory introduced by Traube in 1904 suggested that substances which lower the surface tension of water pass more readily into the cell and cause narcosis by decreasing metabolism. He was able to demonstrate that a parallelism exists between the ability of some drugs to lower the surface tension of water and their narcotic potency. However, his experiments were done on air-water interfaces at room temperature, whereas the true interface is a liquid-colloid affair at body temperature. Additionally, some very powerful narcotics, such as chloroform and ethyl alcohol, do not lower the interfacial tension; conversely, some agents which do lower interfacial tension, such as soap and detergents, have no narcotic properties.

Close relatives of the Absorption Theory are the Permeability Theories of Hober, Lillie, and Winterstein, which propose that the permeability of cell membranes is decreased by narcotic concentrations of aliphatic and other central nervous depressants, and that the cell membrane is less capable of undergoing electrical depolarization, so that the cell is inhibited in its function. However, many cells do not regularly decrease permeability, and some even increase it. Furthermore, the Permeability Theories are vague and indefinite as to what happens after the permeability of the cell membrane has been changed. If narcotics do, in fact, decrease permeability of the cell membrane, then some other reactions must occur to effect narcosis, and these are not defined by the theories.

The Lipoid Theory (often referred to as the Meyer-Overton Theory) is based on the fact that the narcotic potency of an aliphatic compound increases as the coefficient of partition between oil and water increases. A vast amount of experimental work has been done in relation to the lipoid solubility of anesthetic and narcotic drugs, and there is no question that the lipoid solubility of an anesthetic agent influences the distribution within the body (particularly the nerve cell); but the Lipoid Theory itself, as an explanation for the mechanism of action of anesthesia, is open to criticism on several counts. It applies mainly to homologous series of aliphatic compounds, and does not explain the narcotic action of, for instance, alkaloids, heterocyclic compounds, or inorganic substances such as bromine and magnesium. Furthermore, there are many fat solvents related to anesthetic drugs which have no depressant action on the nervous system. Finally, solubilities in water and olive oil cannot really be compared to biological systems, since lymph, blood, and body lipids are quite distinct from water and oil.

The failure of all of these theories to explain the mechanism of anesthesia has not prevented scientists from continuing to ask the question, however, nor from continuing the search for the answer. One recent proposal has been the microcrystal theory of Dr. Linus C. Pauling, which was published in the July 7, 1961, issue of *Science* (*134:* 15, 1961) under the title of, "A Molecular Theory of General Anesthesia,"

and it is reprinted below with the kind permission of the author and the publisher.

A MOLECULAR THEORY OF GENERAL ANESTHESIA
PAULING, L.
Science, 134:15–21, 1961

Based on theoretical considerations alone and without any experimentation, Pauling developed the theory that anesthetic agents interact with water molecules in brain cells to form hydrate microcrystals, which decrease the energy of electric oscillation of protein side chains producing the state of anesthesia. He noted the striking correlation between potency of anesthetic agents and partial pressure necessary to form hydrate crystals, but recognized that any theory based on van der Waals attraction of anesthetic molecules for other molecules would show similar correlation.

Published December, 1981

Probably the earliest—and almost assuredly the most tritely quoted—reference to resuscitation occurs in the Old Testament, II Kings, 5, 32–34:

"And when Elisha was come into the house, behold, the child was dead and laid upon his bed.
"He went in therefore, and shut the door upon them twain, and prayed unto the Lord.
"And he went up, and lay upon the child, and put his mouth upon his mouth, and his eyes upon his eyes, and his hands upon his hands; and he stretched himself upon the child; and the flesh of the child waxed warm."

Whether or not this was true mouth-to-mouth resuscitation, or simply "the laying on of hands," is impossible to tell, although the description of "his eyes upon his eyes, and his hands upon his hands" certainly smacks more of the metaphysical than the physiologic.

By the 16th century, however, Vesalius very clearly described the restoration of life by "an opening . . . attempted in the trunk of the trachea, into which a reed or cane should be put; you will then blow into this, so that the lung may rise again and the

animal take in air. Indeed, with a slight breath in the case of this living animal the lung will swell to the full extent of the thoracic cavity and the heart become strong . . . "

There are references to the use of bellows, mouth-to-mouth, and even mouth-to-nose breathing scattered through the writings of the 17th century; and, indeed, Mayow, in the great English medical classic, *Tractatus Quinque Medico-Physici*, came close to putting the whole thing together when his experiments showed that dark venous blood changed to bright red by taking up certain ingredients in the air and that the object of breathing was to cause an interchange of gases between the air and the blood.

It was the drownings which attracted the public's imagination and interest, however, and it was the drownings that led, during the 16th century, to the first concerted attempts at organized resuscitation, what could by a stretch of the imagination be termed the first inklings of CPR. One of the foremost and most famous of these, instituted in the year 1767, was the Society at Amsterdam for the Recovery of Drowned Persons. Huston has described it as follows: "The Society to Restore Drowned Persons was formed by a group of wealthy merchants at Amsterdam in an attempt to aid in the resuscitation of the many drowned in their waterways. Until this time, anyone taken from the water was deemed dead. The Society offered money to those who would follow their rules of resuscitation and more money if they were successful. The success rate was high, leading to the formation of similar organized resuscitation efforts, and was the spiritual founder of all the other humane societies."

The extensive coastline of the British Isles, and the frequent squalls and storms that arise there, provided no lack of clinical material on which the arts of resuscitation could be practiced. From 1774 onward, The Royal Humane Society published official reports of the Society for the Recovery of Persons Apparently Drowned. These contained detailed instructions for resuscitation and stressed the point for the need of utmost speed if attempts were to succeed.

Rasnekov has stated:

"Not only was the society concerned with victims of drowning but, in addition, readers were advised to use the methods described for resuscitating any person who collapsed suddenly, apparently dead. A description was given of a successful resuscitation of a child who was brought back to life by 'electricity.'

"The problem of how to proceed if ordinary methods of ventilation, eg., mouth-to-mouth breathing or use of tobacco smoke as described, ('another should throw the smoke of tobacco up by the fundament into the bowels by means of a pipe') failed, was also considered and advice given to use a 'tube inserted through the mouth or nostrils to which could be attached a pair of bellows'. If this method also fails, 'it may be necessary to make an opening into the windpipe' into which the breathing tube can be inserted. The reader is cautioned that this method 'should not be attempted unless by persons skilled in surgery.'"

The necessity of ventilation of the lungs in the performance of resuscitation can thus be said to have been established since biblical times, but the problem of the heart was another problem altogether. The November 29, 1902, issue of *The Lancet* gave a rather complete history of the progress up until that time in an Annotation entitled, "Resuscitation in Syncope due to Anaesthetics and in Other Conditions by Rhythmical Compression of the Heart" (*Lancet*, 2: 1476 (Nov. 29), 1902):

"In 1874 Schiff showed that dogs apparently killed by chloroform might be resuscitated by rhythmical compression of the exposed heart. In 1899 Prus independently discovered that dogs apparently killed by asphyxia, chloroform intoxication, or electricity might be resuscitated in this manner. Opportunity has occurred of applying this method to man in a case of suicide. Though two hours had elapsed since death a few flickering contractions of the heart were obtained. In the *Hospitalstidende*, 1900, p. 1217, an extraordinary and unique case was published, in which, after stoppage of respiration and pulse during the administration of chloroform, and failure of ordinary methods of resuscitation, the heart was exposed, rhythmic compression was performed, and after a short time spontaneous contractions were evoked. Perflation of the lungs was simultaneously performed. The cardiac movements gradually increased and after half an hour feeble spontaneous respiration began. After three hours the patient was breathing deeply, then respiration again ceased. Artificial respiration was maintained for eight hours until the heart ceased to beat. A complete account of this case had been published.[1] The *Revue de Chirurgie* for October contains an interesting review of the whole subject by Dr. Maurice Boureau. He finds that rhythmical compression of the heart has been employed in 12 cases, never with final success. M. Tuffier[2] has recorded the following case. He happened to be near when a man died suddenly on the fifth day of an attack of appendicitis, apparently from embolism. Not more than two or

[1] *The Lancet*, April 13th, 1901, p. 1092.

[2] Bulletin at *Mémoire de la Société de Chirurgie*, 1898, p. 937.

three minutes had elapsed when he examined the patient. The body was already flaccid, the pupils were dilated, respiration had stopped, and the heart showed no signs of movement. Having tried all ordinary methods suitable in such a case M. Tuffier rapidly made an incision in the third left intercostal space and pressing on the pericardium with the index finger rhythmically compressed the ventricular region for one or two minutes. The heart first undulated irregularly and then contracted definitely. The pulse reappeared, deep respirations took place, the eyes opened, and the pupils contracted. The wound was covered with an antiseptic pad. The pulse failed again and the circulation was again established by the same means for some minutes, but it then ceased in spite of all efforts. Until the present year surgeons have reached the heart by resecting the fifth and sixth ribs and opening both pleura and pericardium, thus necessarily creating pneumothorax. But in 1902 Porrier, following a method recommended by Mauclaire,[3] adopted the *voie diaphragmatique*, thus avoiding the production of pneumothorax.

"An incision four or five centimetres long is made through the diaphragm. It begins at the middle of the concavity of the diaphragm and is directed a little obliquely from right to left towards, but not as far, as the apex of the heart. In two cases this method has been employed without success. Dr. Boureau thinks that Silvester's method of artificial respiration and Laborde's method of rhythmical traction of the tongue should always be employed in the first instance in cases of syncope from chloroform. If after 10 minutes respiration has not recommenced he recommends the surgeon as a last resource to perform rhythmical compression of the heart. Since the publication of Dr. Boureau's paper the first successful case of resuscitation by rhythmical compression of the heart has been recorded. At the last meeting of the Society of Anaesthetists Dr. E. A. Starling reported the case of a man, aged 65 years, whose appendix vermiformis was removed

[3] *Gazette des Hôpitaux*, 1901, No. 145.

under nitrous oxide and ether. During the trimming of the stump both pulse and respiration stopped together. Artificial respiration and traction on the tongue were performed without success. Then the surgeon, Mr. W. Arbuthnot Lane, introduced his hand through the abdominal incision and felt the motionless heart through the diaphragm. He gave it a squeeze or two and felt it re-start beating, though no radial pulse was discernible. As voluntary respiration was still suspended artificial respiration was continued and other restorative measures were adopted. Artificial respiration had to be continued for about 12 minutes when natural respiration recommenced with a long, sighing respiration, while at the same time the pulse became perceptible. The operation was completed without any more anaesthetic and a good convalescence followed, though there was some diaphragmatic tenderness. It should be noted that the method adopted by Dr. Starling and Mr. Lane, whom we congratulate, differs from those previously employed. Instead of incising the diaphragm as recommended by Mauclaire he adopted the simpler method of compressing the heart through the diaphragm. The previous results of manual compression of the heart are not very encouraging, but Mr. Lane's success by such a very simple and easy procedure justifies us in saying that if during laparotomy the patient's heart stops the case should never be abandoned as hopeless until manual compression of the heart through the diaphragm has been performed."

During the first half of the present century, there were sporadic reports of the restoration of cardiac action by direct compression of the heart through a thoracotomy wound; by compression of the heart through the intact diaphragm during laparotomy, or by an actual incision of the diaphragm during such an operation; by forced flexion of the legs on the abdomen; and even, on at least one occasion, by compression of the thorax. The fundamental problem of the maintenance of cardiac flow during cardiopulmonary resuscitation, however, was in fact solved by a meticulously astute observation by trained scientists who were working on an entirely different problem.

Dr. William B. Kouwenhoven was an electrical engineer and for many years had been the Dean of the School of Engineering at Johns Hopkins University. Much of his career had been devoted to high-voltage measurements and the development of other precise electrical measurement techniques, and studies of magnetic and dielectric materials. During the latter part of the 1950's, Dr. Kouwenhoven's laboratory was working on a grant from the Edison Electric Company of New York and the National Institutes of Health in an attempt to answer the problem of electrocution among power company linemen, which always occurred in the field, away from hospitals where it might be possible to defibrillate the heart in an emergency room.

In the spring of 1958, a typical and quite routine experiment in Dr. Kouwenhoven's laboratory became the crucial and history-making study in terms of cardiopulmonary resuscitation, and has been described with terse, clinical precision by Dr. James Jude:

"An anesthetized dog was strapped to the research table in the supine position with an EKG attached and the femoral artery cannulated and connected to a recording transducer and strain gauge amplifier. The animal's thorax was shaved so that the defibrillator electrodes could be applied. The trachea was intubated and artificial respiration was maintained. A low-voltage alternating current across the chest induced ventricular fibrillation. The experiment was to attempt to prolong the period of reversibility of the ventricular fibrillation. As Dr. Kouwenhoven observed, Guy Knickerbocker applied the heavy electrodes to each side of the highly angled breast of the dog and pushed. The strain gauge recorded a blip of vascular pressure. A relaxation and push caused additional recording of pressure. The defibrillator was discharged and spontaneous action returned. A review of the records revealed the possibility that externally applied rhythmic pressure to the chest wall over the heart might have put pressure on the heart and caused it to empty, thus resulting in some degree of circulation. Together with the artificial ventilation, this would allow circulation of oxygenated blood . . .

". . . further experiments followed, where the hand was substituted for the defibrillator electrode and rhythmic pressure given on the lower sternum over the heart; and . . . even after 15 or 20 minutes of such maneuvers they could still defibrillate the heart and the dog would awaken with an apparently intact central nervous system. Together they all then conducted further studies and the time of reversibility of ventricular fibrillation by cardiac massage extended. The effects of epinephrine, calcium chloride, sodium bicarbonate, and other drugs were recorded under the conditions of external cardiac massage for cardiac arrest."

Within a matter of short months, the method was applied to patients, mostly in the operating room and to patients who had suffered cardiac arrest during operation, and in no instance was it necessary to open the chest for direct cardiac massage. The cases were gone over in detail as they presented themselves; and additional laboratory studies were carried out, especially on the effects of rate, depth of compression, employment of various cardiac stimulating drugs, mechanical cardiac massage, and the direct-current defibrillator. A preliminary paper (Kouwenhoven, W. B., Jude, J. R. and Knickerbocker, G. G.: Closed chest cardiac massage. *J.A.M.A.*, *173:* 1064, 1960) was published in July of 1960. The definitive and classic publication appeared in the December 16, 1961, issue of the Journal of the American Medical Association (Jude, J. R., Kouwenhoven, W. B. and Knickerbocker, M. S. E.: Cardiac arrest. Report of application and external cardiac massage on 118 patients. *J.A.M.A.*, *178:* 1064–1070 (Dec. 16) 1961) and is reprinted below with the kind permissions of the authors and the publishers. Copyright 1961, American Medical Association.

CARDIAC ARREST. REPORT OF APPLICATION OF EXTERNAL CARDIAC MASSAGE ON 118 PATIENTS.

James R. Jude,
William B. Kouwenhoven
and
G. Guy Knickerbocker

Department of Surgery,
The Johns Hopkins University
School of Medicine and Hospital
Baltimore, Maryland

J.A.M.A., 178:1064, 1961

*   *   *   *

"A new method of producing artificial circulation by external sternal compression without thoracotomy—thus being able to apply it rapidly and without trauma—was evaluated in 138 episodes of cardiac arrest in 118 patients: 76 arrests occurred outside the operating room and recovery areas. Seven out of every 10 were in asystole; the remainder were in ventricular fibrillation. Cardiac action was restored in 107 (78%) of the 138 cardiac arrests. In 84 (60%) of the 138, the prearrest status of the central nervous system and heart was regained: 28 (24%) of the 118 patients survived the arrest and inciting disease to leave the hospital."

1962

Published June, 1980

In 1937, Arthur Guedel included in his classic little monograph, *Inhalation Anesthesia*, just over a page on the subject of hyperthermia related to anesthesia:

"It would seem that this small and rather indefinite series of postoperative hyperthermias might be due to the anesthesia although this cannot be certain.

"During the past twenty years the author has had six such cases on his own services and has had perhaps as many more reported to him by others. In all of these cases the anesthesia was ether, usually by the open drop method. They were all elective abdominal operations except one, a brain tumor. There was nothing apparently wrong with the anesthesias, the element of asphyxia which was especially noted, being absent.

"The development of the hyperthermia and its progress was similar in all cases. Within four to six hours after the patient was returned to the ward the temperature registered in the neighborhood of 104°F., following which it rose rapidly and progressively to 108°F. or 110°F., death occurring within the first twenty-four post-operative hours.

"It is interesting to note that four of these cases occurred in the same hospital during a period of one month and with the same shipment of ether. In these the open drop method was used and close investigation failed to disclose anything wrong with the technique. The ether was investigated by the manufacturer but nothing unusual was found.

"Necropsy in these four cases showed only a cerebral edema. No histological study of the brain was made.

"We may assume, in these cases, the cause to be an interference with the heat regulation center in the hypothalamic area but that is as far as our assumptions may be carried at the present time.

"In the matter of treatment, thorough ice packs and, because of the cerebral edema, the intravenous use of hypertonic glucose would be indicated.

"It is highly probable that many cases of this sort have occurred in which the pathological progress halted and turned back before death occurred."

Today, a great deal more is known about this syndrome, which is now called malignant hyperthermia or malignant hyperpyrexia in humans, and is referred to as pork stress syndrome in the pig. In both species, the paroxysmal hypercatabolic reactions of skeletal and heart muscle may be due to the same underlying molecular defect, the variations in clinical expressions being due to species difference itself, or to the site of the defect, the severity of the defect, to environmental factors, or to various combinations of these. In any event, much of the knowledge gained in the past 2 decades has resulted from the fact that the syndrome has achieved the status of a "glamour disease," and as such has commanded not only intense clinical interest, but also a vast amount of investigative activity. Much remains to be learned, of course; but improved understanding of the clinical and chemical features of malignant hyperthermic reactions, and of the management of this potentially lethal disease, has led to a reduction in the mortality rate from more than 70 per cent before 1970 to 28 per cent in 1976, according to the records kept in the Toronto registry of cases of malignant hyperthermia maintained by Dr. Beverly Britt at the University of Toronto.

Most of the affected individuals exhibit bulky and excessively strong muscles and may complain of muscle cramps with localized muscle weaknesses such as hernias, club foot, spinal curvature, joint hypermobility, ptosis, and strabismus. The disease is rare in infants under 2, and in adults over 50, years of age. It is more common in males than in females, which again may be related to muscle development, bulk and strength, or perhaps to sex hormone differences. Some of those who have developed malignant hyperthermia had undergone previously uneventful general anesthesia; conversely, there are some who had exhibited malignant hyperthermia on a previous occasion who have subsequently undergone uneventful general anesthesia.

The earliest presenting sign of malignant hyperthermia is a cardiac arrhythmia, usually tachycardia, although, if succinylcholine has been used at induction for endotracheal intubation, an abnormal response to that drug may serve as a prodromat in the so-called "rigid type" of the disease. A generalized erythematous flush occurs also in the early stages, with areas of mottling which acquire a cyanotic hue, and are accompanied by dark blood in the surgical wound. Hypertension may develop at this stage, and a marked tachypnea and hyperpnea will be noted in the patient who has not been fully paralyzed with muscle relaxants and is breathing spontaneously. The skin is warm to the touch, even before the core temperature begins its rapid and inexorable rise; the soda lime cannister (if a circle system is in use) will also become hot; and the soda lime will discolor rapidly.

The syndrome, if undetected or untreated at this point, progresses rapidly. Muscle rigidity, if it was not observed following succinylcholine, develops subtly, the muscles being in a state of contracture, not spastic contraction, and the muscle bellies are firm and hard. The body temperature increases very quickly ($1°F$ every few minutes) and to high levels ($115°F$. has been recorded); but this is an effect, not a cause, of the disorder—and in that sense it is a late sign. Excessive oozing may develop in the surgical wound, or from previously dry edges of the incision, as coagulopathy develops. Pulmonary edema from left ventricular failure develops in the late stages of the acute crisis.

These physical signs reflect the fundamental biochemical aberrations. The pH falls early and markedly due to the vast CO_2 production in the skeletal muscles, and to this respiratory acidosis soon is added a metabolic component due to lactic acid production, as the metabolic demands of the skeletal muscles exceed the available O_2 supply. Serum potassium is elevated initially, as is the calcium, but the latter soon falls below normal as the high blood gradient pushes the ion across the impaired membrane into the muscle cell. Hemolysis, thrombocytopenia, and lowered levels of fibrinogen and Factor VIII represent the coagulopathy mentioned above; enzyme levels (creatine phosphokinase, lactic dehydrogenase, and glutamic oxalacetic transaminase) may reach high levels during the acute episode, but generally are highest 24 to 48 hours afterwards in patients who survive.

Treatment must be prompt, vigorous, and persistent. Anesthesia must be stopped immediately and surgery terminated as rapidly as possible: this is no time for discussions of if's, and's, or but's. Blood gas measurements give the definitive diagnosis. The lungs must be hyperventilated with 100 per cent O_2. Cooling must be undertaken by every available means: although the py-rexia in children has been controlled by surface cooling alone, adults will require iced saline by gastric lavage, by rectal in-stillation, and by bladder irrigation; if the peritoneal and/or pleural cavities are open, cold saline should be poured directly into these. Extracorporeal circulation and a heat exchanger is the most efficient method of controlling the hyperpyrexia, of course, but are seldom available at the ready in most hospitals. Massive amounts of bicar-bonate are necessary to combat the com-bined respiratory and metabolic acidosis and to reverse the severe hyperkalemia by driving the potassium into the cells. Urine output must be maintained at 2 ml. per kg. per hr. by using Mannitol and Lasix, since myoglobinemia and myoglobinuria will not be harmful to the kidney if flow is main-tained. Procainamide in large doses is as-sociated with a 70 per cent survival rate, and Dantrolene has been associated with survival in 12 of 14 patients in whom it was used. Regular insulin in a bolus of hyper-tonic glucose has been advocated as a method of providing an energy source to the cell.

Malignant hyperthermia has commonly been regarded as an anesthetic complica-tion, an iatrogenic disease caused by anes-thesia—and, indeed, the list of anesthetic drugs and supplementary agents which have been implicated as triggering the syn-drome is appallingly long and frighteningly complete. At one time or another, every type of general anesthesia which is, or has been, in common use has been regarded as the triggering agent, as have many of the skeletal muscle relaxants, and some of the amide local anesthetics: halothane (60 per cent of the cases of malignant hyperther-mia), succinylcholine (77 per cent of the cases), N_2O-O_2-meperidine, spinal, me-thoxyflurane, ether, chloroform, ethyl chloride, trichlorethylene, cyclopropane, ethylene, gallamine, d-tubocurarine, iso-flurane, enflurane, lidocaine, and mepiva-caine have all been implicated.

Figures as to the number of times that these anesthetics trigger an acute crisis vary greatly, the attack rate running as high as 1 : 15,000 in anesthetized children to as low as 1 : 50,000 for a general hospital popula-tion. Of paramount concern has been the predisposition which allows the triggering agent to precipitate an attack. The patho-physiology of malignant hyperthermia is unknown in precise terms, but it is a form of defect in calcium transfer that leads to an increased intracellular calcium level and a resulting fulminant hypermetabolism in the muscle. Many of the patients who are susceptible to malignant hyperthermia have an underlying disease of muscle, and at least 2 predisposing myopathies have been identified. It is now well established that in many of these patients the predis-position has an undeniable genetic basis. There appears to be good evidence that the predisposition is an autosomal domi-nant trait, although, in the instance of one of the predisposing myopathies, it is inher-ited as a recessive characteristic.

The first intimation that the syndrome was not an anesthetic disease, in the sense that was referred to by Guedel in 1937, but rather was in fact a true pharmacoge-netic process which was dependent upon both an abnormal gene and a triggering factor (which, of course, could be an anes-thetic), came from Denborough and his colleagues at the Royal Melbourne Hospital and Royal Women's Hospital in Australia. Their first report was a short Letter To The Editor which was published in *Lancet* on July 2nd, 1960, and was subsequently republished in a more complete version in the anesthetic literature under the title, "Anaesthetic Deaths In A Family," in the June 1962 issue of the *British Journal of Anaesthesia* (Denborough, M. A., Forster, J. F. A., Lovell, R. R. H., Mapleson, P. A. and Villiers, J. D.: *Br. J. Anaesth.*, *34:* 595, 1962). It is reprinted below with the kind permissions of the authors and the publish-ers.

ANAESTHETIC DEATHS IN A FAMILY

M. A. Denborough,
J. F. A. Forster,
R. R. H. Lovell,
P. A. Maplestone
AND
J. D. Villiers

Royal Melbourne Hospital and
Royal Women's Hospital,
Melbourne, Australia

Br. J. Anaesth., 34: 595, 1962

A case history is presented in which a 21 year old male, requiring an anesthetic for a compound fracture of the tibia and fibula, was concerned because several of his relatives had died following the administration of ether anesthesia.

Following administration of nitrous oxide, oxygen and halothane for 15 minutes, he developed hypotension, tachycardia to 160 per minute, and cyanosis. The skin was hot and sweaty. He was rubbed down with ice-cold cloths and gradually recovered over the next 90 minutes. About one year later he had an uneventful spinal anesthetic for removal of a ureteral calculus.

Enquiries showed that 10 of the 38 relatives of the patient had died in association with ethyl chloride and ether anesthetics, the course of events having been similar. In two, the body temperatures were found to be 43°C and 42°C, respectively.

The pattern of inheritance of the abnormality is compatible with that due to an incompletely penetrant dominant gene or genes. The nature of the inherited anomaly is not known.

1963

Published December, 1974

One of the leading concerns of the anesthetist from the very beginning has been judging, or recognizing, or measuring, the degree or depth of anesthesia. Indeed, the mythology of anesthesiology has it that one of the reasons that Crawford Long was deterred from further use of ether anesthesia was the fact that he misjudged the dose which he administered to a young boy, almost with fatal result. Concern with the depth of anesthesia was apparent, too, in the first administration of nitrous oxide anesthesia, on the occasion of the extraction of Horace Wells' aching wisdom tooth, December 11th, 1844: John M. Riggs, who had performed the extraction, said of the operation, "Our agreement, the night previous, was to push the administration to a point hitherto unknown."

The earliest—and still the most common—method of evaluating the depth of anesthesia was the observation of physical signs, the anesthetist using his own 5 senses in combination with his experience as to what any given set of physical signs meant by way of the depth of anesthesia. The evaluation was on the basis of the rate and quality of the pulse; the depth, character, and rate of respiration; the color of the skin and mucous membranes; the tone or relaxation of the muscles; and the responses to painful stimuli.

It was, in fact, the response to painful stimulation which turned the demonstration of nitrous oxide anesthesia by Horace Wells at the Harvard Medical School during early February of 1845 into a complete fiasco. A groan, as the tooth of the subject to whom Wells had administered the nitrous oxide on that occasion was being extracted, led to cries of "Humbug," "Charlatan," "Imposter"; and Wells returned to

Hartford a broken man, eventually to become a chloroform addict and commit suicide at the age of 33.

During the ensuing century and a quarter, "painful stimulation" was regarded more as a surgical joke and an indication of incomplete anesthesia than as a sign of depth of anesthesia itself. When the surgeon plunged knife into belly with the roar, "Is he asleep, Mr. Anaesthetist?", there was vast amusement in the operating theater, and equally vast humiliation at the head of the table if the patient, indeed moved. The "good" anesthetist came to be known as one to whom such humiliation never occurred; and in retrospect he was also, obviously, one who kept his patients deep.

Balanced anesthesia has changed all that, of course, and today movement in response to painful stimuli is a recognized—and valued—sign of anesthesia. Movement of the eyes during the administration of the older agents like ether has been used for 2 generations to denote the depth of anesthesia; and the development of pediatric anesthesia has also seen movement of the extremities become an important indication of depth. Neuroleptanalgesia and intravenous narcotic anesthesia have brought prominence to the grimace as a sign of the level of anesthesia; and the statement, "he's moving," is no longer a source of humiliation, but of reassurance, to the anesthetist.

The past decade has also seen movement in response to painful stimulation used by some workers as a method of comparing the potencies of anesthetic drugs. The minimal alveolar concentration, or MAC, at which movement in response to painful stimulation occurs during the administration of an inhalation anesthetic, is considered far more reliable than physical signs to compare potencies. The traditional physical signs for depth of ether anesthesia, as enunciated by Guedel, for instance, hardly apply for halothane; and, in fact, may even vary from patient to patient during ether anesthesia itself. MAC, however, is remarkably constant for any given inhalation anesthetic agent; and if the same multiple of MAC (1, 2, 3, 4, and so on) is chosen for physiologic and pharmacologic measurements during the administration of different agents, the latter can be compared in regard to respiratory, circulatory, neuromuscular, or reflex responses at the same "depth" of anesthesia.

The biologic constancy of MAC within a given species is apparently quite remarkable, and the variability is small: the standard deviation from the average MAC in the dog is but 10 to 20 per cent. Not only is this constancy apparent within a given species, but even the variability between species is surprisingly small: MAC for halothane at one atmosphere is 0.87 in the dog, 0.75 in man, 0.82 in the cat, 0.95 to 1.1 in the rat or mouse, 0.76 in the goldfish, and 0.76 in the toad. The constancy of MAC extends to time, also, and the value for MAC determined on the same dog on successive weeks varies only 8 per cent. The same is true of the duration of anesthetic administration, for the MAC at the end of 1 or 2 hours of halothane anesthesia is not significantly different than that after 10 hours. Sex also makes no difference, and MAC is the same in both the male and female within the same species.

There are factors which change MAC, and many of these are known to the clinical anesthesiologist on the basis of empirical experience. Extreme changes in acid-base balance represent a stress which produces a decrease in anesthetic requirement, and hence in MAC. Elevation of the Pa_{CO2} to above 90 mm. Hg decreases MAC, and so does hyperventilation to below 10 mm. Hg—the former possibly by an anesthetic effect of CO_2 relating to cerebrospinal fluid hydrogen ion, and the latter possibly due to a fall in cerebral blood flow. A fall in Pa_{O2} below 40 mm. Hg will also decrease the anesthetic requirement, (and MAC), as will reduction in blood pressure to one-third or one-half of control values. Aging and lowered body temperature will reduce MAC, while elevation of temperature will increase it. These are logical effects from the point-of-view of the perceptive clinician.

So, too, are the effects of depressants such as narcotics and other anesthetics, which lower MAC in simple, additive fashion. More subtle are the effects of reserpine and alpha methyl dopa, which deplete central catecholamines and reduce MAC; while iproniazide and dextroamphetamine, which release central catecholamines, raise MAC. The clinician must allow for the changes introduced by the effects of these drugs on anesthetic requirement lest he give too much or too little.

The significance of MAC has been, and is, argued endlessly. There can be no doubt, however, that the concept has dominated the anesthetic literature in this country for the better part of a decade. It was introduced by Merkel and Eger in an article entitled, "A comparative study of halothane and halopropane anesthesia including method for determining equipotency," which was published in the May–June issue of *Anesthesiology* (Merkel, G. and Eger, E. I., II: *Anesthesiology*, *24:* 346–357, 1963) and is reprinted below with the kind permission of the authors and the publisher.

A COMPARATIVE STUDY OF HALOTHANE AND HALOPROPANE ANESTHESIA INCLUDING METHOD FOR DETERMINING EQUIPOTENCY

GILES MERKEL, M.D.,
AND
EDMOND I. EGER, II, M.D.

Anesthesiology, 24: 346–357, 1963

*   *   *   *

SUMMARY

"Two fluorinated hydrocarbon anesthetics, halopropane and halothane, were compared in dogs during spontaneous and controlled respiration. Anesthetic equipotency was defined in terms of the minimal alveolar anesthetic concentration required to prevent muscular response to a painful stimulus. Halopropane was found a less potent anesthetic than halothane, with a narrower range between minimal anesthetic concentration and that required to produce respiratory or circulatory failure. Arterial pressure and cardiac output became depressed at relatively lower alveolar halopropane concentrations. Respiratory arrest also occurred at lower halopropane concentrations. With neither agent did the dogs demonstrate a significant tendency to compensate for increasing anesthetic depression."

Published June, 1975

The day in 1656 when Sir Christopher Wren injected opium into the vein of a large, lean dog by means of a quill and a pig's bladder was not only the beginning of i.v. anesthesia, but also the beginning of narcotic anesthesia.

Anesthesia was, of course, quite unknown as such at the time; and it was not Sir Christopher's intention to produce it, as is demonstrated by the catholic structure of his experiments, which also included the injection of wine and beer intravenously into the same big, black dog! Nine years later the first earnest (and successful) attempt to produce anesthesia by i.v. administration was made by Sigismund Elsholtz, who injected a solution of opiate and did indeed produce narcosis.

It was almost 250 more years before narcotics became an integral part of the anesthesia scene in the form of the basal narcosis known as "Twilight Sleep." This mixture of morphine and scopolamine attained great popularity among patients as a form of pain relief for labor in obstetrics, but its unfortunate effects upon uterine contractions and the fetus turned obstetricians against it. It has persisted as a form of premedication, however, in the 25:1 ratio advocated by Waters.

The first really documented widespread use of i.v. narcotics came with the report by Neff and his colleagues of the use of the combination of nitrous oxide-meperidine-*d*-tubocurarine in the February, 1947, issue of *California Medicine*. This is certainly not to say that others had not used i.v. narcotics as part of their anesthetic regimen—indeed, both the group at the University of Wisconsin under Ralph Waters at Madison and the group at Bellevue under Rovenstine in New York City had been using i.v. morphine during anesthesia some 10 or more years earlier. The article by Neff and his colleagues, however, did identify the technique in the literature, and their work therefore is a form of landmark.

The next chapter on the use of narcotics as a major component of the anesthetic administration was written by the two Frenchmen, Laborit and Huguenard, when they introduced the technique of "Artificial Hibernation" in the early 1950's. This was based on an astoundingly complex conglomeration of drugs; an almost ritualistic procedure for their administration; and—to touch all the bases of the time—hypothermia. The concept of "Artificial Hibernation" was that it would approximate the state of hibernating mammals: hypotension; hypothermia; hypometabolism; reduced capillary permeability; muscular relaxation; and "disconnexion," a state of twilight sleep. This objective was to be achieved by the administration of a series of "lytic cocktails": "Melange M_1" (Largactil 0.05–2 cm.^{3}, Phenergan 0.05–2 cm.^{3}, Dolosal 0.10–cm.^{3}); "Cocktail No. 1" (Largactil 0.05–0.15; Phenergan 0.05–0.15; Dolosal 0.10–0.20; 0.25 on Hydergine 2–3 cm.^{3}, Liquide de perfusion q.s./1000 cm.^{3}); "Cocktail No. 2" (Sulfate de Sparteine 0.20–0.30; sulfate de magnesie 6 gm.; Procaine 2–5 gm.; Liquide de perfusion q.s./1500 cm.^{3}); and a variety of other supplements and maneuvers.

In retrospect, it was a ridiculous concept and an incredible technique; but it served two important purposes in terms of the history of anesthetic progress in that it introduced the phenothiazines to the anesthetic community, and it firmly established the usefulness of the combination of a narcotic and a tranquilizer.

The technique of "ataralgesia" was a logical progression and came fast on the heels of "Artificial Hibernation." It stripped the pomposity from the latter, and got right down to the fundamentals of a narcotic and a tranquilizer (or, as they preferred to call the latter, an ataraxic drug). Its ingredients were Demerol, amiphenazole (Daptazole) and Pacatal, to induce a state of "ataralgesia"—that is, of "calmness and freedom from pain," during which operations could be performed without anesthesia. The problem was that, like mesmerism, hypnosis, Read's "childbirth without pain," and now, acupuncture, it is hard to do surgical operations without anesthesia in a lot of patients. And when the excitement of newness wore off, most anesthesiologists fell back to older techniques with greater reliability and more controllable depression. As Orkin has put it, "Nothing is more disconcerting to a patient, surgeon or anesthesiologist than to await an anesthetic procedure which fails to produce adequate conditions for surgery. Our own experience with ataraxic or tranquilizing drugs is that they have additional unreliabilities. Some patients remain remarkably awake and others need practically no anesthesia. A few may show excitement instead of sedation."

The most recent significant development in the use of narcotic anesthesia has also had its basis in the combination of a narcotic with a tranquilizer, or so-called neuroleptanalgesia, this time in the form of Innovar, a wedding of fentanyl and droperidol. There are indications that the proportions of the two drugs in the marriage is not necessarily a happy one, and that perhaps fentanyl, the potent and short-acting narcotic, may be the ultimate survivor. Nevertheless, it is true that, in many an anesthesiologist's practice, Innovar to produce neuroleptanalgesia has brought a substantial end to the Decade of the Halogenated Hydrocarbons. The clinical use of Innovar (or Innovan, as it was then called) was reported in the May–June, 1963, issue of *Anesthesiology* (Holderness, M. C., Chase, P. E. and Dripps, R. D.: *Anesthesiology*, *24*: 336–340, 1963) in a paper titled, "A Narcotic Analgesic and a Butyrophenone with

Nitrous Oxide for General Anesthesia," and it is reprinted below with the kind permissions of the authors and the publisher.

A NARCOTIC ANALGESIC AND A BUTYROPHENONE WITH NITROUS OXIDE FOR GENERAL ANESTHESIA

MARGARET C. HOLDERNESS, M.B., CH.B.,
PATRICIA E. CHASE, M.D.,
AND
ROBERT D. DRIPPS, M.D.

Anesthesiology, 24: 336–340, 1963

* * * *

SUMMARY

"A technique of general anesthesia using phentanyl, a potent analgesic, and dehydrobenzperidol, a butyrophenone derivative, intravenously, together with the inhalation of nitrous oxide has been utilized to anesthetize 400 patients for general surgical procedures. The method affords excellent analgesia and hypnosis for operations not requiring muscular relaxation. For the latter a relaxant must be added. Circulatory stability was impressive during and after operation. Respiratory depression resembled that seen when other narcotic analgesics are used as adjuvants to anesthesia, but was of lesser duration than with most. Rigidity of skeletal muscles, occasionally making pulmonary ventilation difficult but responding promptly to small doses of relaxants, was seen primarily when excessive amounts of the mixture had been given by vein.

"Profound analgesia, minimal hypotension, probably protection against epinephrine-induced ventricular arrhythmias, and a smooth postoperative course constitute some of the appealing features of this technique with non-explosive agents which appears to merit further exploration."

1964

Published December, 1978

For a great many years, the Professor of Pharmacology taught, and the Pharmacology Textbook stated, that thiopental sodium was an ultra short-acting barbiturate. For clinical purposes, the barbiturates had been classified into 4 main groups, depending upon their duration of action: long-acting, such as phenobarbital; intermediate action, of which amytal and pentobarbital were examples; short-acting, such as secobarbital and similar compounds; and the ultra short-acting thiopental and hexobarbital (Evipal), which could be administered intravenously for anesthesia.

Thiopental was classified in this schema as ultra short-acting because, if a dose was given intravenously, the patient rapidly lost consciousness; but if no further thiopental was administered, the patient also would wake up in a short period of time. The logical explanation for this sequence was that the drug had been destroyed in the body at a very rapid rate and therefore, *ipso facto*, was ultra short-acting.

Furthermore, (the Pharmacology Textbook continued), it appeared possible to relate chemical structure to duration of pharmacologic action: "In general, barbiturates with alkyl radicals are relatively stable in the body, while those with complex cyclic radicals, such as Evipal, are unstable and readily destroyed. Derivatives of thiobarbituric acid are likewise rapidly decomposed in the body and therefore are short in duration of action."

There were. however, some clinical experiences which were disturbingly at odds with these reasonable-sounding explanations. It was true that thiopental would produce anesthesia of only short duration following the administration of a small dose, and in that respect the drug appeared to be ultra short-acting. However, if the patient was maintained under prolonged anesthesia by successive injections of thiopental, the duration of the subsequent continuing narcosis could be very prolonged: in other words, thiopental no longer acted like an ultra short-acting drug. This unpleasant fact (in that it did not fit the concept of rapid destruction in the body) was conveniently explained away by ascribing this unusual activity to the production and accumulation in the body of less active metabolic transformation products of thiopental which had a very long duration of anesthetic action and a slow rate of detoxification. In fact, even when sensitive methods of measuring plasma-decay curves of thiopental became available by utilizing ultraviolet spectrophotometry, and showed thiopental concentrations falling rapidly at first and then more slowly, the data were still misinterpreted as indicating speedy destruction of the drug.

The classical work of Brodie and his colleagues in 1950 demonstrated that the early sharp decline in plasma concentrations represented not rapid detoxification of the drug but, rather, a shift of thiopental from brain to other tissues during the process of redistribution of the drug following its initial injection. Further, they recognized that the rate of metabolism of this drug is actually slow, amounting to only some 10 to 15 per cent per hour; and the continuation of their investigations, together with the work of Price and his co-workers, led to a coherent, unified explanation of the clinical behavior of the so-called ultra short-acting barbiturates which, in oversimplified terms, can be stated as follows.

Sleep occurs promptly after a small intravenous dose because of the swift entry of the lipoid-soluble drug into the brain. Return of consciousness is also prompt following a single intravenous dose due to the rapid fall of the concentrations in the brain and plasma below anesthetic levels as the drug is redistributed from vessel-rich organs to the lean body mass and the fat depots. The entry of the drug into the tissues of the lean body mass peaks about half-an-hour after the initial administration and serves to cushion the early impact of the drug on the brain; and then for an hour or so the drug enters the fat depots, which serve as a secondary cushion and become dominant in the termination of anesthesia. However, if larger doses are used or the administration is continued over a longer period of time, the ultra short action is not seen, and awakening is delayed beyond the period of major uptake by fat. Under these circumstances, plasma concentrations remain at or above anesthetic levels and fall slowly because of the slow metabolism of the drug, and postanesthetic depression can be markedly prolonged.

The same Professor of Pharmacology who was teaching that thiopental was an ultra short-acting drug was also teaching that inhalation anesthetics were chemically inert within the body and were exhaled in the same form, and in the same amount, as they had been inhaled into the lungs. This was the accepted doctrine for over a century, and was reinforced by the only really scientific investigation into the matter: that by Haggard in 1924 concerning the absorption, distribution and elimination of diethyl ether. Haggard concluded from his work that the drug "is not destroyed or utilized in the body" but "is all excreted unchanged." The concept that anesthetic molecules remain unaltered during their stay in the body was thus apparently established on a firm scientific basis.

There had been, however, hints in the literature that perhaps occasional exceptions existed to this universally held concept that inhalation anesthetics were totally inert and left the body completely unchanged—but the hints were not sufficiently blatant to command the attention of those dealing with matters anesthetic at the clinical level. As early as the 1880's, for instance, there were independent studies by two Germans, Zeller (1883) and Kast (1887), investigating the urinary excretion of chloride in dogs maintained on a sodium chloride deficient diet. They found that chloroform given orally or by inhalation resulted in a fourfold increase in urinary chloride excretion. It was to be another 80 years before the significance of these findings were appreciated by the anesthetic community.

Another known exception was the metabolism of trichlorethylene. In 1938, Barrett and his colleagues noticed that "not only was trichlorethylene changed by the organism" but that 5 to 8 per cent of the trichlorethylene absorbed by dogs during anesthesia could be recovered from the urine as trichloracetic acid. A few years later, Powell made a more precise study of trichlorethylene metabolism in man, and showed that it was partly excreted by the lungs within 24 hours of anesthesia, but was also partly metabolized to trichloracetic acid, which she measured in the blood and urine for several days after anesthesia. The change of trichlorethylene into trichloracetic acid was an unusual one from the chemist's viewpoint, since although it was possible that intermediary compounds were formed, what these might be were not known. Butler subsequently found trichlorethanol in larger amounts than trichloracetic acid in the urine of dogs anesthetized with trichlorethylene, and he believed that chloral hydrate might be the precursor of both. Much of this work was reported in such journals as the *Journal of Industrial Hygiene* and the *British Journal of Industrial Medicine*, because until the introduction of trichlorethylene as an anesthetic during the Blitz of London in 1941, it had been mainly employed in industry for the removal of grease from metal and machinery, particularly by German heavy industry during World War I. Thus, although these facts were known to those employing trichlorethylene as an anesthetic, they were regarded more as a hazard to those in industrial medicine than to those administering anesthesia.

Finally, although Haggard (as noted above) had determined that most of the inhaled ether was excreted unchanged, some 13 per cent of the inhaled ether was not accounted for in his studies. Little if any attention was paid to this fact because it was accepted that this amount of ether was within the range of laboratory error of the methods available to Haggard at the time. In retrospect, of course, this is almost precisely the amount of ether now known to undergo transformation in the body.

These available clues, therefore, were entirely ignored in favor of the wholly accepted doctrine that inhalation anesthetics are biochemically nonreactive and exhaled unchanged by the lungs. It came as quite a shock, therefore, when, in the early 1960's, these cherished beliefs and dogmas were rudely negated by 2 series of critical investigations into anesthetic metabolism, which established that not only was diethyl ether metabolized, but that other volatile anesthetic drugs were also biodegraded to identifiable and not always inert metabolites. A landmark article from these studies was entitled, "Metabolism of Volatile Anesthetics. I. Conversion in vivo of Several Anesthetics to $^{14}CO_2$ and Chloride," by Van Dyke and his colleagues, and was published in the 1964 volume of *Biochemical Pharmacology* (Van Dyke, R. A., Chenoweth, M. B. and Van Poznak, A.: *Biochem. Pharmacol., 13:* 1239, 1964). It is reprinted below with the kind permissions of the authors and the publisher.

METABOLISM OF VOLATILE ANESTHETICS— CONVERSION IN VIVO OF SEVERAL ANESTHETICS TO $^{14}CO_2$ AND CHLORIDE

RUSSELL A. VAN DYKE,
MAYNARD B. CHENOWETH
AND
ALAN VAN POZNAK

Biochemical Research Laboratory,
The Dow Chemical Company,
Midland, Mich., and
Department of Anesthesiology,
Cornell University
Medical College,
New York, N.Y.

Biochem. Pharmacol., 13: 1239, 1964

This paper presents evidence that diethyl ether, chloroform, methoxyflurane, and halothane are metabolized.

The study was carried out in rats selected on a weight basis (200 ± 15 g.). Administration of the anesthetics was by intraperitoneal injection of 0.1 ml. doses. Immediately after the injection the animals were placed in an all-glass metabolism cage designed to allow the recovery of the expired gases and separate collection of urine and feces. The animals remained in these containers for periods up to 96 hours and were given access to food and water. As a rule the animals were narcotized by the anesthetic injection.

DIETHYL ETHER.

The total $^{14}CO_2$ collected from the expired air in 24 hours was 4 per cent of the amount injected. The urine contained 2 per cent of the injected radioactivity.

CHLOROFORM

The total amount of $^{14}CO_2$ collected was 4.5 per cent of the ^{14}C-chloroform injected.

HALOTHANE

The only labeled halothane available was ^{36}Cl-halothane. The total ^{36}Cl recovered in the expired air in 30 hours was 85 to 90 per cent of the administered dose. At the end of 14 days the ^{36}Cl was still appearing in the urine as inorganic chloride and at that time amounted to 2.9 per cent of the injected dose.

METHOXYFLURANE

The amount of exhaled $^{14}CO_2$ in most animals was 1 to 2 per cent. The amount of ^{14}C metabolites in the urine was 3 to 5 per cent of that injected.

The intermediates arising in the conversion of these anesthetics to CO_2, when identified, should reveal interesting information concerning the pathway of metabolism of these and other similar materials.

1965

Published February, 1972

1957 was quite a year.

No historian worthy of his salt would ever try, from a vantage point of a mere 15 years, to assess the historic significance of events; but an amateur can be pardoned for remembering, very clearly, that cold New England November morning when the World was informed of the chilling news that *Sputnik II*, with a dog named Laika aboard, was traveling around the earth once every 103.7 minutes at a rate of 17,840 miles per hour in an orbit ranging from 194 to 1,056 miles from our planet. Sputnik—a word that had been previously unknown outside of the Soviet Union, but which United States readers came to learn means "something that is traveling with a traveler"—both fascinated and frightened humanity; people all over the world looked for a glimpse of it in the sky, and listened transfixed to the beep-beep-beep of its transmitter. The satellite radio was reporting data on such things as cosmic rays, solar radiation, temperature, space composition and density, the danger of meteors, navigation problems, the earth's gravitation and magnetic field, and Laika's pulse, breathing, blood pressure and electrocardiogram. Scientists everywhere believed that the U.S.S.R. had developed a new type of fuel to accomplish the feat of pushing such heavy objects as the *Sputniks* into space, and Soviet authorities confirmed that "new sources of power" were employed. Laika lived for several days, probably about a week, but the Russians would reveal only that the dog had died.

The Space Race was on, and this event was one of transcending significance.

Meanwhile, back on earth, there were other reasons why 1957 was quite a year. Dwight David Eisenhower was President of the United States, and as such, of course, he made headlines all year long—the most important two concerning Little Rock and his own health.

The latter was a constant worry to the nation. A cold and a cough in March affected his hearing, but a six day, 700 mile cruise to Bermuda and a 10 day golfing vacation cured him. Then in June he was confined to bed with a "mild stomach upset", but he got back to his desk within a couple days. Finally, in November, right after a thorough physical examination had given him a clean bill of health, he suffered a slight stroke; and although the illness was sufficiently severe to affect his speech, he recovered rapidly and attended the NATO meeting in Paris in December. None of these illnesses were important, but the people were conditioned to worry themselves silly over the health of the Chief Executive during the short time that they lasted.

The nation's worries over Little Rock, on the other hand, did concern an important illness, and were to last much longer— they have been going on for 15 years, in fact, and there is no end in sight. Governor Orval E. Faubus of Arkansas refused to integrate Little Rock Central High School, despite a federal court order. Eisenhower talked to Faubus in Newport, Rhode Island, on September 14, but to no avail; and finally in late September federal troops were sent to Little Rock to control the riots and enforce integration. "The troops are there", the President explained, "pursuant to law, solely for the purpose of preventing interference with the orders of the court". Northern Congressmen criticized the President for delaying so long before sending in the troops; Southerners were infuriated by what they called an "irresponsible and dictatorial act"—but integration of the school was accomplished and violence was averted.

There were headline events throughout

the rest of the world, too. By the end of the summer, the Hungarian Communist government of boss Janos Kadar had presided over a blood bath of some 5,000 executions of strikers and other "enemies of the state" who had been involved in the October 1956 revolt. The Soviet Union cast its 80th veto in the United Nations Security Council to block a U.S. plan for UN-India-Pakistan talks on Kashmir; and, in Russia itself, Nikita Khrushchev won a Kremlin struggle for power and sent his three chief rivals—Georgi Malenkov, Vyachelav Molotov, and Lazar Kaganovich— packing to minor posts far from Moscow. Eamon de Valera, 74 years old, became prime minister of Ireland for the third time; and the government of 81 year old Chancellor Konrad Adenauer won a smashing victory at the polls in Germany. In Cuba, a young rebel by the name of Fidel Castro directed raids and bombings against the widely despised government of Fulgenico Batista from a mountain hideout; while in Indonesia, Achmed Sukarno threw the Dutch out—after confiscating their businesses, of course—and took over the country lock, stock, and barrel. The Suez was reopened, after being cleared of 50 ships sunk during the British-French-Israeli invasion of Egypt; and the last British troops left Jordan under agreements which ended the British-Jordan defense pact. France wavered constantly on the brink of disaster, while three different governments tried to lead the nation beyond crisis after crisis; and next door in Italy, the government finally gave the body of dictator Benito Mussolini to his widow—it had been held in a secret place for 11 years to prevent his followers from making it a shrine.

It was the year that *Kukla, Fran and Ollie*, once one of television's leading shows, finally went off the air; and that "Music Man" and "West Side Story" took Broadway by storm. Paris fashion designers introduced "the sack silhouette"; but American women, proud of their figures, eschewed the new shapeless style that had no waistline. Arturo Toscanini, the great maestro, died and was much mourned; and Senator Joseph R. McCarthy also died, and was hardly mourned at all. *Iron Liege* won the Kentucky Derby after veteran jockey Willie Shoemaker, aboard *Gallant Man*, misjudged the finish line and pulled up his mount too soon. People were reading "Peyton Place", "By Love Possessed"; "Atlas Shrugged", "Rally Round The Flag, Boys!", and "On the Beach"; and going to the movies to see "Les Girls", "Funny Face", and "The Bridge On The River Kwai". Oklahoma finally lost a football game after 47 straight wins, and the Detroit Red Wings won the National Hockey League title for the eighth year in nine. The top individual sports accomplishments were turned in by Lew Burdette, who pitched the Milwaukee Braves to three victories over the New York Yankees to win the World Series; and by Althea Gibson, who became the first negro in history to win the Wimbledon women's tennis title and the U.S. women's tennis title.

There were other less publicized, but nevertheless important, events in 1957. A lion and tigress became the proud parents of four *ligers* at the Victoria Garden Zoo in Bombay, where the superintendent pointed out that a *liger* is much rarer than a *tigon*, the offspring of a tiger and a lioness. An Alexandria, Virginia, city record book was discovered which revealed that George Washington was delinquent 9 pounds in his 1794 local taxes. Portugal planted its flag on a new volcano created island in the Azores on October 12; but on October 30 the island slipped quietly into the sea and disappeared. A paper shortage in September forced indefinite postponement of Nepal's first general elections. The Brooklyn Public Library reported that one of its staff members helped a private secretary to help her employer to help a committee chairman to write a speech on "How To Do It Yourself". The main bell in Canterbury Cathedral, tolled by hand since 1498, began operating by push button in 1957. When Queen Elizabeth II visited France in April, she brought 230 pieces of luggage, weighing 2½ tons, in three planes: it took five trucks and a bus to haul the luggage

through Paris. Doria Shafik, an Egyptian feminist leader, went on a "hunger strike to the death" to protest the dictatorial regime, and did not eat anything at all for 11 days. And the Soviet radio, continually throughout the year, referred to Asian Flu as Australian influenza.

But in a few quarters the most significant event of 1957 was the beginning publication of a new journal, *Survey of Anesthesiology*, which is just 15 years old today. "Classical File", as has been its wont every five years, offers as a birthday present a departure from its usual sequential plan and its strict concern with history and musty archives to reprint a thought provoking contribution titled, "I Think, Therefore:", which was written by Dr. Richard H. Strauss and was published in the Summer, 1965, issue of *Perspectives in Biology and Medicine*. *Survey* and its readers are indebted to the late Dr. James H. Matthews, Professor of Anesthesiology at the University of Minnesota, for calling attention to this essay, which is reprinted below with the kind permissions of the author and the publishers.

I THINK, THEREFORE:

RICHARD H. STRAUSS, M.D.

Perspectives Biol. Med., 8: 516, 1965

A whimsical tale in which a 75 year old biologist, with failing kidneys and heart, had these vital systems replaced with artificial mechanisms. To assist him with his research, he was provided with an all-encompassing computer by name of John. Eventually John, in addition to his scientific duties, could win at chess, reply to telephone messages, and even take over the thought processes of his master. One day the artificial heart gave out, and then John assumed full functions, of course with the knowledge and assent of his master. When John was assigned to other duties, his master in fact was then murdered!

Published December, 1972

Until 2 years ago, acupuncture was just another word as far as most anesthesiologists were concerned—and one without either any very perceptible connotation or even denotation, at that. And then along came Ping Pong.

Ping Pong parted the Bamboo Curtain, albeit ever so slightly, when Premier Chou En-lai of the People's Republic of China invited the United States table tennis team to Peking. He could hardly have startled the world more had he ordered Shanghai to bid against San Diego and Miami for the Republican National Convention. "Ping Pong diplomacy" had begun, and maybe was going to usher in an era which one cold war and two hot ones had been unable to produce. It was a type of diplomacy which would have flabbergasted a Talleyrand, sent a Disraeli off on the dead run to the palace, or prompted a Metternich to turn in his diplomatic pouch.

The whole thing was the more astounding in that almost no one knew that the United States even *had* a table tennis team, let alone one that was capable of international matches with a world Ping Pong power such as China. But the team turned out to be as American as apple pie: it had (1) a hippie; (2) a college professor; (3) a housewife; (4) a chemist; (5) a black; (6) a Wall Streeter; (7) a computer programmer; (8) a collegian; and (9) a Detroit automobile executive. The team's record was completely unknown to the sports world, and more than one rank-and-file sports fan was fairly sure in his heart of hearts that he would have been much more comfortable if the Chinese had invited, say, the UCLA basketball squad, the Indiana swimming team, or even the Baltimore Orioles.

The results of the Ping Pong tour hugely validated these suspicions. "We had the impression that the Chinese were trying not to embarrass us by lopsided scores," commented Tim Boggan, the team's professor from Long Island University; and it became clear—as the Chinese swept to victory—that the world's champions were playing well within themselves. It also became equally clear that the table tennis was

a means, not an end; and as Premier Chou shook hands with the United States team, he told the visitors, "We have opened a new page in the relations of the Chinese and American people."

Thus the 1971 United States table tennis team, comprised of the world's most improbable—and perhaps most naive—group of diplomats, accomplished something that nobody else had accomplished over the course of the past 25 years; it paved the way for a small but steady trickle of American citizens into the People's Republic. One of the spin-offs was a vast popular interest in acupuncture.

The Ping Pong Incident took place in April 1971. During the summer, the next step in the American awareness of, and general public excitement over, acupuncture came when New York Times columnist, James Reston, one of the first to go to China as part of that small trickle, was operated upon for acute appendicitis at Peking's Anti-Imperialist Hospital. Reston's appendectomy was performed with standard Western surgical techniques and the administration of conventional Western chemical anesthesia. In retrospect, Reston has considered the possibility of the coincidence in the timing of his appendicitis attack as implicating Presidential Advisor, Henry A. Kissinger: "The first stab of pain went through my groin," he wrote, when Chinese officials disclosed that Kissinger's secret visit to Peking to set up President Nixon's Chinese Summit had occurred at a time when Reston himself was being kept out of the Chinese capital. "In my delirium," the columnist wrote, "I could see Mr. Kissinger floating across my bedroom ceiling grinning at me out of the corner of a hooded ricksha."

The patient did well for about 36 hours, at which point he developed an ileus and was "in considerable discomfort if not pain" from gas pressure distending his intestines. With Reston's full approval, an acupuncturist was called in and inserted 3 slender needles into the right elbow and below the knee, twirling them "to stimulate the intestine." Reston later reported that they "sent ripples of pain racing through my limbs and at least had the effect of diverting my attention from the distress in my stomach."

In short order, stories of other VIP's who had been treated with acupuncture began to come to light. Prince Bernhard of the Netherlands had been involved in an auto accident back in 1937 and suffered a recurrence of the severe pain in his back, left shoulder, and arm 2 years ago while visiting Singapore. He was treated by Yong Keng-ngoh, a Chinese acupuncturist, and immediately felt better. Ten months later the Prince, afflicted again, wrote to the Singapore acupuncturist, and was referred to Yong's son, Dr. Yong Chai-siow of London's Harley Street. The younger Yong diagnosed the problem as constipation and not the remnants of the auto injury. He proceeded to insert and twirl his needles over the course of a 2 day treatment, at which time Bernhard, a middle-aged 60, proclaimed that he felt at least 10 years younger.

Another such was Marshal Lon Nol, the Premier of Cambodia, who suffered a massive stroke during the winter of 1971. Lon Nol was flown to Honolulu, where he received all of the indicated therapies offered by the best in Western medicine. He made a good, but incomplete, recovery, and when he returned home to Phnom-Penh, he was treated by a Taiwanese acupuncturist, Dr. Wu, who inserted needles as deep as 3 inches into Lon Nol's muscles and joints, with further improvement in the patient's condition. Whether that improvement was due to the good Dr. Wu's needles or to the natural history of the disease—which is often characterized by progressive recovery—is a moot point.

In addition to the VIP's, a number of athletes also sought the magic of the acupuncturist's needles to relieve their assorted aches, pains, and bruises. "Sudden Sam" McDowell, a star pitcher with the Cleveland Indians (now with the San Francisco Giants) underwent acupuncture in the spring of 1971: "The muscles of my left shoulder have a tendency to tighten up because of inactivity during the winter. It takes two or three weeks of hard work to break the adhesions and loosen up the arm.

Last spring because I was so late going to camp I didn't have time to follow my normal routine." McDowell appealed to the trainer of the Tokyo Lotte Orions when they came to play an exhibition game against the Indians, and underwent acupuncture: "The next day, believe me, the arm was as loose as it ever had been. Amazing, really." Now, since the San Francisco Giants train with the Tokyo Lotte Orions, there are a whole raft of Giants addicted to acupuncture: Chris Speier thinks that it helps his back spasms; Juan Marichal believes that it helps his arm; Jerry Johnson is sure that it helps his elbow; and Willie McCovey submitted to the technique last spring for the pains in his hip—but has not ventured a verdict. Many Japanese baseball players, particularly pitchers, swear by acupuncture to relieve their sore forearms, elbows, shoulders, and waists. Norboru Akiyama, the pitching ace of the Taiyo Whales, is a particularly dedicated convert: one day in 1963 he had such excruciating elbow pain that he failed to finish the first inning; the Whales' trainer applied acupuncture, and the next day Akiyama pitched a full nine innings and won his ball game. Alvin Dark is another convert: when he was managing the Giants, his own bursitis was so improved by two acupuncture treatments that he wanted to hire a Japanese specialist for the team, but was talked out of it by American doctors.

Football players have benefited, too. Ed Lothamer, the 270 pound defensive tackle for the Kansas City Chiefs, had suffered stiffness and recurrent pain in his lower back for some 8 months after he felt something snap there while he was lifting 500 pounds from a squat. He met Dr. Kunzo Nagayama, president of the Pain Control Institute of Kyoto, Japan, who was in Kansas City visiting a chiropractor friend, Dr. Richard D. Yennie; and Drs. Nagayama and Yennie suggested that Lothamer try acupuncture for his aching back. "I was skeptical about it," Lothamer said, "but then I decided, why not? First Dr. Nagayama said he wanted to take my pulse. 'Take off your shirt', he told me. It turned out he wanted to take my pulse not on my wrist but at various places on my back. He patted it all over and said I had good circulation in my upper back but that it wasn't so good down lower. He started by sticking one needle in my hand. I hardly felt it. Then he began probing my back with his hands and every time he'd find a spot where I reacted because of soreness he'd mark an X on it with a pen. He marked about 25 places and then he picked out 20 of them and began inserting needles. They looked like they were made of gold and silver and were about the size of the filament in a light bulb. I hardly felt them going in. He left them in for from three to five minutes, occasionally vibrating them.

"Next he put two larger needles in my back and drew about 2 cm of blood. He withdrew these needles and where they had gone in he placed two small silver balls, taping them in place with small squares of pink tape. He told me to leave the balls in place for three days but didn't explain why. Then he put one in the middle of the stomach and when he took that one out later he taped one of the silver balls where the needle had made a small hole. After that he put three needles in each of my arms. While he was inserting them in the outer side of my right forearm I suddenly felt my whole right hand go dead. This sort of upset me but he said this effect was perfectly normal."

When the needles were removed, Lothamer felt "more circulation in my back than I've had for years. My back has taken quite a beating in four years of college and eight years of pro ball and for a long time that area hadn't felt very much alive." It does now, though, and Lothamer can get up in the morning without feeling stiff, and can jog his 2 miles without tightening up, the way he used to after just half a mile. He thinks that every pro football team should have access to acupuncture.

Not all athletes give acupuncture high marks, however. Chi Cheng, the world's fastest female runner, developed tendonitis in her thigh and was not improved by standard Western medical treatments. She returned to her native Taiwan for treatment by traditional Chinese medicine. She had undergone acupuncture fruitlessly 8 times in California; but when 2 sessions a day for 2 weeks with a Chinese specialist in massage and osteopathic manipulation failed to help her, she was referred to an acupuncturist who stuck myriad needles, some several inches long, into her legs, hands, and lower back. Chi Cheng found the needling and subsequent twirling of the needles "excruciating." "They say it shouldn't hurt," she said, "but I call it my Chinese torture"; and she would not hear of a second session, scheduled for the next day. She settled for Western type surgery on the muscle of her thigh.

These tales and anecdotes might have been dismissed as little more than interesting gossip, but Reston, who actually is both an editor and a vice-president of the New York Times, was quick to provide an autobiographical scoop on his appendectomy and joust with acupuncture, and the summer issues of such important medical journals as Time and Life were full of short prose recaps of the technique of acupuncture, photographs of patients with needles sticking out of them like porcupine quills, and pictures of Ming Dynasty Medical Charts of the various acupuncture "points." Medical librarians who had never even heard of the volume were requested to order The Yellow Emperor's Classic of Internal Medicine, the title given to a series of translations of writings on acupuncture by Dr. Ilza Veith, Professor of the History of Health Sciences at the University of California. The mystique of acupuncture was building, but the technique was still being dismissed lightly in many medical circles as superstition and folklore.

An abrupt change in this attitude began to occur in September, 1971, when a distinguished group of American doctors, including Dr. Paul Dudley White, the internationally famous cardiologist, and Dr. E. Grey Dimond, Provost for the Health Sciences at the University of Kansas, were invited to the People's Republic of China by the China Medical Association. The visitors were asked to indicate areas of their special interests, and Dr. Dimond, who had become interested in the subject several years previously during a visit to Vietnam, specified acupuncture. His observations in Vietnam had been on the use of acupuncture for the treatment of a variety of medical problems (Ward Rounds with an Acupuncturist, *New England J. Med. 272:* 575, 1965), but the trip to China produced a startling new development—acupuncture anesthesia, which had also been reported the previous month by Reston (the *New York Times,* Sunday, August 22, 1971). Dimond and his colleagues watched such major surgery as thyroidectomies, gastrectomies, and craniotomies performed under acupuncture anesthesia and came home impressively awed and enthusiastic. These physicians were clearly competent and qualified observers, and their report of successful acupuncture anesthesia in 90 per cent of the patients in whom it was applied (Dimond, E. G.: Acupuncture anesthesia. *J.A.M.A., 218:* 1558, 1971) could scarcely be dismissed as idle gossip.

President Nixon's Summit Trip to Peking in February of 1972 served to commit American medicine firmly to a serious and detailed investigation of acupuncture anesthesia. The President was accompanied by White House Physician, Dr. Walter Tkach, who went into Communist China sharing the skepticism of many American physicians about the technique, but came away just short of being ecstatic about the potential inherent in its future use: "It could open the door to fantastic possibilities if we could eliminate general anesthesia. There is no doubt in my mind that acupuncture deserves an in-depth look from a strictly objective and scientific approach." Such a statement, coming from such a quarter, appears certain to guarantee an extensive study in the immediate future.

Acupuncture is said to have originated from the observation many centuries ago by Chinese warriors that, when they were pierced by arrows in certain parts of their bodies, they felt better in other parts which were remote from the site of the arrow puncture. The early Chinese medicine men kept track of these puncture points, and eventually described 12 Ching Lo channels or meridians, connecting them all along the path which the universal energy *chi* is said to travel. There are 365 of these points (or 1000, according to whom you read— mod-

ern acupuncturists have added several hundred points, just as they have added sterilization of the needles) at which the insertion of a needle will have a physiologic effect, and the points do not follow any anatomic system recognized by Western medicine. The Chinese explanation for acupuncture is that the forces of Yang and Yin flow through the 12 Ching Lo channels and must be precisely balanced if good health and well being are to be maintained. Yang is variously translated as good, positive, and "on the sunny side," whereas Yin is bad, negative, and "on the shadowy side." If a patient has too much Yin at some site, the traditional acupuncturist will jab a gold Yang needle into a selected point to counteract. Diagnosis of an ailment is made by taking six pulses in each wrist, and it may be quite a problem since there are 27 possible qualities for each pulse.

It is difficult for the Western medical mind not to attach a certain element of witchcraft to all of this, and the aura of mystique is not lessened by the accoutrements of acupuncture: the mannikan with blue meridian lines connecting black dots; the importance attached to the manner in which the needles are "twirled" or "vibrated"; the special qualities attributed to needles of different lengths, diameters, and materials (gold, silver, or stainless steel); the concomitant "moxibustion" or burning of herbs to transmit heat down the needle shaft to increase stimulation and extract dampness (modernists have substituted a low voltage electric current for moxibustion); and the use of the small silver balls.

Nevertheless, it is imprudent to judge a healing craft born more than 2500 years ago against the fledgling standards of Western medicine. Over the centuries, acupuncture had spread in various forms throughout Asia, and within the last 30 or 40 years it has attained some status in Russia, England, Germany, and especially France— there are over 600 acupuncturists in France who give more than a million treatments a year, and several reputable French hospitals permit acupuncture to be prescribed and administered. There are practitioners of acupuncture scattered even in the United States, although they are mainly congregated in the Chinatowns of New York and particularly San Francisco.

There remains the major problem of a serious explanation of the mechanism of acupuncture which is acceptable to the Western trained medical mind. It has been suggested that hypnosis or self-hypnosis may well be the basis for the technique; but at least in the case of acupuncture anesthesia, this explanation is probably not creditable, since the Chinese claim that over 400,000 cases have been done in the past few years with an 80 to 90 per cent rate of success, which is far higher than the usual rate of success expected with hypnosis.

Reston has suggested (and he is the first to point out that he is a newspaperman, not a scientist) that it may be a special form of hypnosis, one with an almost religious quality or overtone. He and his wife spent 4 hours at the Han Shan Hospital in Shanghai watching acupuncture anesthesia:

"The interesting thing here . . . is that, while they cannot agree on the theory of how needle anesthesia works, they are increasingly convinced that it does work, and are operating on the pragmatic evidence and not waiting for theoretical justification.

"One troubling diversion in all this for a visitor is that the impressive objective evidence of the medical uses of acupuncture is always mixed up here with subjective psychiatric and even ideological explanations.

"For example, all the patients we saw on the operating table were clutching their little red books of Chairman Mao Tse-tung's philosophic and moral teachings. And the doctors and surgeons, after participating in the operations, were explaining that the success of this system depended importantly on trust between doctor and patient and on a common faith in 'Mao Tse-tung thought.'"

Dimond makes very much the same point: "The practice of medicine and the national policy of China are inseparable and this report can only be rational if the political reality is identified." And again, on the subject of acupuncture anesthesia, "The stoicism of the Chinese and the cur-rent ideological indoctrination play a role"; then he adds "but do not seem adequate explanations for the effective anesthesia."

Another explanation is the "gate control" theory of pain, which has now been extended by Drs. Pang L. Man and Calvin H. Chen into a 2 gate theory (the so-called Man-Chen Theory) to explain acupuncture anesthesia—1 gate being postulated in the spinal cord and 1 in the thalamus. The original "gate control" theory of pain was advanced by Professors Ronald Melzack of Montreal's McGill University and Patrick D. Wall of University College in London. Their paper was published in the November 19, 1965, issue of *Science* under the title "Pain Mechanisms: A New Theory" (*Science, 150:* 971–979, 1965) and is reprinted below with the kind permission of the authors and the publisher.

PAIN MECHANISMS: A NEW THEORY A GATE CONTROL SYSTEM MODULATES SENSORY INPUT FROM THE SKIN BEFORE IT EVOKES PAIN PERCEPTION AND RESPONSE

RONALD MELZACK
AND
PATRICK D. WALL

Science, 150: 971, 1965

* * * *

GATE CONTROL THEORY OF PAIN

"Stimulation of the skin evokes nerve impulses that are transmitted to three spinal cord systems: the cells of the substantia gelatinosa in the dorsal horn, the dorsal-column fibers that project toward the brain, and the fine central transmission (T) cells in the dorsal horn. We propose that (i) the substantia gelatinosa functions as a gate control system that modulates the afferent patterns before they influence the T cells; (ii) the afferent pattern in the dorsal column system acts, in part at least, as a central control trigger which activates selective brain processes that influence the modulating properties of the gate control system; and (iii) the T cells activate neural mechanisms which comprise the action system responsible for response and perception. Our theory proposes that pain phenomena are determined by interactions among these three systems."

*   *   *   *

1966

Published April, 1977

When halothane was the Prodigal Son and methoxyflurane just an infant, the halogenated hydrocarbons were at the top of the heap. Everybody was for them, and why not? They were potent; they were nonflammable and nonexplosive; they provided a rapid and pleasant induction; they were followed by a recovery that was free from nausea and vomiting, and other such unpleasant phenomena; they produced a degree of muscle relaxation if carried to a sufficient depth of concentration; and all of this without deleterious respiratory and cardiovascular effects.

Within a matter of a few years, however, it became apparent that unpleasant things could occur following the administration of these drugs. These were not direct toxic effects in the instance of either drug, but untoward complications were reported after anesthesia conducted with both of them.

The first reports of so-called "halothane hepatitis" began to occur in 1958 and the flood of reports reached disturbing proportions in 1963 when 46 cases of liver dysfunction and/or damage (including 20 deaths, most of which were the result of massive hepatic necrosis) were reported. Since then, there has been a steady addition of anecdotal case studies in the literature. In point of fact, however, all that turns yellow is not halothane. There are a dozen factors other than the anesthetic agent which produce changes in liver function in the surgical patient: the dose of the drug,

the duration of exposure to the drug, repeated exposures, the nutritional status of the patient, hypoxia, hypotension, hypercarbia, the site of surgery, blood transfusions, disease states and metabolic disturbances, and a number of the drugs and therapeutic agents employed in the surgical patient. Halothane is certainly not a direct hepatotoxin in the sense that carbon tetrachloride is: it does not invariably provoke hepatic damage in all individuals at even high dose levels; it does not produce a lesion that is of a severity directly related to the dose; it does not produce a lesion that can be reproduced in the experimental animal; and it does not have a predictable or necessarily short latent period between acute exposure and the occurrence of the lesion.

The hypothesis that halothane produces hepatic injury on the basis of allergy is also untenable in the light of present knowledge. If it were an allergic phenomenon, a great many more operating room personnel (anesthesiologists, nurse anesthetists, circulating and scrub nurses, and the like) should have developed the lesion.

The current hypothesis, therefore, is that the liver damage is on the basis of the metabolites which are produced when halothane undergoes biotransformation within the body. This theory is attractive, because it is certain that the drug is indeed broken down in the body, and to a considerable extent (20 per cent). The end product is a dehalogenated oxidized compound, trifluoroacetic acid; but the intermediate metabolites have not been conclusively identified. So the hypothesis, while attractive and comforting to our sense of ignorance, remains neither established nor disproved. Perhaps there are genetic factors involved in the individual patient.

Methoxyflurane produces a nephrotoxicity in the form of high output renal failure which has a clinical picture similar to diabetes insipidus. This nephropathy *is* dose related, but it is not the methoxyflurane itself which causes the lesion, but rather a breakdown product, the free fluoride ion. The metabolism of methoxyflurane in the body can run as high as 50 per cent, which would produce a lot of free fluoride ion; and it is also possible that the oxalic acid, which is another metabolite, may contribute to the overall toxicity of methoxyflurane. Again, the capability of converting the anesthetic into these metabolites depends on the drug-metabolizing enzymes of the patient, which in turn are determined by the person's genetic makeup.

None of the above points were lost upon the pharmaceutical houses, the research chemists, and the clinical investigators in the medical centers; and the halogenated hydrocarbons (of which ether, with a birthday dating from October 16th, 1846, is the granddaddy) began to receive renewed attention. One of these, Ethrane (or enflurane) has made it into clinical practice, and may prove to be one of our best weapons against the contingency-fee lawyers. We should have about 5 years before enough cases of obesity, or hang-nail (remember Hannah Greener?), or gross surgical hemorrhage from a cut cystic artery, are attributed to Ethrane, and attract the lawyers to malpractice suits like honey attracts bees. Maybe we will have longer than that, since Ethrane is metabolized to a far lesser extent than either halothane or methoxyflurane, which could be a factor if the metabolite theory of the toxicity of inhalational anesthetics holds true. And, of course, it will be another 5 years before that sterling Federal Bureaucracy, the F.D.A., pontificates that it had told us so all along (if any are still using the drug after the contingency-fee

onslaught by the lawyers) and proceeds to ban the drug.

Krantz had done pharmacologic studies of Ethrane in animals as early as 1963, but the drug's clinical introduction was reported by Virtue, Lund, Phelps, Vogel, Beckwitt, and Heron in a paper entitled, "Difluoromethyl 1,1,2-trifluoro-2-chloroethyl ether as an anaesthetic agent: results with dogs, and a preliminary note on observations with man," which was published in the May, 1966, issue of the *Canadian Anaesthetists' Society Journal (Can. Anaesth. Soc. J.*, 13:233–241, May, 1966), and which is reprinted below with the kind permissions of the authors and the publishers.

DIFLUOROMETHYL 1,1,2-TRIFLUORO-2-CLORETHYL ETHER AS AN ANAESTHETIC AGENT: RESULTS WITH DOGS, AND A PRELIMINARY NOTE ON OBSERVATIONS WITH MAN

ROBERT W. VIRTUE,
LAWRENCE O. LUND,
MCKINLEY PHELPS, JR.,
JOHN H. K. VOGEL,
HENRY BECKWITT
AND
MICHAEL HERON

University of Colorado
Medical Center,
Denver, Colorado

Can. Anaesth. Soc. J., 13:233–241, 1966

The above-mentioned drug, now known as enflurane (Ethrane), was investigated in dogs, human volunteers (8), and in patients (11) undergoing operations.

This new anesthetic agent, administered to dogs by the open-drop technique, produced smooth anesthesia without salivation, irritation or nausea. Enzyme studies before, at the end of, and two days following hour-long administrations showed no significant changes. In three of 16 dogs anesthetized with enflurane, ventricular fibrillation followed injections of epinephrine.

The concentration of enflurane required for surgical anesthesia in dogs was about twice that with halothane. When the animals were sufficiently anesthetized to show burst suppression on the EEG, there frequently appeared spontaneous twitching motions.

In the volunteers, anesthesia induction was pleasant. Blood pressure dropped, as did cardiac output, when anesthesia was deepened. The degree of analgesia was similar to that seen with halothane. Two subjects carried to "burst suppression" showed brief spontaneous twitches that disappeared quickly on removal of the agent.

In the surgical patients, systolic blood pressure fell an average of 25 mm. Hg following induction. Relaxation was adequate for abdominal surgery. Ten of the 11 patients were awake by the time they reached the recovery room. One vomited moderately.

Enflurane appears to be similar to halothane, with the exception that, in deeper planes of anesthesia, spontaneous movements may be observed.

Published April and June, 1974

When halothane was introduced as an anesthetic agent in 1956, it did not go unnoticed that it was a halogenated hydrocarbon which was at least partially related chemically to chloroform and carbon tetrachloride (the prototype of a true hepatotoxin), and that it might, therefore, be capable of liver damage. Such suspicions of hepatotoxic effects have greeted all new halogenated hydrocarbon anesthetics as the latter have made their clinical debut, and careful studies of hepatic function have been a routine part of their investigative screening.

Observations of liver function and morphologic structure in laboratory animals, and tests of hepatic function in man, indicated that, although halothane, in common with all of the general anesthetic agents, has an effect upon the liver, it is a mild and transient effect; and that the morphologic changes which the drug produced, such as fatty infiltration and vacuolization, were completely reversible. Indeed, Johnstone, in the first clinical report of the use of halothane in anesthesia, described its administration to 8 jaundiced patients, 7 of whom made uneventful recoveries and one of whom died postoperatively of widespread carcinomatosis. In addition, in a number of patients who received halothane anesthesia and subsequently came to autopsy, lesions of the liver were conspicuously absent. This finding was even true of very massive and prolonged doses of the drug: Haid maintained a 5 year old boy with tetanus under nitrous oxide-oxygen-halothane anesthesia continuously for a total of 6 weeks of treatment, using 1500 ml. of halothane during the first 3 weeks alone. The patient ultimately died of gross hemorrhage resulting from erosion of the innominate artery, but examination of the liver at autopsy revealed that there was neither abnormal pathology nor any degenerative hepatic changes indicative of necrosis: "The liver was enlarged with some opaque swelling and on section showed a completely maintained lobular structure. The liver cells were rather poor in glycogen content at the lobular periphery, particularly around the periportal areas where there were some slight fatty infiltrations. There was moderately copious pigment in the Kupffer cells reacting positively to a test for iron." At no time during the course of the illness did the patient show any clinical signs of liver damage.

Despite all this reassuring evidence of a comforting absence of liver pathology following halothane anesthesia, Burns and his coworkers in the British Isles, in 1957, described jaundice, fatty degeneration, and liver cell necrosis in a patient who had received halothane. However, the patient had a malignancy, and the portal areas of the liver were grossly infiltrated by neoplastic cells, which could easily account for the findings.

The following year, in 1958, Burnap, Gall and Vandam reported 2 patients in whom liver disease worsened after halothane anesthesia, and both showed structural changes in the liver, one at autopsy and the other on liver biopsy. There were again, however, a great many mitigating factors involved in each of these patients, and the conclusion was that there was no direct evidence of hepatic toxicity. The authors were constrained to raise the question as to whether halothane might intensify hepatocellular disease, and they advised caution in the administration of the drug under these circumstances.

A few months later, Virtue and Payne reported a death from acute yellow atrophy of the liver and pancreatitis in a healthy, middle-aged woman 11 days following an elective cholecystectomy performed under halothane anesthesia. This case also was complicated by additional contributing factors; but Virtue and Payne pointed out that, except for the fact that the syndrome did not appear until the sixth postoperative day, the clinical course and autopsy findings were consistent with those of the delayed chloroform poisoning of an earlier generation.

The next year, 1959, Barton made a brief note in the *Lancet* of 2 patients who developed postoperative jaundice 48 hours after the administration of halothane. He was disturbed by the occurrence of these complications, but the jaundice apparently cleared without the development of further signs or symptoms of liver injury, and nothing more was heard of the matter.

In 1960, Vourc'h and his colleagues described an acute, fatal hepato-nephritis following a simple herniorrhaphy performed under halothane anesthesia in a young man who had been in excellent health prior to operation. In the first direct statement as to the involvement of the drug in postoperative liver damage, they firmly attributed the complication to halothane.

Another instance of massive hepatic necrosis was reported by Temple, Cote and Gorens, in 1962, in a patient who suffered massive hepatic necrosis after the second of 2 administrations of halothane for 2 relatively straightforward surgical operations. There was an interval of 21 days between the 2 administrations, but the postoperative course following the first anesthesia and operation had been entirely uneventful. This death was the first which occurred following a second exposure to halothane, and in retrospect it is worth noting that the first postoperative course was indeed unremarkable. The authors did not attach any great importance to the fact that there had been 2 exposures to the drug, but did take note of the great number of etiologic factors which can be involved in the production of acute massive hepatic necrosis in the surgical patient, and concluded that the problem in their patient was not necessarily related to the anesthetic drug.

Not too much attention was attracted by these few isolated reports of hepatic complications until 1963, when some 46 new cases of liver dysfunction and/or injury were reported, including 20 deaths, most of which were the result of massive hepatic necrosis, and several of which occurred in middle-aged women undergoing biliary tract surgery. This sudden flood of hepatic complications, coming so soon after the thalidomide tragedies, drew the attention of the press; and on March 13, 1963, the *Wall Street Journal* carried banner headlines of a report which began, "Questions about whether a widely-used gas anesthetic can cause life-threatening damage to the liver were raised by *The New England Journal of Medicine*. The anesthetic is halothane, a nonexplosive gas developed in England by Imperial Chemical Industries, Ltd., and sold in this country under the trade name Fluothane by Ayerst Laboratories, a division of American Home Products Corp."

The article touched off a furor throughout the country which approached hysterical proportions; and the following week the news magazine *Time* picked up the story and under the headline, "A Gas and the Liver," ran a detailed article on "Anesthetics": "When halothane was introduced as an anesthetic in 1956, it seemed nearly perfect. Unlike ether and cyclopropane, it is both nonflammable and nonexplosive—a valuable asset in the modern operating room crammed with electronic gadgetry. It causes patients a minimum of discomfort and, it seemed, could do them no harm at all. It rapidly became widely used. But last week doctors were disturbed by reports in *The New England Journal of Medicine* that halothane might have caused as many as ten deaths by damaging the patient's liver."

Time's article was far more dispassionate than the scare headlines in the *Wall Street Journal* and many a hometown newspaper, and it went on to explain, "At least 6,000,000 Americans have had operations in the last five years under halothane. Even if all the deaths and illnesses now charged against the gas were proved, its safety record would still be impressive: in the previous five years about as many patients were killed or severely injured in operating room explosions of anesthetics." *Time* concluded, "Some claims for halothane may have been too good to be true, but the anesthetic is still too good to lose."

Nevertheless, despite this refreshing objectivity on the subject, the great Halothane Liver Controversy had begun, and it was destined to occupy a dominant amount of time and attention in anesthesia circles for some time to come. In fact, in the minds of some, it has not been resolved completely to this day.

The unfortunate publicity, coupled with the established fact that liver deaths had occurred following the administration of halothane, aroused the interest and anxiety of the National Academy of Sciences—National Research Council's Committee on Anesthesia. A Subcommittee on the National Halothane Study was formed, and plans for a countrywide study of liver injury following anesthesia and surgery were developed. The first report of this million dollar investigation was entitled, "Summary of the National Halothane Study: Possible Association between Halothane Anesthesia and Postoperative Hepatic Necrosis," and was published in the September 5th, 1966, issue of the *Journal of the American Medical Association* (*JAMA, 197:* 775–788, 1966). It will be republished in 2 parts

in this and the June, 1974, issue of *Survey*, with the kind permission of National Academy of Sciences—National Research Council and the Editorial Board of the J.A.M.A.

*   *   *   *

This investigation came to be known as the National Halothane Study and, in all, data from 856,500 patients undergoing surgery and general anesthesia in 34 institutions from 1959 through 1962 were examined. The study demonstrated that massive hepatic necrosis was a rare postoperative complication: only 82 cases were collected (an incidence of approximately one in 10,000 administrations of general anesthesia), and all but 9 of these could be explained on the basis of circulatory shock, sepsis, or previous hepatic disease. Massive hepatic necrosis did occur more frequently in patients who had 2 or more operations while under general anesthesia in the same or consecutive months, however, and this was particularly true of halothane. Of the 9 unexplained instances of massive hepatic necrosis, 7 had received halothane for the final operation, and 4 had received the drug on 2 or more occasions. Contrary to expectations, an increased incidence of massive hepatic necrosis following biliary tract surgery did not occur, and it was concluded that there was no evidence to support the imputed risk of halothane in operations performed on the gallbladder or bile ducts.

SUMMARY OF THE NATIONAL HALOTHANE STUDY

POSSIBLE ASSOCIATION BETWEEN HALOTHANE ANESTHESIA AND POSTOPERATIVE HEPATIC NECROSIS

Subcommittee on the National Halothane Study of the Committee on Anesthesia, National Academy of Sciences-National Research Council

J.A.M.A., 197:775–788, 1966

SUMMARY AND CONCLUSIONS

"A retrospective survey of the incidence of fatal massive hepatic necrosis and overall death rate following general anesthesia in 34 hospitals for the four-year period from 1959 through 1962 was undertaken. Special attention was paid to a comparison of halothane and other commonly used anesthetics with respect to hepatic necrosis and postoperative death generally. The main conclusions are:

"1. Fatal postoperative massive hepatic necrosis was a rare occurrence. It could usually be explained on the basis of circulatory shock, sepsis, or previous hepatic disease. The possible rare occurrence of halothane-induced hepatic necrosis following single or multiple administrations could not be ruled out.

"2. Halothane, rather than being a dangerous anesthetic, had a record of safety as reflected in an overall mortality of 1.87%, compared to an average for all anesthetic practices of 1.93%. This overall parity of halothane holds up when imbalances in patient populations are taken into account by detailed statistical adjustments. No evidence was found to support the imputed risk of halothane in operations performed on the gall bladder or bile ducts, or in craniotomies.

"3. In the middle-death-rate operations cyclopropane and "other" were associated with reliably higher mortality than were halothane and nitrous oxide-barbiturate; in terms of crude death rates there was a nearly twofold contrast. After statistical adjustment to compensate for differences in the populations exposed to the various agents, cyclopropane and "other" had death rates 2.5% or more, compared to approximately 2% for halothane and nitrous oxide-barbiturate, roughly 25% greater.

"4. Ether deserves more systematic study; although the death rate following ether administration was lowest of all, the result is unreliable because so few hospitals in the study used it extensively, and so no further conclusions can now be drawn.

"5. Of special interest and concern were the large differences in postoperative mortality occurring among the participating institutions. These differences could not be accounted for by the variations among hospital populations by any of the criteria measured in this study. This matter is discussed further in the full report."

1967

Published April, 1981

The almost constant parade of new muscle relaxant drugs onto the clinical scene during the course of the past 40 years or so can really mean only one thing: the ideal neuromuscular blocking agent for clinical use has yet to be found.

Curare itself, of course, was the first and led the parade. Introduced into clinical practice by Griffith in 1942, the drug revolutionized the practice of anesthesia for all time by permitting utter muscle flaccidity without resort to deep and dangerous levels of general anesthesia; and it became the standard of comparison by which each of the subsequent muscle relaxants was evaluated. Curare has been a wonderfully serviceable drug, and remains one of the most widely used muscle relaxants almost 4 decades after its clinical introduction. Time and use, however, revealed a number of flaws and side effects (histamine release, ganglion blockade and hypotension), and within a short time the search was on for other drugs which might replace it.

One of the major aims was to find a drug of sufficiently rapid onset and brief duration of action that it might be applied for short procedures such as endotracheal intubation (or extubation) and endoscopy in general; for the reduction of fractures and dislocations; for the amelioration of the impact of electroshock therapy (and now, cardioversion) on the skeletal system; for the treatment of laryngospasm during general anesthesia; for relaxation during certain types of obstetric delivery, or external rotation of breech presentations; and for similar situations in which the duration of action of curare far exceeded the need for muscular relaxation.

A second major aim was to find a synthetic muscle relaxant which might replace curare, which was an expensive drug in a post-war, dollar poor Europe. The pharmaceutic firms were quick to recognize that muscle relaxants could be a whole new branch of the industry, with large (not enormous) sales potential; and they were equally quick to mobilize their research facilities for the search. Any substance, synthetic or occurring naturally, which had neuromusuclar blocking properties, was assured a pharmacologic, and usually a clinical, hearing. This search led to trials of such unlikely candidates as dihydrobeta-erythroidine, which produced a well defined decrease in blood pressure in anesthetized man, and mephenesin (Myanesin, Tolserol), which produced muscular relaxation only as a secondary effect to its blocking action at the level of the internuncial neurones in the spinal cord itself. Most of the effort, however, was directed toward finding a short-acting synthetic muscle relaxant which had no toxic effects.

Gallamine triethiodide (Flaxedil) was one of a series of synthetic curare substitutes first reported on extensively by Bovet and his coworkers in 1947. Their work in this field began with the synthesis of structures related to, but less complicated than, d-tubocurarine. They then further simplified the structure of the active members of their various series, and found that the bis-choline ethers of phenols and polyphenols had potent curare-like actions. Gallamine is a nondepolarizing blocking drug: its neuromuscular effect is counteracted by neostigmine, edrophonium, and pyridostigmine, and is potentiated by ether and other fully potent inhalation anesthetics. The average

duration of its action is shorter than that of d-tubocurarine, in the order of 20 minutes. Excretion is by the kidneys, and it should be used carefully, if at all, in patients with decreased renal filtration. It also shows an atropine-like vagal blocking effect on the postganglion nerve endings of the heart, which results in tachycardia, even with small doses, and has led to the recommendation by some that it should not be used in the presence of cardiovascular disease or hyperthyroidism.

The polymethylene bis-trimethylammonium series, referred to by the generic term methonium compounds, was developed simultaneously and independently by Barlow and Ing, and Paton and Zaimis, in 1948. These workers, acting on the recognition by Crum-Brown and Fraser back in 1869 that there is a relationship between the quaternary ammonium groups of curare and its neuromuscular transmission, prepared and tested a number of simple bis-quaternary ammonium salts in which the nitrogen atoms were directly attached to the terminal carbons of polymethylene chains of different length. Potency was greatest in the bis-trimethylammonium series, and unusually high activity was found when the chain contained 10 carbon atoms (decamethonium). This drug causes neuromuscular block by prolonged depolarization of the postjunctional membrane of the motor endplate in skeletal muscles. It is not antagonized by the anticholinesterases such as neostigmine; and as a matter of fact, anticholinesterases, by causing acetylcholine to persist, may actually increase the paralyzing effect of decamethonium. A tachyphylaxis may develop with repeated doses; and repeated doses may also lead to the depolarizing effect at the endplate giving place to a nondepolarizing effect, the so-called phase 2 block. For these various reasons, but particularly because of the development of more admirable depolarizing drugs, decamethonium is no longer manufactured.

Diacetylcholine (succinylcholine) was first synthesized by Hunt and Taveau in 1906, but the use of curarized animals in their experiments prevented them from observing the neuromuscular blocking activity of the drug, and this property went unrecognized until 1949, when it was described independently by Bovet and his coworkers in Italy, and Phillips in this country. Succinylcholine is a depolarizing muscle relaxant with a rapid onset and brief duration of action, the latter being due to the fact that the drug is almost completely hydrolyzed in the organism by plamsa cholinesterase, at first fairly rapidly to succinylmonocholine and choline, and then more slowly to succinic acid and choline. It has enjoyed almost universal acceptance in clinical anesthesia for short periods of relaxation, and has been used for more prolonged muscular relaxation in the form of a titratable continuous infusion. There is no useful antagonist to terminate its action; and in situations in which the levels of plasma cholinesterase are low (liver disease, severe anemia, hypoproteinemia, cachexia due to malnutrition, malignancy, or chronic infection), the duration of relaxation may be considerably longer than might oridinarily be expected. In patients with atypical forms of plasma cholinesterase, termination of the succinylcholine activity is by a slow alkaline hydrolysis. Other unwanted side effects can include postanesthetic muscle pains, alterations in cardiac rhythm, increased intraocular and intragastric pressures, and exaggerated hyperkalemia in patients with severe burns, neurologic damage, muscular dystrophies, and massive trauma.

Benzoquinonium (Mytolon) is a neuromuscular blocking agent obtained by quaternization of a compound originally synthesized as a candidate antibacterial substance by Cavalitto and his collaborators in 1950; investigated pharmacologically by Hoppe that same year; and studied clinically by Arrowood, and by Foldes and his associates, in 1951. In contrast to d-tubocurarine and gallamine, which produce a typical nondepolarization block that can be antagonized by cholinesterase inhibitors, the activity of benzoquinonium is less uniform. Its neuromuscular block in man is little if at all antagonized by neostigmine. Furthermore, the drug stimulates the vagus nerve, causing marked increase in salivary and bronchial secretions and a tendency to bradycardia. Its use is therefore contraindicated in acute or chronic respiratory disease or in patients with disturbances of cardiac conductivity. The drug is no longer used in clinical anesthesia.

Laudexium (Laudolissin) was introduced into clinical anesthesia in 1952 by Bodman, after having been synthesized and studied pharmacologically by Collier and his colleagues in 1950. It is a heterocyclic decamethylene (bis-quaternary ammonium compound) which is a true nondepolarizing myoneural blocking agent, one-half as potent as d-tubocurarine, not always completely antagonized by anticholinesterases, acting longer than d-tubocurarine, and with greater cumulative effects. It is no longer available for clinical use.

It is obvious that, despite this continuous stream of new neuromuscular blocking compounds prepared by the chemists and screened as muscle relaxant drugs by the pharmacologists, the ideal relaxant has yet to be found. There is fairly widespread agreement, however, as to the properties of such a drug. It should have a brief, noncumulative, nondepolarizing blocking action, with rapid onset and recovery; it should be readily reversible by an appropriate and nontoxic antagonist; it should cause neither histamine release nor ganglion blockade; its breakdown products should have no neuromuscular blocking effect; and it should give rise to minimal cardiovascular side effects.

The search continues, and one of the more recent areas investigated has been the bis-quaternary aminosteroid drugs. In 1964, Hewett and Savage synthesized a diacetate dimethobromide compound of this series; and 3 years later, in the October, 1967 issue of the British Journal of Anaesthesia, Baird and Reid reported a pilot study in man under the title, "The neuromuscular blocking properties of a new steroid compound, pancuronium bromide" (Baird, W. L. M. and Reid, A. M.: Br. J. Anaesth., 39: 775, 1967), which is reprinted below with the kind permissions of the authors and the publisher.

THE NEUROMUSCULAR BLOCKING PROPERTIES OF A NEW STEROID COMPOUND, PANCURONIUM BROMIDE. A PILOT STUDY IN MAN.

W. L. M. BAIRD

AND

A. M. REID

Department of Anaesthetics,
Royal Infirmary,
Glasgow, Scotland

Br. J. Anaesth., 39: 775, 1967

Six healthy female patients undergoing minor gynecologic surgery were studied. Anesthesia was provided with thiopental 350 to 400 mg. and nitrous oxide-oxygen-halothane.

In doses of 2 to 3 mg. i.v., pancuronium produced a degree of blockade similar in intensity and duration of action to that of 10 to 15 mg. of *d*-tubocurarine. Electromyography showed a rapid fall-off in tetanus followed by post-tetanic facilitation, which would point to the blockade being of the nondepolarizing type. Of particular interest was the fact that the injections caused no changes in pulse rate or systolic blood pressure. Moreover, there was no evidence of histamine release such as the formation of skin wheals or bronchospasm.

INDEX